Chronic Mercury Toxicity

New Hope Against an Endemic Disease

A topic of importance to doctors of <u>every</u> health speciality, as chronic mercury toxicity may be an underlying factor in all diseases.

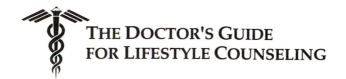

THE DOCTOR'S GUIDE FOR LIFESTYLE COUNSELING

Volume I

Chronic Mercury Toxicity

New Hope Against an Endemic Disease

H. L. Queen

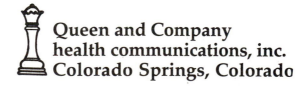

Queen and Company
health communications, inc.
Colorado Springs, Colorado

Queen and Company health communications, inc., Post Office Box 49308, Colorado Springs, Colorado, 80919-9938

Made in the United States of America.

All quotes preceding each chapter are taken from:
Familiar Medical Quotations
Maurice B. Strauss, M. D., editor
Little, Brown and Company, Boston, 1968.

Library of Congress Catalog Card Number: 88-90637

International Standard Book Number (ISBN): 0-9620479-1-0

Table of Contents

Chronic Mercury Toxicity:
New Hope Against an Endemic Disease

PART II
IV-C SAFETY

PART III:
The IV-C Mercury Tox Program

Figures and Illustrations

Tables

Forms

Books Recommended

Acknowledgements

Chronic Mercury Toxicity: New Hope Against an Endemic Disease was
the culmination of findings that were important not only to solving my own
personal battle with this disease, but also important to the treatment of all
diseases in general.

In writing this book I was not at all familiar at the outset with a number of topics with which I was forced to deal, so the process of researching and
writing was an educational one for me. In order to better assure the reader that
the health care information in this book is accurate, credible, and up-to-date,
consultation and critical reviews were solicited from the authorities. I am,
therefore, indebted to the following who helped me bridge the knowledge gap,
and who comprise the book's medical, scientific, and legal advisory staff:

Consultant	Specialty
Lewis A. Barness, M. D. Department of Pediatrics University of South Florida College of Medicine Tampa, Florida	Pediatrics International authority on vitamin C safety
Gerald Brunzie, M. D. Vice President of Regulatory Affairs Steris Laboratories Phoenix, Arizona	IV-C manufacture
Robert F. Cathcart, M. D. Los Altos, California	Environmental, ortho- molecular medicine
S. B. Elhassani, M. D. Director, Intensive Care Nursery Professor of Pediatrics Medical University of South Carolina Spartanburg, South Carolina	Neonatology International authority on treatment of neonatal mercury poisoning
Bengt Fellström, M. D., Ph. D. Associate Professor of Nephrology Department of Internal Medicine University Hospital Uppsala, Sweden	Urology International authority on kidney stones Vitamin C researcher
Warren M. Levin, M. D., FAACP, FACN World Health Medical Group New York, New York	Treatment of mercury- toxic patients
Burton A. Miller, D. D. S. Anchorage, Alaska	Treatment of mercury- toxic patients
Walter J. Murphy, Jr., Esquire Welch, Murphy & Welch Law Offices Wheaton, Maryland	Medical/legal affairs Authority on informed consent

Tadao Takeuchi, M. D. Emeritus Professor, Kumamoto University Kumamoto, Japan	Pathology Internationally recognized authority on mercury poisoning
James S. Woods, Ph. D. Senior Research Scientist Battelle Seattle Research Center Research Professor University of Washington Seattle, Washington	Environmental toxicology Researching the development of the porphyrin fingerprint
Jonathan V. Wright, M. D. Tahoma Clinic Kent, Washington	Nutritional medicine Author, educator, and major prescriber of IV-C

Collectively and individually, these professionals have made a significant contribution to the book, and their services are greatly appreciated. In the final analysis, however, the responsibility for the accuracy and the context in which their comments are used is mine.

The following people also deserve recognition for their instruction, critical advice, and encouragement: Dennis Adair, Ph.D., Schering Plough, Kennelworth, New Jersey; E. Cheraskin, M.D., D.M.D., MetriScience, Vestavia, Alabama; Sandra C. Denton, M.D., Tahoma Clinic, Kent, Washington; Howard C. Elliott, Ph.D., Baptist Medical Centers, Birmingham, Alabama; Barbara Hannah, R.N., Tahoma Clinic, Kent, Washington; Pat Hayes, R.N., Anchorage, Alaska; Hal A. Huggins, D.D.S., Huggins Diagnostic Clinic, Colorado Springs, Colorado; Robert Jenness, Ph.D., New Mexico State University; Linus Pauling, Ph.D., Linus Pauling Institute of Science and Medicine, Palo Alto, California; G. Fred Reynolds, Ph.D., professor of chemistry (retired), Colorado Springs, Colorado; John D. Walsh, D.D.S., Anchorage, Alaska; and Kenneth E. Warner, M.D., Ph.D., State Medical Examiner, Tuscaloosa, Alabama.

A heartfelt thank you is extended to my wife, Betty, for her love, her steadfast faith in this project, and for the dedication and perseverance that she aptly demonstrated as managing editor.

A special thank you to my very dear friend, H. B. Wallace of Scottsdale, Arizona. A director of the Wallace Genetic Foundation, and curator of one of the finest personally-owned collections of cacti in the southwest, H. B. provided constant encouragement and technical support. In addition, he and his wife, Jocelyn, funded the research and development of this book, which extended over a period of several years.

Finally, because a great deal of energy, time and money was spent on this project, which might have been spent in quite a different way, I would like to thank my parents, family, and friends for their patience, and for respecting this choice.

H.L. Queen

Notice to the Reader

The writings contained in this book are meant as a source of information to the medical professional, and are not intended to provide individual medical advice for the layman. Such advice must be obtained from a qualified practitioner.

To the Health Care Professional:
Chronic Mercury Toxicity: New Hope Against an Endemic Disease was written as a means of assisting the doctor in his or her treatment of the mercury-toxic patient. It is not intended as a treatment for mercury poisoning (please see the Glossary). Much of the regimen suggested requires that the doctor alter a patient's lifestyle accordingly. Yet we recognize the limitations of such a recommendation—ultimately, only the doctor can fully judge what lifestyle regimen should be followed for any particular patient. Additionally, while believed safe and effective when administered as suggested, the treatment regimen (referred to herein as the **IV-C Mercury Tox Program**) has not before been officially tested in a controlled, clinical setting. Generating an interest in such future testing is one of the many goals of this work, as this book was purposefully constructed to satisfy most of the demands for establishing a clinical research protocol.

Foreword
by Dr. Tadao Takeuchi

In view of increasing public awareness and fear of mercury contamination, as well as of the recent discovery of mercury in foods, the publication of the book, **Chronic Mercury Toxicity: New Hope Against an Endemic Disease**, is timely and important.

Various scientific investigations have broadened our understanding of the kind and extent of mercury contamination in the environment. The human and animal intoxication of mercury has also been clarified, because of the unexpected causes of Minamata disease in Japan since 1956, and of the similar situations in other countries. Although inorganic mercury poisoning has been known since early time, the importance of organic mercury poisoning has recently been recognized. The organic mercury contamination may result from 1) mercury residue produced during the manufacturing process in chemical plants, 2) agricultural chemicals used widely on the farm, 3) erratic use of disinfectants and fungicides for medical supplies, and 4) other factors. Methyl mercury, which may most frequently cause the poisoning, may result from inorganic mercury through so-called food chains. There may be dangerous situations in and around the mercury-contaminated areas.

For instance, our Japanese have had a great deal of experience with mercury subjects. We still have over two thousand patients of mercury poisoning in Minamata. There are so many unhappy and miserable people, who have had experience with noneffective treatments tried frequently and repeatedly. We have no other acknowledged treatment for the disease right now. Mercury remains in the patients' body, especially in the brain, for long periods of time.

Therefore, it would be wonderful if the prescription of a large amount of intravenous vitamin C, as discussed in this book, has any effect on removing mercury from the body, particularly nerve cells in the brain.

Under the circumstances this book is timely published. Though I personally do not certify the result, such a new medical treatment should be tried to ease the patients' pain. In this respect, it is not too much to say that this book is a long-awaited one for people in the medical field who are forced to face the debilitating, longer-term consequences of mercury poisoning (chronic mercury toxicity).

Tadao Takeuchi, M. D.
Professor Emeritus of Kumamoto University
President of Junior College of Shokei, Kumamoto
Kumamoto City, Japan
December 1987

PREFACE

Precautions, Limitations, and Qualifying Remarks

From the viewpoint of one who regularly reads technical manuscripts, I appreciate most the authors who disclose the strengths and limitations of their books up front. Such a statement is especially helpful in reading <u>this</u> book, since there are particular precautions, qualifying remarks to the treatment regimen, and certain limitations that relate to indications and contraindications. Such remarks will guide the doctor in determining who should, or should not, be allowed access to the proposed treatment program, and under what set of circumstances. The format also gives me the chance to do a short synopsis. Before reading any further, however, you will find it helpful to read and study the Glossary, and to consult the Glossary often as you go through the book.

This book, **Chronic Mercury Toxicity: New Hope Against An Endemic Disease**, is intended not to treat acute mercury poisoning, but to introduce a promising new treatment for chronic mercury toxicity, for which there has not previously been a safe and effective treatment.

While the proposed therapy, referred to throughout the book as the **IV-C Mercury Tox Program,** is believed safe and effective when administered as suggested, <u>the treatment regimen has not been officially tested in a controlled, clinical setting</u>. Generating an interest in such future testing is one of the many goals of this book, as the program was purposefully constructed to satisfy most of the demands for establishing a clinical research protocol.

Although mercury in its various forms represents different types of hazards with different toxicities, the various chemical species were sparingly differentiated throughout the book, mainly because the treatment program being suggested is believed effective against all forms of chronic mercury toxicity—without regard to the source and chemical species of mercury.

People who have been exposed to elemental mercury, mercury salts, or organomercurials readily develop hypersensitive reactions (allergic and idiosyncratic) which may occur without the typical dose/response curve. It is equally a fact that neither the nephrotic syndrome of chronic mercury toxicity, nor acrodynia, shows a typical dose/response relationship. Thus, if doctors limit their diagnosis of chronic mercury toxicity to those mercurial effects that show a well defined dose-response relationship and treat only those who demonstrate the traditional dose/response relationship, many people who are mercury-toxic will go unidentified and improperly treated. In practice this happens all too often.

Doctors who specialize in industrial medicine typically support the validity of the atypical, dose/response thesis. They report that many people working with organomercurials become sensitized: Severe dermatitis forces them to halt their exposure from the workplace, and they soon learn to become especially alert to other potential sources of mercury in their environment. Therefore, the standard means of identifying those who should be treated for mercury exposure—by establishing first a dose/response curve, and focusing too intensely on the chemical species of mercury involved—simply doesn't apply when considering the **IV-C Mercury Tox Program.** Nor does the standard means of evaluating treatment outcome through a demonstrated change in the body burden of mercury apply. Because these practices no longer satisfy, a newer means of identification and evaluation are necessarily discussed.

Realization of the fallacy of relying totally upon the standard dose/response curve for determining who is mercury-toxic, leads to the necessity of questioning the role that even the smallest exposure to mercury might play in the onset of disease. For this reason, and because of extensive worldwide use among dentists, a portion of the attention is focused on the potential contribution of mercury from dental amalgam fillings to the onset and exacerbation of chronic mercury toxicity, and to the many diseases that it mimics. Involvement in this controversy is not for the purpose of pointing a finger at the dental profession, but a result of the belief that *the total amount of mercury from all chemical species has grown in our world environment to the point that chronic mercury toxicity is now an endemic disease.* The fact that mercury from dental amalgam fillings adds unnecessarily to the growing environmental problem, as well as the mounting evidence that dental amalgam fillings potentially and significantly contribute to the body burden of mercury, makes the practice of placing mercurial amalgam fillings more susceptible to criticism today than ever before. Thus, I feel an in-depth discussion of the dental amalgam debate is necessary. Let it be known, however, that this book does not advocate the indiscriminate replacement of mercury amalgam fillings. Rather, the doctor and patient must make that decision together based upon the evidence of mercury exposure and the patient's medical history.

The **IV-C Mercury Tox Program** is also being proposed for the treatment of patients with chronic methylmercury toxicity, particularly those who survived Minamata disease, who were poisoned after eating fish contaminated with mercury from the discharge of a local factory—and the groups of people in Iraq and other countries who have become ill from eating seed grains pretreated with a mercurial fungicide. Special consideration for treatment should be given to these people, whose health conditions have progressed pathetically to disorders involving nerve, brain, or neuromuscular dysfunction. These conditions, which ultimately contribute to the cause of death, are the inevitable consequence of exposure to methylmercury.

It is likely that many people throughout the world suffer even today from chronic methylmercury toxicity without knowing it. This happens mainly when doctors fail to connect their patient's symptoms with methylmercury exposure. Yet these people are most definitely candidates for this treatment. Without the information in this book, however, it is unlikely that they will ever be recognized—let alone treated properly—since a large percentage of them will express a dose/response curve that is atypically low.

People rarely suffer from chronic exposure to inorganic mercurial salts, mostly because acute intoxication from this chemical species of mercury is most often fatal. Yet those who may be rescued would probably benefit from the **IV-C Mercury Tox Program**, just as any other victim of chronic mercury toxicity. There are some exceptions not to receive this treatment: patients suffering from the nephrotic syndrome or some other contraindicated condition, as is explained in PART II of the text.

There are several mechanisms responsible for the decision to use megadose vitamin C—and particularly intravenous vitamin C—to improve the patient's condition in cases of chronic mercury toxicity. While much is known of the antioxidant effects of vitamin C in preventing trace metal effects, very little has been reported on the remedial effects of vitamin C in recovery from metal toxicity. Although the evidence is not conclusive, it indicates strongly that vitamin C therapy stimulates repair of damage done by viruses and environmental chemicals. While further verification is necessary, proving this theory will depend, I believe, partially on the outcome of the work being done at the Battelle Seattle Research Center and elsewhere. Researchers at the Battelle Seattle Research Center are currently studying a means to determine the extent of damage attributable to mercury. Once developed, this test may assist the clinician to evaluate the physiological effect of the treatment, rather than depending solely on a change in symptoms and the body burden of mercury.

A significant improvement in the patient's well-being, which is the likely outcome of the **IV-C Mercury Tox Program**, would mean more to him than a reduction in body burden of mercury, although this too is expected. Ultimately, therefore, it is anticipated that this test will prove useful in monitoring the efficacy of the **IV-C Mercury Tox Program**. Once the test is operational I see no reason why laboratories could not begin monitoring exposure of patients in the vitamin C treatment program to determine if they recover more quickly, or completely, from the biological effects of mercury than patients receiving an alternate form of therapy. The test may also be useful to the clinical researcher in determining at what point megadose vitamin C is most effective following rescue from mercury poisoning, and at what point it should initially be administered. We are all looking forward to the time when these possibilities can be explored.

Chapters 5 and 6, which provide an in depth look at vitamin C safety, are designed to (1) make the doctor thoroughly aware of risks involved in administering megadose vitamin C; (2) serve as an aid in identifying high-risk patients; and (3) establish a preventive diet and lifestyle program for reducing such risk. A protocol is suggested to help the doctor in risk/benefit analysis. I advise the doctor to read and put these steps into practice before administering megadose vitamin C, even if treating a patient for a condition other than chronic mercury toxicity. While high-risk patients are generally denied access to the **IV-C Mercury Tox Program** and megadose vitamin C therapy, a pre-treatment program is suggested for those patients whose potential for benefit outweighs the risk.

Chapter 6 extensively addresses factors important for the development and prevention of kidney stones, particularly hyperoxaluria, hypercalciuria, and hyperuricosuria. Contrary to popular opinion, a review of the literature indicates that the association between kidney stones and megadose vitamin C is not a cause/effect relationship. Yet stones do form predictably in certain high-risk people who can be readily identified through the questionnaire and tests suggested, and thereby denied access to the treatment program. Those who are not at high risk are instructed to follow the preventive program, which is generally all that's required for their protection.

Some doctors who regularly treat patients for kidney stones report discouraging results when prescribing a corrective diet and lifestyle for difficult patients. Diet and lifestyle changes, they say, are extremely difficult to encourage in some people. Many doctors, therefore, are inclined to rely on drug intervention rather than lifestyle counseling for certain difficult patients. To overcome this objection I have suggested the use of informed consent, which involves the patient's family as well as the patient himself.

The intent of informed consent is to get the patient actively involved (with his family's support) in his own treatment program, and it <u>works</u>. It works because it builds a bond of trust between the patient and doctor, thereby improving patient compliance. Thus, if the patient at risk closely follows the lifestyle treatment suggested here, based upon results of his work-up, the chance of getting a successful result is quite good. As an added benefit, the diet and lifestyle program suggested here is far more complete for preventing kidney stones than any previous program—more reason to get the patient actively and personally involved, and to adopt this program rather than resort to drug therapy.

It is through this concept of informed consent that the doctor finds it convenient, and natural, to incorporate lifestyle counseling into his health and medical practice. In fact, *I recommend that the doctor not administer megadose vitamin C, or the* **IV-C Mercury Tox Program,** *to <u>anyone</u> without informed consent.* This better ensures a positive treatment outcome while also satisfying professional liability.

After saying this, a qualifying note is in order. The limitations of such a recommendation are well recognized—ultimately, only the doctor can fully judge what lifestyle regimen should be followed for any particular patient.

Additionally, I am hopeful that the evidence presented will stimulate, in the very near future, the reporting of individual case studies and clinical trials—involving critically ill people, certain population groups, and cohorts of test subjects who have been chronically exposed to <u>all</u> of the various chemical species of mercury. Judging from the results I've already witnessed, the potential benefit to human health is endless.

GLOSSARY

Interpretation of Certain Terms
Pertinent to the Understanding
of this Book

Before reading **Chronic Mercury Toxicity: New Hope Against an Endemic Disease**, it is important that certain words and phrases be defined. Megadose intravenous vitamin C, for instance, is being proposed for use in the treatment of chronic mercury toxicity, but not for treatment of mercury poisoning. (In fact, megadose vitamin C may be contraindicated in acute mercury poisoning, in which case an adequate course of therapy is already available—see Appendix G).

Endemic: A disease of low morbidity that is constantly present in a human community, but clinically recognizable in only a few.

IV-C: Intravenous vitamin C.

The IV-C Mercury Tox Program: The registered name assigned to the program herein suggested for the treatment of chronic mercury toxicity.

The Three Forms Of Mercury:

Inorganic Mercurial Salts: Bichloride of mercury is one of the most common salts of mercury, and certainly the most toxic. When ingested it is quickly ionized and highly corrosive. If the patient is to live, appropriate action must be taken in the first 10 to 15 minutes after ingestion. While the mean lethal dose ranges from 1 to 4 grams, people have died from consuming as little as half a gram. Chronic mercury toxicity from this form, therefore, is rare. When it <u>does</u> occur, some patients are peculiarly susceptible to developing the nephrotic syndrome—a delayed, indiosyncratic reaction. Such patients are generally not candidates for the treatment program described within this book.

Elemental Mercury: Also known as quicksilver, elemental mercury is highly volatile and is transported throughout the body attached to proteins. Since proteins in blood circulate both singularly and as an integral part of lipoproteins—which transport fats through the blood—elemental mercury may be transported either alone or in combination with fats. Therefore, mercury is capable of reaching nearly every tissue type. Poisoning occurs mainly, however, through inhalation of vapors, as it is almost completely absorbed through the alveolar membrane. Thereafter the central nervous system is most affected, as elemental mercury easily crosses the blood/brain barrier, where it is quickly oxidized by brain tissue to mercuric ion, which is then readily attracted to the brain's many sulfhydryl protein molecules. Patients suffering from this form of mercury toxicity are generally prime candidates for the treatment program outlined in this book. The exceptions would include those few people who develop a delayed, idiosyncratic nephrotic syndrome reaction, similar to what may occur following exposure to mercurial salts.

Organic Mercury Compounds: All organic mercurials are highly toxic. The degree of toxicity varies, however. The simple organic, alkyl mercurials—such as methylmercury and ethylmercury—are the most toxic, followed by the complex aryl compounds and the organomercurials used in medicines. **The IV-C Mercury Tox Program** is best suited for treating these, and for treatment of chronic mercury toxicity from elemental mercury and its vapors.

Toxicology: Dr. Thomas J. Haley, Honorary Professor of Pharmacology at the University of Arkansas for the Medical Sciences, Little Rock, Arkansas, has defined toxicology as "the science of poisons, their effects on the body, various antidotes for their action, and their detection in body fluids and tissues."[1] In toxicology the words "acute" and "chronic" are used in reference to the extent and duration of exposure.

 Acute, according to Haley, "implies a single exposure to a toxicant (measured in seconds, minutes, or hours) that may result in unconsciousness, shock, collapse, severe damage to pulmonary tissues, and even sudden death."

 Chronic, he states, "implies exposure to sublethal quantities of mercury over a prolonged period of time (measured in days, months, or years) with very few clues as to what the toxicant is doing to vital organs and tissues." Before symptoms of intoxication can occur, mercury must accumulate in vital organs to critical concentrations. "Chronic" may also equally imply (1) the longer-term consequence of acute mercurialism, following rescue, or (2) the development of hypersensitivity to mercury. One or the other would be the case when referred to in this book as "the mercury-toxic patient".

Chronic Mercury Toxicity: "Toxicity" generally refers only to the quality, state or degree of being toxic, or poisonous. Nevertheless, the term "chronic mercury toxicity" is proposed in this book to represent generically any mercury-toxic state other than acute mercurialism. In this text, "chronic mercury toxicity" encompasses all unfavorable symptoms produced by exposure to any form of mercury, regardless of the duration of the initial exposure, and whether the initial exposure was acute or chronic. Strictly speaking, even an acute exposure to mercury will eventually produce chronic illness. Chronic mercury toxicity begins immediately following the rescue of the acutely-poisoned patient. In other patients, such as those with dermatitis, acrodynia, and the nephrotic syndrome, it can readily produce reactions that do not follow the usual dose/response curve.

Chronic Heavy Metal Toxicity: This term, like "chronic mercury toxicity," has been coined to represent generically any heavy metal toxic state other than acute poisoning.

---

[1] I. Sax and T.J. Haley, et al., eds., *Dangerous Properties of Industrial Materials*, Sixth Edition, Section I, Vos Nostrand Reinhold Company, N.Y., 1984.

The Mercury-Toxic Patient: This term refers to anyone who has a condition that fits the description of chronic mercury toxicity, which may include those people who originally suffered from acute mercurialism as well as those who demonstrate an allergy or hypersensitivity to mercury, with or without a previous, significant exposure.

The Mercury-Sensitive Patient: Similar to "the mercury-toxic patient", this term is a subclassification of the mercury-toxic patient. It strictly refers to anyone who has developed a hypersensitivity to mercury (allergic or idiosyncratic) over a long period of time. Once established, minute quantities of mercury—less than the amounts normally required to cause a toxic reaction—can precipitate an attack. Although allergic and idiosyncratic hypersensitivity to mercury are specific, there is speculation that cross-sensitivity may also occur with other metals and chemicals. Thus, the mercury-sensitive patient, if not treated, may become a universal reactor (one who literally becomes allergic to his total environment).

Minamata Disease: The name given specifically to methylmercury poisoning; named for the bay in Japan near where the condition was first observed. Ironically, the acute stage is not treatable partly because acute methylmercury poisoning is rarely diagnosed clinically. If recognized and treated in the early stage, the body burden of mercury may be decreased. It is supposed that, by this action, the progress of the disease is mitigated. However, because of the severity of the Japanese people's exposure, it is unlikely that any treatment would have had an effect on those who died within a few weeks of the onset of disease in Minamata. Even if they had been rescued there has not—until now—been a means of treating the chronic stage of Minamata Disease, which eventually and inevitably causes disability and death due to brain and neurological damage, as well as congenital defects.

IV-C is being suggested only for chronic mercury toxicity. Since mercury poisoning and chronic mercury toxicity are often confused, the following are terms that are interchangeably used in differentiating the two conditions:

Synonyms of Conditions for which Intravenous Vitamin C (IV-C) is Indicated:
    Acrodynia (pink disease, erythredema polyneuropathy) is typically an early childhood disease caused by repeated contact or ingestion of mercury.
    Chronic mercury toxicity
    Chronic mercurialism
    Low-level mercury toxicity
    Mercurial hypersensitivity (allergic and idiosyncratic reactions)
    Mercury sensitivity
    Micromercurialism: Symptoms of mercury toxicity due to low-level, chronic exposure, demonstrated by an atypical, idiosyncratic dose/response relationship
    Subacute mercury toxicity

Synonyms of Conditions for which Intravenous Vitamin C (IV-C) is <u>Not</u> Indicated:

Acute mercury poisoning (also called hydrargyria)

Acute mercurialism (or hydrargyrism)

Macromercurialism: Significant, acute exposure to mercury, in which there is a pronounced dose-response relationship

INTRODUCTION

Why It Became Necessary to Write this Book

"Work which is useful may receive approbation and become a standard for others. Work which excites opposition and criticism is also valuable if it leads to ideas of permanent value. Even if wrong in conception or execution it may be valuable if it directs thought and action into new and previously unexplored paths."

~William E. Tanner [1889-   ]

The need for this book has emerged from several directions:

From the realization that there is currently no known, effective treatment for chronic, subacute mercurialism, without which thousands of people worldwide must face the inevitability of prolonged suffering, disability, and death;

From the realization that the amount of mercury in our environment is on the rise, and that the risk of becoming mercury-toxic is growing proportionately, due mainly to the combined effects of industrial exposure and a recent increase in consumption of foods (such as fish) that are potential sources of mercury;

From the long-standing use of mercury in dentistry as a component of silver amalgam fillings, resulting in a growing number of dentists who believe that mercury-laden fillings are a source of many health problems;

From the realization that dentists and physicians alike are generally unfamiliar with the symptoms of chronic mercury toxicity;

From the recognition that ridding the body of mercury and other heavy metals is an important first step in preventing heart disease, and many other diseases as well;

From the growth in interest in the use of megadose vitamin C, particularly intravenous vitamin C (or IV-C), as adjunct therapy in a wide assortment of diseases, including chronic mercury toxicity;

From the need for a source book on the safe and effective use of IV-C; and,

From the exciting revelation that steps necessary to ensure the safety of administering IV-C uniquely form a basis for inclusion of lifestyle counseling in the doctor's professional practice.

Controversy has been the rule throughout the 150-year history of the use of mercury in dentistry. The opinion of authorities, who feel that dental amalgam is safe and effective for the patient and presents no health risk except to the doctor and staff, has changed very little throughout the years. They note that dental amalgam is extremely durable and can withstand many (10-20) years of the daily chewing and grinding required of molar teeth. Most importantly, proponents say, the amalgam restoration is affordable, with gold being an alternate choice only for a few. On the other hand, opponents contend that the health risk to patients far outweighs the obvious benefit.

With today's technical improvements in detection of oral mercury vapor, and with an accompanying surge in suspicion of the effect dental mercury might have on health, a significant number of dentists have excluded amalgam fillings from their dental practice. Others have turned to replacement of old amalgam fillings with alternative materials that are less toxic—a practice that has been reported to benefit the health of select patients, but which has also become a focal point for criticism. The prospect for health advantage has stimulated many practitioners—dentists and physicians alike—to focus on methods of recognition and treatment of the mercury-toxic patient relating to chronic mercury toxicity in general. It is this group of concerned professionals who will find this book most useful.

Other health professionals (nurses, dieticians, medical technologists, and health counselors) who must deal with the mercury problem through their allied health specialty will also find this book of interest, especially since there has not previously been an effective method for treating the patient who suffers from chronic mercury toxicity. Researchers, particularly, will benefit, as **Chronic Mercury Toxicity: New Hope Against an Endemic Disease** aids in highlighting important considerations for developing a research protocol.

The positive association of vitamin C with dental health has played an important role in the choice by doctors of megadose, intravenous vitamin C as a significant part of their therapy for chronic mercury toxicity. These doctors note that IV-C was popularly used only a few short years ago as an effective antidote for mercury intoxication due to overdose from organomercurial drugs. Thus, this sudden rise in popularity for the use of IV-C in treating the dental patient suspected of being mercury-sensitive has come not only from the heightened level of awareness of such need, but from successful past experiences in medicine and dentistry.

Prior to this volume there was only fragmented instruction available for the proper use of IV-C. Research indicates that several precautions are necessary, most of which center around the need to screen patients for kidney dysfunction. In addition, it is clear that particular patient lifestyle practices must precede and follow the IV-C infusion to ensure its safety and effectiveness. These same lifestyle steps are the primary steps to be taken by anyone seeking optimal health, and by those striving to avoid heart disease. This book, therefore, is ideally designed to provide a basis of instruction for conducting a professional lifestyle counseling practice. The reader should bear in mind that this book lays the intentional groundwork for a planned lifestyle series—THE DOCTOR'S GUIDE FOR LIFESTYLE COUNSELING—each volume of which will build upon the previous one.

The ultimate goal of this lifestyle series is to provide the doctor with a plan for prevention of heart disease; the number one cause of premature death in the Western World. Patients' interests will be served with improvement in health and a better quality of life—regardless of their initial health condition.

One might logically ask how the correction of chronic mercury toxicity relates to the task of solving heart disease. The answer is quite simple: An accumulation in the body of heavy metals (mercury, lead, and cadmium in particular) has the unfortunate propensity for interfering with cellular function through alteration of cell membranes and enzyme systems. For instance, lead and cadmium absorption are associated with high blood pressure, which, in turn, is associated with heart attack and stroke. Likewise, mercury may cause an interruption in heart rhythm, and may act in other indirect ways to adversely affect the heart.

An interesting aspect of this tendency is the negative mental effect experienced by mercury-toxic patients whose total serum cholesterol is lowered suddenly by diet and drugs. This group, I believe, has accounted for the unusual number of violent deaths (murders, auto fatalities, and suicides) noted in the now-famous, $ 150 million Lipid Research Clinic (LRC) study of the effects of cholesterol lowering on the incidence of heart attacks.

The effect of mercury and other heavy metals, however, is not limited solely to heart malfunction and mental disturbances. They may contribute also to the onset and progression of all degenerative diseases. In fact, the data to be presented demonstrates that these heavy metal intruders have such an adverse effect on human health that solving the problem of heavy metal toxicity, particularly chronic mercury toxicity, is basic to any program for improved health. This becomes even more pertinent when one realizes that as many as 70 percent of adults in the Western World are believed to have dental amalgam fillings.

A doctor may rightfully ask, "Why should I get into lifestyle counseling? My practice is going just fine, so how can lifestyle counseling enhance my professional goals?"

The average layman today has an acute awareness of, and enthusiasm for, healthful living habits; an attitude that did not exist 20 years ago. This can be attributed to the information explosion that has since occurred. Today's health consumer knows more and demands more. They ask more questions and want thorough explanations for a particular course of action. They want to know alternatives and, perhaps most importantly, they want to know WHAT CONSTITUTES HEALTH? All of this is occurring while the majority of doctors of every health specialty continue to emphasize only diagnosis and treatment in their professional practices. So it isn't surprising that the majority of lifestyle counseling services available today are provided by people who are not health professionals. Patients who seek this service haven't found satisfaction within the health care system, so they are seeking their health needs and medical needs in different quarters—a trend that is not ultimately in the best interest of health.

This book, as well as forthcoming volumes in the series, is drafted with the premise that doctors of both medicine and dentistry have the best possible background of experience and education for lifestyle counseling, but lack only the specialized training. **QUEEN AND COMPANY HEALTH COMMUNICATIONS, INC.**, has taken the responsibility of leading in this direction; providing training through this lifestyle series of books. The doctor's interest in this specialty is coming at a perfect time.

It became apparent while conducting research for **Chronic Mercury Toxicity: New Hope Against An Endemic Disease** that by age 40, many dentists admit to having reached the point of professional "burnout". Complaints that vacations are too infrequent are heard. Most of those interviewed stated that they would like to get away, but when their vacation starts their income stops. So, many dentists continue working rather than take time off, and become even more discontented. Those who identify with this scenario have additional reason to read this book. The information provided can completely change one's dental practice. Of greater importance, perhaps, it can improve one's outlook, providing an additional mental stimulation that every health professional seeks.

By becoming proficient in lifestyle counseling, and by training key personnel, particularly the registered dental hygienist, the dental office staff can continue to operate effectively and profitably in the doctor's absence, making it possible for him to enjoy the beach and still pay the bills! Additionally, the entire office staff will enjoy the rewarding stimulation that lifestyle counseling provides—knowing that the time spent with each patient can positively affect not only the life of the patient, but his or her whole family as well. Everyone benefits.

Physicians are faced with a special problem. While there are still too few physicians for the poor, the elderly, and the institutionalized,* the doctor shortage of recent years is fast becoming a doctor surplus. There were 334,000 doctors licensed to practice in the United States in 1970. Today the figure is up to 490,000. By 1990 there will be 536,000 practicing physicians. That will be 63,000 doctors too many.

There are presently 470 people for every doctor. The ratio is smaller in large cities (i.e., Denver, where the ratio is 210 to 1). By 1990, Denver's ratio will decrease to 150 to 1; a time when a major surplus will surface throughout the United States in many medical specialties.

The full impact of the excess hasn't yet hit. When that happens we are going to see many changes, beginning with the doctor/patient relationship. Doctors will raise their fees to substitute for fewer patients, says Stuart Wesbury, past President of the American College of Hospital Administration. In turn, the cost of all health services will rise even higher, to the point that health consumers will demand to know, even more, WHAT CONSTITUTES HEALTH? They will want to know what they can do personally to prevent and correct health problems through lifestyle changes. In fact, the trend is already here. So what's the answer for professional survival?

An age-old axiom in successful marketing demands that the service match the needs of the people. That's pretty much what I've tried to do in this volume, and what is planned for succeeding volumes in the series. There is an immediate and potential health problem from dental fillings that needs a solution, and there are thousands currently suffering from the chronic effects of mercury from other sources for which there has not before been an effective therapy. The **IV-C Mercury Tox Program**, which will be outlined in this book, is designed to fill this need and offer these people hope. Even so, there are limitations and a danger in administering IV-C without being fully informed. A remedial protocol is herein provided for this as well.

There is also the patient's ongoing need to rely on a lifestyle professional he can trust. The expertise of select reviewers and the scientific advisors for this and future books offer the credibility needed to build such trust. Thanks to these dedicated professionals I know that doctors, researchers, allied health professionals, and patients alike will enjoy a new beginning together.

---

* Excerpted from an interview conducted with a spokesman of the Graduate Medical Education, National Advisory Committee to the federal government, by *U. S. News & World Report*, p. 62-64, December 19, 1983.

PART I

IV-C Rationale and Efficacy

CHAPTER 1

The Mercury Controversy

"A critical and flexible judgement comes of a familiarity with, and an appreciation of, the relative value of ideas, present and past."
~Sir Clifford Allbutt [1836-1895]

Controversy surrounding the use of mercury in dentistry began over 150 years ago when silver amalgam fillings were first introduced. During most of the years that followed, the dental profession managed to keep its differences contained within the borders of scholarly debate. In the last seven to eight years, however, order has given way to quarreling and chaos. There has been a growing tendency to defend viewpoints with unfounded opinion. While this could be interpreted as a decaying state of affairs—a cataclysmic evolvement within an otherwise respected profession—a more accurate and correct assessment might be gained from examining the comment of Sir F. M. R. Walshe, who reasoned that "controversy is dead only in fields of knowledge that are not advancing."[1] Within the field of dentistry, therefore, it can perhaps more accurately be stated that the heated condition of today's controversy is a positive symptom that one can expect when standing on the threshold of a profession experiencing rapid, intellectual advancement.

Today, doctors and patients alike recognize multifactorial causes for many disease conditions. Oral disease, diseases of the nervous and immune systems, and cardiovascular disease are just a few examples. A growing number of people now suspect that mercury from "silver" amalgam fillings is in some manner involved in the onset and progression of many of these same diseases. Mercury comprises 50 percent of the contents of amalgam fillings (silver totals no more than 30 percent). The remainder is a mixture of copper, zinc, and tin bonded together as an inorganic metal alloy. Mercury is dominant because it is naturally in a liquid state before the amalgam is prepared, and aids in mixing the compound before placement in the tooth cavity. Once in place, it also serves to facilitate hardening of the restoration.

Dental authorities have generally always believed that mercury in the amalgam filling is inert and essentially harmless, leading to its widespread use. In the United States alone dentists now use over one hundred tons of mercury each year.[2] It is believed that over one hundred million Americans (at least 40 percent of the population) have amalgam fillings in their mouths; many of these have multiple fillings. This recognition of its widespread use, and the growing number of reports that it may be toxic, is indication enough for a thorough investigation.

In essence, the controversy is centered around:
- Whether or not mercury is released from dental amalgam
- Whether or not dental amalgam is capable of causing chronic mercury toxicity
- Whether or not amalgam fillings are a cause of disease

• Whether or not amalgam fillings are capable of causing disease by a mechanism other than heavy metal toxicity, but nonetheless related to mercury

In order to understand this controversy, it is necessary to understand the nature of mercury.

CHARACTERISTICS OF MERCURY AND MERCURY POISONING

Mercury is a potent human poison that has long been a source of serious health problems whether ingested, inhaled, or absorbed through the skin. While acceptable limits are often quoted by the federal regulatory agencies and health agencies, mercury is a poison at any level, whether the level of intoxication is sufficient to cause recognizable symptoms or not. Inorganic salts are recognized as the most toxic form of mercury. Next are the simple organic, alkyl compounds, such as methyl mercury and ethyl mercury. These organic forms are followed closely by elemental mercury vapor. The least toxic, perhaps, are the more complex organic compounds, the organomercurials, from which some medicines are derived. For all practical purposes, however, all mercury forms are a potential cause of disease. The findings of Swedish scientist Arne Jernelov, who demonstrated that certain microbes can change inorganic mercury to the methyl form, substantiated this.

Symptoms for acute and chronic poisoning differ considerably. Acute mercurialism may arise from a single, significant exposure to any form of mercury. The patient complains at once of a harsh metallic taste, followed quickly by burning pain in the mouth, throat, and stomach. Severe gastroenteritis follows with abdominal pain, salivation, and vomiting.

Chronic mercurialism, on the other hand, is much more difficult to recognize. Gingivitis and mental disturbances (erethism) were among the first signs attributed to mercury. Ramazzini, in his work on the diseases of workers in 1700, confirmed that the miners' teeth usually fell out, and that a gilder who was not careful to protect himself from the fumes of mercury had mental stupor. Symptoms are often obscure and misleading, and as a result the condition is often improperly diagnosed. Prolonged exposure can result in damage to the immune system, cardiovascular system, brain, and nervous system, as well as other conditions that have only recently been attributed to mercury (to be discussed in greater detail in Chapter 3). In such cases the doctor is more apt to treat the symptoms rather than suspect mercury as the underlying cause, particularly mercury from dental amalgam fillings. The exception would occur in individual case histories where repeated exposure to mercury was more obvious and the effects more severe. This, as was demonstrated in 1972 during the worldwide investigation by *National Geographic* reporters John Putman and Robert Madden,[3] is not that uncommon.

Putman made mention of the classic example of chronic, but severe, mercurial poisoning which occurred in the 19th century. At this time, makers of felt hats were routinely dipping their material into mercuric nitrate before shaping. In so doing, they assimilated mercury as the result of inhalation of mercury vapor and direct contact, thus poisoning themselves. Their symptoms were diverse, and highlighted—as in acute poisoning—by a metallic taste in the mouth, a feeling of numbness or soreness of the tongue, difficulty in walking, tremors, loss of teeth, incoherent speech, and feeblemindedness. They were forever immortalized in the phrase "mad as a hatter" and characterized by the Mad Hatter in *Alice in Wonderland*.

MERCURY IN NATURE

Mercury is not alien to mother earth; but is as natural as silver and gold. In all likelihood, prehistoric man first used the sulphide ore of mercury—cinnabar—to draw on the walls of caves. Rainfall extracts cinnabar from the soil, releasing mercury into streams, lakes, and oceans in small amounts, where it is absorbed from the water by small, aquatic plants and fish. Terrestrial plants, on the other hand, are remarkably resistant to mercury in the soil, and thereby resist contamination.

Mercury enters into the food chain at the plankton level, and reaches us at the end of the chain in the form of tuna, larger swordfish, halibut, and Pacific blue marlin. Crustaceans, or bottom feeders, such as lobster, clams, and shrimp, are also vulnerable to acquiring a significant amount of mercury. However, the concentration of mercury in fish depends usually on age and weight of the fish. The largest and oldest fish always seem to have the most. Mercury has been found even in remains of prehistoric fish, which seems to show that the heavy metal has always been a contaminant of the food chain. It also indicates that sea life long ago developed an effective method of coping with low-level intoxication.

Mercury-related health problems did not occur until man learned to mine and isolate mercury for industrial and proprietary purposes. We are reminded by Magos,[4] for instance, that Pliny in the first century B.C. described the disease of slaves employed in mercury mines. Putman, upon visiting Earth's richest mercury mine, in Almaden, Spain (a mine that accounts for roughly 15 percent of the world's mercury output), found that the same health problems persist today among miners.

The process of manufacturing paints and plastics, the manufacture of fungicides, and the burning of fossil fuels, all release additional mercury into our air and water in quantities that our sea and animal life have never before experienced. As a consequence, isolated incidences and occasional outbreaks of poisoning have occurred throughout history—always a result of man's carelessness and our general lack of understanding of the hazards. On the positive side, our current, heightened level of understanding was derived through a detailed study of these outbreaks. To explain the origin of the program, it will perhaps help to retrace the road map that led to this level of understanding.

Mercury Poisoning Chronicled

Drawing upon both the writings of Pliny and the effect of mercuric nitrate on hatters, Edwards,[5] in 1885, became the first to describe fatal methylmercury intoxication. Hunter and Russell,[6] in 1940, then described the syndrome of methylmercury poisoning. McAlpine (who had previously seen Hunter's patients in London) and Araki,[7,8] after being shown patients with mysterious symptoms in Minamata Bay, Japan, suggested that the disease may be caused by thallium. Because mercury poisoning was thought to be a secondary, underlying factor of thallium poisoning, they further recommended that thallium poisoning be differentiated from mercury poisoning. A second conclusion was arrived at independently, in 1956, by Dr. Tadao Takeuchi. Dr. Takeuchi, who was assigned to study the disease affecting the Minamata Bay-area people, was first to develop the theory that the unknown disease was in fact methylmercury poisoning.[9] His conclusions were based upon his own findings of significant brain atrophy and lesions on autopsy, chemical evidence, and reproduction of Minamata disease in cats. He also established that the poisoning in Japan was derived from eating contaminated fish. Thereafter, "Minamata disease" became the official name of methylmercury poisoning.

The contamination in Minamata Bay has since turned out to be one of the two largest outbreaks of methylmercury poisoning ever recorded. (The other major outbreak occurred in Iraq.) While significant but less extensive outbreaks have occurred elsewhere, the information gained from these two major epidemics has provided modern medicine with the bulk of what is known today about methylmercury poisoning, mercury poisoning in general, and chronic mercury toxicity. Let's examine what occurred with these:

Minamata Disease. From 1932 to 1968, the Chisso factory in Minamata used mercury as a catalyst for making acetaldehyde (acetic acid); between 1941 and 1971 it was used for vinyl chloride production. During these periods the factory dumped an estimated 100 tons of mercurial wastes into the coastal bay of Minamata. This resulted in acute mercurialism of the people who ate fish that were caught there. The families most affected were the poor, who consumed an average of three meals of fish per day.

Minamata disease, as it became known, demonstrated to the world the hazards of dumping mercurial waste without regard to the consequences. In 1976, long after the practice of dumping raw mercurial wastes had been halted, 126 deaths in the Minamata Bay province could be attributed to this disease, and there were over 800 people with severe brain damage. By 1982 a total of 1,773 residents of Minamata Bay had been declared victims of Minamata disease, and 456 of those had died.[10]

The statistics don't stop there. The gravity of the problem continues even today. At last count, only 50 people with the disease are able to be processed each month, while 5,000 with various neurological complaints wait to be evaluated. Even so, their suffering will continue long after the diagnosis and a two-year wait for testing, since there is no known means of correcting their conditions.*

Through the experience at Minamata Bay, people everywhere came to realize that methylmercury poisoning, as well as the "mad as a hatter" (poisoning from elemental mercury) symptoms, described a very real condition that could happen also to them. Worldwide, governments responded with protective legislation that outlawed indiscriminate dumping of mercury-containing waste. Led by the World Health Organization (WHO), standards and safeguards, set before the Minamata incident, were more rigorously enforced in the workplace. This action led health and environmental scientists to reexamine all possible sources of mercury contamination.

In Sweden in the late 1950's, naturalist Erik Rosenberg stimulated a wide scale investigation, after noting that birds and other wildlife dependent on freshly-sown seed grain were falling ill with neuromuscular disorders, in a manner similar to the occurrences at Minamata Bay. It was learned that Swedish farmers had been planting seed grain pretreated with a fungicide comprised of methylmercury—a practice widely followed throughout the world. Furthermore, some of the seed was being fed to animals intended for human consumption. Through this common practice of using methyl mercurial

---

* I believe, however, that the **IV-C Mercury Tox Program** has the potential to greatly improve their conditions, even those with mercury-induced congenital defects.

fungicides, mercury was finding its way into the food chain.

It was soon realized that contamination was occurring in many ways, not just through treated seed grains and isolated violations of industrial dumping. The content of mercury in the general environment was on the rise. Consequently, the Swedish government led the world in restricting the use of mercury in general, and specifically banning the use of methyl mercury in agriculture. The leading seed corn company in the U. S.—Pioneer Hybrid of Des Moines, Iowa—recognized the wisdom of the Swedish government's lead and reverted to a safer fungicide (thiol, or mercaptan-based). This practice has since become a worldwide standard, but has been slow in coming.

The Iraqi Experience(s). The most frequent and serious outbreaks occurred in Iraq in 1956, 1960, 1970, and 1972. The first group which reported details of the Iraq epidemics was a collaborative study group consisting of scientists from Rochester, N.Y. and clinicians from Baghdad.   Their findings, revealed first by Bakir, et al.,[11] detailed the use of thiol resins in the treatment program. A report by Rustam, et al.[12] followed, detailing the neuromuscular disorder that is a part of the process of Minamata disease. Together, the study group learned that the 1972 outbreak was the most catastrophic ever recorded.

Officially, 6,530 cases were admitted to hospitals, and 459 deaths were attributed directly to methylmercury poisoning. The victims had eaten homemade bread made from seed grain intended for planting that had—again—been treated with methyl mercurial fungicide. The seed bags were properly labeled, and a warning was stamped clearly on each bag, but many of the people couldn't read, or believed the poison could be removed by washing. Initial symptoms began from two to eight weeks after the bread was eaten. The deaths happened generally within two weeks of the onset of symptoms. Others died gradually, while some remain ill even today, similarly to the plight of the people of Minamata Bay. The point to be made, however, is that some lessons are learned slowly. The disaster need not have happened at all had the Iraq officials followed the Swedish decision to ban mercury-based fungicides as a treatment for seed grain.

And More Contaminations. An experience similar to that in Minamata again occurred in the mid-1960's in Nigata Province, Japan. Seven deaths resulted from eating poisoned fish and shellfish before industrial dumping of mercurial wastes was again halted.

An isolated, non-fatal outbreak occurred during the period from 1961 to 1970 in northwestern Ontario and Quebec in Canada. In this case, Indians who ate fish from the English River were purportedly poisoned, causing a great deal of controversy. While there was not a single death or clinically-confirmed intoxication, and while epidemiological studies produced conflicting results, there were nevertheless many illnesses among the Indians that were never otherwise explained. Swedish and Japanese scientists had found that inorganic mercurial waste is quickly transformed in fish muscle to methylmercury (mercury's most toxic form), but the company responsible had ignored these previous discoveries.

Outbreaks of methylmercury poisoning from treated seed grain (used by companies and by countries that were slow in adopting the use of thiol-based fungicides) continued throughout the world: in Pakistan in 1963, in Guatemala in 1966, and in the United States in 1970.

MERCURY IN MEDICINE

Ironically, the very toxic nature of mercury is a feature that has made it useful in the practice of medicine. Variations of the heavy metal and its salts have been incorporated for hundreds of years in therapeutics such as laxatives, anti-inflammatory drugs, treatment for unwanted intestinal bacteria, disinfectants, and agents for wound closure. For over three hundred years mercury was the principal drug used in the treatment of syphilis (See Figure 1:1).

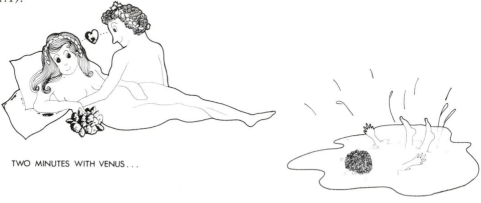

TWO MINUTES WITH VENUS...

TWO YEARS WITH MERCURY.

Figure 1:1 (Courtesy of S. B. Elhassani, M. D., "to emphasize the arduous treatment of syphilis with mercurial compounds")

In recent years organic mercurials have been used as purgatives, and especially as diuretics. In some parts of the world the umbilical stump is still being painted with merbromin (Mercurochrome 2%) as an antiseptic.[13] While seldom used today, organic mercurial diuretics are still available for cirrhotic patients who have low potassium intake, because mercurial diuretics tend to promote reabsorption of potassium; or for patients with congestive heart failure, particularly those in whom acute potassium loss might precipitate digitalis toxicity. On a positive side, its common use in medicine has allowed professionals in every field of health care to better understand, and become cautiously aware of, some of its long-term, undesired effects which might best be construed as symptoms of chronic mercury toxicity.

Chronic, low-level exposure can result in an accumulation of mercury in particularly vulnerable tissues, such as the kidneys, liver, brain, and heart muscle. The highest concentrations are in the kidneys, with the liver only slightly less affected. The central nervous system (CNS) is particularly sensitive to mercury, due, perhaps, to its high lipid content and to the slowness of nerve tissue in releasing mercury. (This will be discussed later.) In a general sense, chronic mercury exposure may cause renal damage, anemia, nonspecific weakness, malnutrition and a profound state of overall ill health.[14]

The Demise of Mercury in General Medicine

Mercury has been with us for a long time and has not been easy to completely replace. It is still being used in thermometers, though alcohol thermometers and heat sensor devices (thermistors) are taking its place. Perhaps the most notable replacement of mercury has occurred in instruments for measuring blood pressure, although the reading will likely always be given in mm Hg. Its use in the clinical laboratory, where it was once routinely used in the Van Slyke apparatus for measuring the blood bicarbonate level (CO_2), has likewise been virtually eliminated.

The use of mercury in medicine did not begin its dramatic decline until the late 1950's and early 1960's, when people throughout the world became concerned with industrial and environmental pollution. To the consumers and providers of health care alike, it became apparent that mercury was not just a funny, silvery-white liquid that beaded and scattered when a thermometer broke. Rather, mercury was something to be feared and respected, and no one could be entirely safe from its effect unless everyone, in every field of endeavor, was committed personally and responsibly to its safekeeping, as well as to its safe use and disposal. Hence, while the world was becoming enlightened about the dangers of mercury abuse, there was a corresponding movement within the health care system to investigate the problem—credited partly to the public outcry and partly to the ongoing and responsive development of improved technology and newer and safer drugs. For the most part the change has been well accepted.

The Demise of Mercury in Dentistry

The departure of mercury from dentistry has not, unfortunately, been so well accepted. Opponents of dental amalgam claim that mercury seeps slowly from a restored tooth over most (if not all) of the life of the filling; an average of 10 years, although some fillings are left in place as long as 40 years. They feel that this continuous, twenty-four hour-a-day exposure to traces of mercury may contribute to many poorly-defined, nonspecific health problems, both mental and physical. The proponents of amalgam fillings, led by the American Dental Association (ADA), present their own plausible argument. They feel the primary health risk is "to the dentist and the dental staff"[15] who must prepare the restorative material before placing it in the patient's mouth, but believe there is little risk thereafter to the patient. In fact, the ADA asserts, "there is no scientifically sound evidence linking amalgam restorations to any general medical disorder, and amalgam restorations continue to be shown safe for the vast majority of dental patients." They do readily admit to exceptions for those few people who are mercury-sensitive.

A problem here is that no form of testing for mercury sensitivity has ever been required prior to placing an amalgam restoration, nor is there presently an accepted, sensibly-priced test for determining patient/amalgam compatibility. There is an urgent need to solve this problem. Those few people, critics assert, could translate to a significant number who may be walking around with amalgam dental fillings and are sensitive to mercury: no one knows for certain what effect this has on general health.

Evidence that Dental Mercury Presents a Potential Health Risk to the Patient. Abraham, et al.,[16] suspecting that dental amalgam was a chronic source of toxicity, noted that blood mercury levels correlated with amalgam surface area. This work led researchers Vimy and Lorscheider[17] to perform serial measurements of intra-oral air mercury, estimating the daily dose of mercury from dental amalgam.   The researchers compared their findings to Threshold Limit Values (TLV's)—an international guide for mercury intoxication developed in West Germany. They compared further their findings to subjects who were free of dental amalgam. Intra-oral air mercury of patients with amalgam restorations, it was discovered, was 9 times that of people having no amalgam restorations. In addition, chewing for 10 minutes (thereby raising oral temperature to a point that enhances mercury vaporization) increased intra-oral air mercury an additional 6 times over the original baseline values. Thus, the amount of mercury released by chewing, in those people with amalgam restorations, exceeded by 54 times (9 x 6) a similar measurement from people who had no amalgam restorations. These findings were based upon an average of 8.6 occlusal amalgams per patient. When the toxic significance is compared with the TLV guideline, "the amount of elemental mercury calculated to be released daily from dental amalgams," said the authors, "either exceeds or comprises a major percentage of internationally accepted TLV's for environmental mercury exposure."

In their conclusion, Vimy and Lorscheider stated that suspected chronic exposure to mercury from dental amalgam should no longer be questioned. The focus instead must be turned to the number and type of amalgam restorations, which make a difference as to the quantity of intra-oral air mercury and the likelihood of toxicity. The focus should also be on methods of countering the problem; and on those people who are mercury-sensitive, because "the amount of mercury released from dental amalgam in some individuals could be sufficient to result in mercurialism."

Brune and Evje,[18] who studied man's mercury loading from dental amalgam, provide further evidence of the potential for causing chronic mercury toxicity. The researchers reported that the amount of mercury that appears daily in food and beverages will average 20 micrograms. While this amount is generally not dangerous to most people (the exception always being those who are mercury-sensitive, those who may already be mercury-toxic, or those who demonstrate adverse physiological changes to unusually low levels of mercury), the amount of mercury vapor released from the teeth of a patient with 20 amalgam restorations may add an additional 180 micrograms daily—nine times what is normally obtained through the diet. This level dangerously approaches the maximum allowed for industrial air quality.

While these works provide adequate reason to believe that dental amalgam presents a threat to human health, it becomes even more evident when one considers that the body has a natural barrier to the absorption of ingested, elemental mercury, but that methylmercury is absorbed by the intestines and the oral mucosa, and that mercury vapor from amalgam restorations is breathed into the lungs.

How Mercury From Dental Amalgam Intoxicates. Drs. Brune and Evje explain that "mercury released from the amalgam surface in the oral cavity may to some extent be ascribed to the effect of biological corrosion," which has been studied by Palaghias and Soremark.[19] These researchers learned biological corrosion was caused by living organisms, such as bacteria, and that a common bacteria in the mouth—streptococcus mutans—was most often responsible. Dr. Orstavik and his team added support[20] when they demonstrated that streptococcus mutans can thrive abundantly on amalgam restorations. They also stated that bacteria-induced corrosion results in the transformation of amalgamated, elemental mercury to methylated mercury that can either be swallowed or vaporized and drawn into the lungs. Therefore, the researchers believe, through the action of bacteria, biological corrosion forms two important chemical species of mercury: methylmercury and elemental mercury vapor.

The rate of intoxication (of elemental mercury vapor) is then influenced indirectly by lifestyle factors—chewing food, drinking hot beverages, and smoking cigarettes, all of which increase the rate of vaporization. When engaged in these activities the affected individual is also more apt to breath inwardly through the mouth rather than the nose, enhancing the entry of mercury vapor into the lungs; possibly the most dangerous point of entry.

Another complicating fact of corrosion, it has been hypothesized, is electrical corrosion due to oral galvanism. Patrick,[21] in 1880, was first to describe oral galvanism, the premise of which is that a leaky, dental amalgam filling is constantly supplying the oral cavity with the necessary ingredients to form a battery (ionizable metals, the warmth of body temperature and the mouth's natural electrolytes [saliva and dentinal fluid]). An electrical current emanates from the teeth twenty-four hours a day, and this abnormality may provide the body with an electrical source stronger than that generated by the brain, thereby contributing to brain disorders and neurological and neuromuscular diseases by interfering with normal brain waves and nerve signals. It has been hypothesized that amalgam fillings and other dental materials may contribute to disease through a mechanism other than chronic mercury toxicity or mercury sensitivity.

While there is currently no instrument approved by the FDA for measuring this phenomena, future development and approval of such an instrument may be important for several reasons. First, a reading above normal would suggest that the patient has amalgam fillings that are leaking, and which are therefore posing a potential risk to health. Second, the association of symptoms of micromercurialism with a positive reading would give the doctor of any specialty reason to suspect mercury as a possible underlying cause of disease.

Fragments of amalgam restorations are at times swallowed, but with limited danger. The mercury in this form is absorbed with great difficulty, since amalgam fragments are generally excreted through the intestine. If excretion is delayed, however, methylation of mercury can occur in the lower intestine just as it occurs on the tooth surface—through bacterial activity—but this action is limited to an isolated incidence. In addition, the intestinal flora are capable of degrading as much or more methylmercury than they can synthesize. Therefore, the significance of dental amalgam in human health is reserved for the sensitivity effect of elemental mercury, the neurological effect of mercury vapor, and the addition of methylated mercury—however slight— to the total body burden. All of these chemical species are likely to enter the body on a daily basis (especially if the patient has a number of old fillings), either through the lungs or by direct absorption through oral mucosal tissue. They can then be transported throughout the body.

The Public's Reaction

In keeping with custom the general public had previously been both forgiving for the use of mercury in medicine, and grateful for the changes. Their anger, if recognized at all, was cast aside. Until the last few years this accepting attitude has always been the people's response to scientific discovery and medical advances. Today, however, this reaction is changing. In the past, the changes that occurred in science and medicine took place over several generations. People were not faced with contradiction upon contradiction within a lifetime. The rapidity of change today has many people feeling helpless and sometimes suspicious of their health leadership. They don't like feeling as if they have been misled, and in turn have misled their families.

As a result, increasing numbers of American consumers of health services are discovering that the U. S. legal system offers a channel for protest, and

subsequently, a sophisticated means for profit. Lawsuits involving either medical or dental malpractice are growing in popularity, and increasing at a rate
that even has lawmakers looking at ways to curb their progression. The consumer sees in the judicial system an avenue for a just and equitable settlement;
their due financial compensation for failure of the health care system to meet
their societal expectations and ever-changing demands. The tendency to sue
and gain revenge rather than forgive and forget is coming at a time when the
issue of "proper use, or mercury abuse" is once again becoming an emotional debate, this time in the field of dentistry. For doctor and patient alike this development is most unfortunate, for the quest for truth in dentistry is currently
roadblocked by motives previously rarely encountered in science.

        In the U. S., because of the legal aspect, dental authorities who today
must set the guidelines of acceptable dental protocol may be reluctant to speak
out against the use of mercury when such action is warranted. They may fear
that dentists who have followed their previous guidelines will become liable.
If this is truly what is happening today then those whose health may be affected now and in the future will continue to have difficulty finding adequate
treatment. Likewise, their insurance companies will be reluctant to reimburse
them for that treatment. An extension of this concern may also affect research.
Whatever progress is made in getting closer to the truth would most likely be
met with a great deal of resistance. For this reason, and because of the recent
official declaration by the Swedish Dental Care System that amalgam is an
unsuitable and toxic dental filling material,* other doctors are pushing
ahead—without official word—to help solve their patient's mercury-related
problems. The purpose here is to help the doctor in as many ways as possible in
setting guidelines that, regardless of the outcome of future research, will aid in
their quest to improve the patient's overall health.

        The first 150 years of the use of amalgam in dentistry has provided no
clear-cut answers to the many questions that have arisen. Considering this, the
reader is encouraged to become familiar with both sides of the issue. In an attempt to be objective, this book will not make claims to defend or discredit the
motive of any individual or organization involved in the mercury amalgam debate.[†] Rather, the purpose is to address an issue that both sides agree upon:
MERCURY IS A POISON. IT IS ONE OF THE MOST POISONOUS ELEMENTS
KNOWN TO MAN, AND MERCURY AMALGAM MAY CAUSE ILL EFFECTS IN
THOSE PEOPLE WHO ARE MERCURY-SENSITIVE.

        Thus, the discussion here will primarily serve the opponents of dental
amalgam who seek background information on how mercury might affect
health. It will explain how the doctor might go about determining if a patient
is mercury-sensitive and mercury-toxic, and give considerations for treatment.
It will also serve those doctors who seek a source of information for the safe and
effective use of intravenous vitamin C in treating this and a variety of
indications.

        * The Bio-Probe Newsletter (see Appendix E) reported the finding of the So-
cialstyrelsen (Sweden's Social Welfare and Health Administration) investigation into
the dental amalgam debate. The Swedish authorities concluded that amalgam is unsafe; that its use shall be discontinued as soon as suitable replacement materials are
produced; and that its use in pregnant women will be stopped immediately.

        [†] The ADA position is found in Appendix A. A list of key doctors and health
organizations opposing the use of amalgam dental fillings can be found in Appendix B.

LITERATURE CITED

[1] Sir F.M.R. Walshe, *Perspectives in Biology and Medicine*, 2:197, 1959.

[2] A. Grollman and E.F. Grollman, Eds., *Pharmacology and Therapeutics*, Sixth Edition, Lea & Febiger, Philadelphia, Ch. 42, Heavy Metals, 1965.

[3] J.J. Putman and R.W. Madden, "Quicksilver and Slow Death," *National Geographic*, 142(4): 506-27, October 1972.

[4] L. Magos, "Mercury And Mercurials," *Br Med Bull*, 31(3): 241-5, 1975.

[5] G.N. Edwards, "Two Cases of Poisoning by Mercuric Methide," *St. Bart's Hosp Rep*, l: 141-50, 1885 (Notes on the termination of the second case of poisoning by mercuric methide. St. Bart's Hosp Rep 2: 211-12, 1886).

[6] D. Hunter, R.R. Bomford, and D.S. Russell, "Poisoning by Methyl Mercury Compounds," *Q J Med N*, S: 9: 193-213, 1940.

[7] D. McAlpine, and S. Araki, "Minamata Disease: An Unusual Neurological Disorder Caused by Contaminated Fish," *Lancet,* 2, 629-31, 1958.

[8] D. McAlpine, and S. Araki, "Late Effects of an Unusual Neurological Disorder Caused by Contaminated Fish," *A.M.A. Archs Neurol*, 1, 522-30, 1959.

[9] T. Takeuchi, "Pathology of Minamata Disease," *Acta Pathol Jpn*, 32 (Suppl l): 73-99, 1982.

[10] O. Gen, et al., "Urinary Beta-2-Microglobulin Does Not Serve as Diagnostic Tool for Minamata Disease," *Arch Environ Health*, 37(6): 336-41, November/December 1982.

[11] F. Bakir, et al., "The Employment of a Thiol Resin in Mercury Poisoning," *Science,* 181: 230-41, 1973.

[12] H. Rustam, et al., "Evidence for a Neuromuscular Disorder in Methylmercury Poisoning," *Arch Environ Health,* 30: 190-5, April 1975.

[13] S.B. Elhassani, "Neonatal Poisoning: Causes, Manifestations, Prevention, and Management," *So Med J,* 79 (12): 1535-43, December 1986.

[14] Grollman, op. cit.

[15] J.H. Berry, Manager of Media Services(*ADA*), Bureau of Communications, 211 East Chicago Avenue; Chicago, Illinois 60611, *Special News Release*, 1983.

[16] J.E. Abraham, et al., "The Effect of Dental Amalgam Restorations on Blood Mercury Levels," *J Dent Res*, 63:71-73, 1984.

[17] M.J. Vimy, and F.L. Lorscheider, "Serial Measurements of Intra-oral Air Mercury: Estimation of Daily Dose from Dental Amalgam," *J Dent Res*, 64(8): 1072-1075, August 1985.

[18] D. Brune and D.M. Evje, "Man's Mercury Loading from a Dental Amalgam," *The Science of the Total Environment*, 44:51-63, 1985.

[19] G. Palaghias, and R. Soremark, "The Electrochemical Properties of Three Amalgam Alloys in Cultures of S. Mutans," *Scandinavian Association for Dental Research*, 66th annual meeting, Stockholm, Sweden, p. 56, August 27-29, 1985.

[20] D. Orstavik, et al., "Bacterial Growth on Dental Restorative Materials in Mucosal Contact," *Acta Odontol Scand*, 39:267-274, 1985.

[21] J.J.R. Patrick, "Oral Electricity and New Departure," *D. Cosmos*, 22: 543, 1880.

CHAPTER 2

Ridding the Body of Heavy Metals:
An Important First Step
to Better Health

"The deviation of man from the state in which he was originally placed by nature seems to have proved to him a prolific source of diseases."
~Edward Jenner [1749-1823]

The evidence seems to indicate that a patient wishing to attain optimal health, regardless of the initial complaint or symptom that brings him to his doctor, may find a barrier to that goal in chronic heavy metal toxicity. The mechanism by which chronic mercury toxicity causes adverse symptoms must be accurately defined in order to find a solution to the problem. The approach in this book will be to outline, first, how most diseases begin: as an initial consequence of the disruption of cell membrane fluidity, leading eventually to impairment of normal cell function. The reader will learn how heavy metals in general—and mercury in particular—are involved in this process, and how chronic mercury toxicity may occur independently of the levels of blood and urine mercury. This will lead to a concluding, three-step program for ridding the body of heavy metals, with an emphasis on the treatment of chronic mercury toxicity. The success of the **IV-C Mercury Tox Program** is dependent on thoroughly implementing these steps before and after IV-C is administered.

Heavy metals such as mercury, lead, and cadmium, are so named to indicate a group of trace metals that 1) are generally of high atomic weight, 2) are normally present in the human diet, and 3) are toxic to humans when present in quantities other than trace amounts. Ironically, copper, iron, zinc, and selenium, which are essential to the diet of humans, are included among the heavy metals. Rarely do they become poisons, mostly because there are systems of checks and balances that occur first and mainly in the gastrointestinal tract. Until recently it was generally assumed that repeated, low-level exposure to heavy metals was of no more than academic importance to human health; the only true threat was acute poisoning.

The revelations of research during the past several years, however, have literally shattered that assumption. One finding, for instance, realizes that all disease (including heart disease), in one way or another involves an alteration in the structure and function of cell membranes, and that chronic, low-level exposure to heavy metals is an important cause of these changes. A second finding by Wedeen[1] revealed that endstage renal disease today accounts for an expenditure in excess of $2 billion per year in the U. S.; that the bulk of this expense is incurred by hemodialysis and transplantation programs almost entirely funded by Medicare; and that the evidence points to heavy metals as the primary, underlying cause. Wedeen's reporting suggests that if doctors would address the issue of chronic heavy metal toxicity in each and every patient, regardless of the presenting symptoms, it is likely that the incidence and expense of endstage renal disease could be greatly reduced.

In a search for the source of environmental heavy metals, it is important to note that the normal human diet seldom contains enough toxic metals to override a natural protection afforded by the gastrointestinal tract. Any excess of heavy metals is routinely excreted before absorption can occur. Diet, therefore, is rarely the source of chronic heavy metal toxicity, although an unbalanced diet may impede the normal protective mechanisms, as will be illustrated later.

Chronic heavy metal toxicity is usually the result of industrial contamination, occupational risk, or the use and misuse of man-made products. The sources of contamination are generally tainted drinking water and polluted air, which intoxicate through ingestion and direct contact with the skin and mucous membranes. Once intoxication has begun, or is imminent, diet and preventive steps become very important, for it is then necessary to safeguard against further contamination and provide the nutritional support needed for detoxification.

This chapter will explain the initial lifestyle steps that are necessary to minimize the potential for disease due to some of the major heavy metals. In order to completely understand the problems of chronic heavy metal toxicity, and particularly chronic mercury toxicity, the reader must fully comprehend the extent to which heavy metals now pollute our environment. The process of heavy metal poisoning, particularly the way it interferes with cell functioning, must also be understood. We will first attempt to provide all the background information necessary for that comprehension.

HEAVY METALS: THE LEAST AND THE MOST SIGNIFICANT

The Industrial Revolution brought with it the need for a large quantity and variety of heavy metals. In turn, people of every country and occupation have since become exposed to heavy metals to an extent that the world's population has never before experienced. While all of these are potential sources of toxicity, some present a greater health risk than others.

Silver, gold, and tin are included among the heavy metals that are potentially toxic but are rarely causes of poisoning. In addition, when present in the diet in normal trace amounts they have been reported to enter into biochemical reactions compatible with human health. Even so, it is still not clear whether in these extremely small increments they are essential for human health, or simply enter into cell reactions that would occur anyway. Regardless, there is a growing concern for their toxic potential, mostly because of their widespread use in recent years as common components of dental materials that are routinely placed in the mouth. The same might be said for aluminum and nickel, which have a much greater potential for toxicity.

Mercury, lead, and cadmium, however, are the heavy metals that we are here mainly concerned with. More than all other environmental pollutants today, these represent the greatest threat to human health. Mercury is the most dangerous, followed by lead and then cadmium (although lead contamination is thought to be the most widespread). Optimal health, as we shall see, is attainable only after the potential for bodily damage from these three heavy metals has been maximally reduced.

From 1965 to 1980 the average levels of mercury, lead, and cadmium in our environment tapered off somewhat, notwithstanding the growing recognition of chronic mercury toxicity from its use in dental materials. Reasons for the decline can be attributed in part to the Clean Air Amendments of 1970; to the workplace safeguards mandated by the National Institute of Occupational Safety and Health Administration (OSHA); and to the Safe Drinking Water Act of 1974.

Yet even with legislative actions of this magnitude, the level of heavy metal pollutants still remains higher today than anytime before 1900. In the U. S. this is largely due to auto exhaust, heating fuel, and extensive metal refining. Other countries have additional problems. In Denmark, for example, spent shotgun ammunition accounts for three times more environmental lead (800 tons annually) than does automobile exhaust.[2] The decomposition products of leadshot are largely in an unbound extractable form, which make their way into streams, dust, and terrestrial plants.

Airborne particles from these various sources settle to earth and contaminate the food chain. Polluted dust settles upon plants that are then eaten by cattle, poultry, and hogs, and later transferred to humans. As dust reaches our lakes, rivers, and oceans, fish may also become contaminated. Only recently, in the U. S., the nation's first major long-term (1974 to 1981) study of water quality was completed.[3] While the level of lead in rivers decreased during the study period, there was a widespread increase reported for nitrate (from fertilizer runoff and acid rain), river salinity (from road salt), and two heavy metals: arsenic and cadmium. To the dismay of many, the heavy metals were found to originate not from direct discharge into the waters by industry, but rather from atmospheric pollution, mostly coal combustion emissions.

We will examine in more detail the three heavy metals we are most concerned with.

Cadmium

Cadmium originates from coal combustion as well as many other sources, and has become a growing pollutant of air and water. It is produced during the processing of zinc, resembling zinc both physically and chemically. In the early 1900's only small amounts of cadmium were manufactured. By 1975, however, the annual world production totaled approximately 15,000 tons. Cadmium is used as a binding agent in the electroplating industry, in production of dyes, and in construction of nickel cadmium batteries. It enters the food chain from edible plants that have been fertilized by sewage sludge, finding its way there from industrial sources.

"Cadmium is mobile," says toxicologist Donald Lisk of Cornell University, in an interview published in *Science News*.[4] "It moves readily from soil to plants to animals."

While smelter workers are the most likely people to be subjected to acute poisoning, a growing concern today is the eventuality of chronic contamination from cigarette smoking, as cadmium tends to "load" in the leaves of tobacco plants. It is difficult, however, to determine a dangerous level of cadmium exposure. While none seems to be ideal, it has been reported that the average American intake is about 70 micrograms daily[5]..."a level that should probably not be exceeded," says Lisk.

Lead

While the concentration of lead is declining in our waterways, lead from a variety of other sources is several hundred times more concentrated in humans now than it was in 1900. Recognizing this trend, The World Health Organization has set a maximum daily limit for human exposure to lead at 430 micrograms (μg). The present average daily intake is already at 300 μg per person, a level which the officials of WHO recognize is much too close to the maximum allowed.

Mercury

Chronic mercury toxicity today is recognized not so much as a consequence of accepted dental practice, but more for the danger that it presents to workers in industry. (A list of high risk occupations will be found in Appendix C.) Many other sources of mercury exposure were disclosed in Chapter 1. These include methyl mercurial fungicides used in treating seed grain, organomercurials used in medicines, and methylmercury in fish caught in polluted water, as well as the mercury found in silver amalgam dental fillings.

Mercury, note the editors of *Pharmacology and Therapeutics*,[6] in spite of its highly toxic effect on all living cells, has continued through the years to be important for industrial and medical use. This seems inexcusable given the facts.

Mercurial salts, elemental mercury, and high-dose methyl mercurials have the potential to cause severe intestinal irritation, and their action precipitates proteins. It is this property that is primarily responsible for the abundance of mucoid threads that appear in the stools of those with acute intoxication. While insoluble mercury is less likely to be absorbed, even the pure metal may be oxidized and absorbed when it is applied to living tissues or allowed to enter the blood in a state of fine division. Methylmercury from contaminated seed grains and fish caught in polluted water, therefore, as well as elemental mercury and mercury vapor from corroded dental fillings, may lead to poisoning or chronic mercury toxicity upon entering the intestines and the lungs. Mercury applied directly to the skin likewise has the same effect after passing into the gland ducts, along the roots of the hairs, and into the blood stream for distribution to all tissues—a scenario which continually happens today in the practice of medicine from the use of Mercurochrome.[7]

An international committee of WHO, in 1969, found it necessary to set guidelines to protect workers, establishing the Maximum Allowable Concentration (MAC),[8] referred to today as Threshold Limit Values, or TLV. It is interesting that for most of the free world, the TLV for metallic mercury vapor is 50 µg mercury per 1.0 m^3 air; for inorganic salt, 100 µg mercury per 1.0 m^3 air. However, the Soviet Union has set a TLV for their workers of 5 µg mercury per 1.0 m^3 air[9] (10 times less than the average limit), suggesting that perhaps the Soviets have become much more aware of the dangers of mercury.

Responding to this difference, in 1972 WHO set the tolerable weekly human intake for mercury at 0.3 mg (300 µg) from all sources, and cut the TLV in half, from 50 to 25 µg mercury per 1.0 m^3 air. This level, according to an assessment by the National Research Council, is easily surpassed even by those who don't work with mercury directly. A predatory fish caught in heavily polluted water, for instance, may contain as much as 4 mg mercury in a six-ounce serving, as opposed to an average of 0.067 mg (67 µg) for the same fish caught in unpolluted water. It is evident, therefore, that any additional, unnecessary pollution of the environment by mercury is a potential negative factor toward general health, and has the possibility of being a causal agent in many disease conditions.

This may be one important reason why the issue of mercury in dentistry is of greater significance today than at any time during its previous history. Because environmental mercury is fast becoming a more widespread threat to our health than ever before, the contribution of mercury from dentistry is becoming more significant, just as the potential for disease from contaminated fish is becoming more significant. Each source of contamination adds to our overall health risk. The answer to solving this problem is to eliminate the use of mercury in every way possible. Dentistry must do its part by researching alternative materials.

ABOUT HEAVY METALS: SOME FACTORS THAT MAY MAKE THE DIFFERENCE BETWEEN HEALTH AND DISEASE

In his book, *Nutrition Against Disease*,[10] Dr. Roger Williams used the term "biological individuality" to explain that every human is genetically and biochemically different from every other individual, and that each of us individually has a biological weakness that makes us different from any other person. His teaching implies that certain people are especially vulnerable to heavy metals in general, and vulnerable to one or another of the heavy metals in particular. Biological individuality also implies that not one of us is truly "normal" and that even while in our normal state of health we are all affected in some way by heavy metal poisoning. Some people are affected more than others.

Biological individuality helps to explain why some people develop symptoms even from low-level exposure to a heavy metal while others do not, and how the symptoms of chronic mercury toxicity can differ so widely from patient to patient. Chronic exposure promotes accumulation in particular body cells according to the patient's genetic and biochemical makeup, which logically may depend upon his current health status. People who are healthiest before being exposed to heavy metals are most likely to have the greatest resistance to its effect.

A unique property of heavy metals is that they are absorbed more easily than they are excreted; particularly true of the early phase of exposure. When *steady state* (bodily absorption vs. excretion) is reached, as much metal is excreted as absorbed; as exposure declines more of the metal is excreted than absorbed until the new steady state is reached. One can see why it is so very important to the treatment process to remove the patient from further exposure as soon as possible.

The opportunity for brain involvement increases if the patient's exposure is prolonged. The mean half life for clearance of methylmercury, for instance, has been estimated by Takeuchi to be 70 days for the body in general, and 240 days for the brain.[11*] It is easy to see how a prolonged exposure can become a serious mental health problem long after the patient has been removed from the source of exposure, and long after the patient's physical health improves. Additionally, due to idiosyncratic reactions those who are most sensitive to mercury, especially elemental mercury, or any other heavy metal may continue to react in ways that do not fit the usual dose/response curve. Due also to chemical and biological differences, each heavy metal differs in its affinity for particular tissues or organs, thereby having the potential to cause a variety

* Takeuchi's calculation of the half life of brain mercury is an estimation. The analysis was carried out after many years of preservation, rather than in fresh tissue. The autopsied patients' exposure to methylmercury was known, but the blood mercury level at the onset of disease was not. Additionally, the only condition of selection was death (the primary cause of death for these patients was not always methylmercury poisoning), so the data was never intended to be anything more than an estimation.

of diseases (Table 2:1).

Wedeen informs that the crucial diagnostic organs (through biopsy) for cadmium, lead, and mercury are, respectively: liver, bone, and the kidneys. Yet these organs are not necessarily the same organs that are most affected by the heavy metal. Table 2:1 aptly demonstrates this fact. Cadmium, for instance, has an affinity for hemoglobin and for lung tissue, thereby contributing to emphysema and fatigue. Lead is found in the gastrointestinal tract, blood, and brain tissue as well, which may make it a factor in fatigue and retardation, as well as in many other diseases that relate to the central nervous system. Mercury, the most harmful of the heavy metals, while most easily detected in the kidney, is more likely to affect the functioning of the CNS, brain, immune system, and the heart. It also affects the teeth, gums, and gastrointestinal tract. Its effect has best been explained by Sami B. Elhassani, M. D., Professor of Pediatrics at the Medical University of South Carolina, and also a member of the reviewing staff for this book. Dr. Elhassani—who has had extensive experience treating the mercury-toxic patient—reports that patients with minor exposure to methylmercury may show signs and symptoms mimicking those of other diseases, especially CNS and psychiatric-related illnesses.

The attending doctor, therefore, in conjunction with his usual diagnostic procedure, would wisely take steps to evaluate the possible role of mercury in any patient with appropriate symptoms, and in any patient who failed to respond to therapy. A study of the cell membrane offers a clue as to how heavy metals, particularly mercury, contribute to disease.

THE CELL MEMBRANE THEORY IN DISEASE: HOW HEAVY METALS MAY CONTRIBUTE TO ALL DEGENERATIVE DISEASES

Every doctor and health professional who reads this will likely have had some training in the workings of the cell membrane. A few will be experts. Regardless, the explanation here will begin with the basic, historical development of our present knowledge. This is needed in order to present a new and changing perspective that will differ somewhat from the contemporary view, and in order to sympathize with those who have been out of school long enough to have forgotten how a cell works. Finally, a return to the basics will help when discussing the topic with patients and colleagues.

The cell membrane theory in disease is important not only in discerning how mercury contributes to disease, but also in explaining an underlying argument of this lifestyle series. What's being emphasized here is not that heavy metals are the cause of all degenerative diseases, but rather that a review of cell membrane function provides an understanding of how heavy metals may contribute to the cause of all degenerative diseases. The cell membrane theory in disease also forms the basis for my own interpretation of an elevated total serum cholesterol (TSC).

The view of cholesterol taken here differs only slightly, but significantly enough, from the contemporary view which was formally presented at the 1986 Scientific Sessions of the American Heart Association;[12] and from the guidelines set forth a year later by the National Heart, Lung, and Blood Institute's Expert Panel on Detection, Evaluation, and Treatment.[13] In both instances a panel of noted scientists made it clear that a severely elevated TSC should be considered dangerous, that a moderately to severely elevated TSC serves as a causal factor in heart disease, and that an elevated TSC should be

Table 2:1

Heavy Metal	Tissues and Organs Most Affected	Diseases That May Result
Mercury	Liver Kidney Teeth and Gums Intestinal Wall Muscle and Bone Lungs Spleen Brain Central Nervous System	Enters every body organ and may contribute to all diseases
Lead	Brain Blood Digestive System Bone Kidney	Headache Irritability Depression Fatigue Gout High Blood Pressure Kidney Diseases
Cadmium	Lungs Kidney Blood Liver	High Blood Pressure Iron Deficiency Anemia Emphysema Hypercalcemia Itai-Itai (ouch-ouch disease) Prostate Hypertrophy Bone Wasting Disease Kidney Diseases: albuminuria hypercalciuria kidney stones
Nickel	Thymus Gland	Cancer Depression of the Immune System
Aluminum	Brain Kidneys	Alzheimer's Disease
Silver	Connective Tissue	Argyria
Gold	Blood Kidneys	High Fever Unexplained Rash and Urine Albumin
Copper	Blood Hemoglobin	Anemia
Iron	Liver Heart	Fatigue Iron Overload Disease

lowered through a low-fat, low-cholesterol diet, or by combining same with appropriate drug therapy.

My own interpretation differs not with the importance of reducing a moderately to severely elevated TSC. Rather, I contend that the program now being promoted to reduce TSC does not address all possible underlying causes, in which case simply reducing an elevated TSC through reduction of dietary cholesterol and fat (with and without drug intervention) will in some patients do nothing more than eliminate an important symptom of disease, while the primary defect remains.

The amended interpretation of an elevated TSC, presented here, lays the groundwork for understanding the basic approach taken in the lifestyle series for preventing heart disease: An elevated TSC should more accurately be interpreted as a symptom, rather than the cause, of arterial disease, and any program for the prevention of heart disease must necessarily address all underlying factors affecting cell membranes, where all diseases begin. Chronic mercury toxicity represents one such possibility.

Although heavy metals in general have the capacity to increase the risk of heart disease, Shaper reports that mercury itself may play a causal role independently of any other factor,[14] raising suspicion that an elevated TSC linked with heart disease may, in many cases, reflect the presence of mercury. Perry and Erlanger demonstrated that mercury may also be a cause of high blood pressure.[15] Looking more closely at the role that mercury might play in heart disease, it is hypothesized in our January 1987 issue of **HEART TALK**[16] (from data derived from the work of two Nobel Prize-winning scientists—Drs. Michael S. Brown and Joseph L. Goldstein), that mercury may interfere with available receptors for LDL (low density lipoprotein) cholesterol, thereby causing an elevated TSC. This would seem to indicate the wisdom of addressing the mercury issue before attempting to reduce a patient's cholesterol through a combination of diet and drugs.

The approach taken here for preventing or correcting any disease draws upon the principle that "a simple solution requires a well defined problem." Before the microscope was introduced, the problem of chronic heavy metal toxicity presented a formidable challenge. The treatment for this as well as other metabolic diseases was mostly accomplished by trial and error through the use of remedial methods, as opposed to today's more scientific approach. The microscope made it possible to study disease at the cellular level, which in turn made it possible to redefine the disease process, and thence to better define the problem.

Disease Redefined: The Modern Concept

The steps required for the modern definition of disease began in 1855 when Carl Nageli became the first to distinguish a difference in the transfer rate of pigments in damaged and undamaged cells. Nageli observed that pigment uptake of healthy cells was much slower, suggesting an external cell barrier, while damaged cells showed little resistance to the same pigment. He reasoned that a discriminating wall separated the healthy cell from its liquid environment, and coined the phrase "plasma membrane" to identify it. Today it is known that a system of plasma membranes is present in each cell. This system serves to compartmentalize the cell and protect its constituents. While the discussion here is limited to the outer cell membrane, factors that affect one plasma membrane will likely affect the entire system. (Figure 2:1)

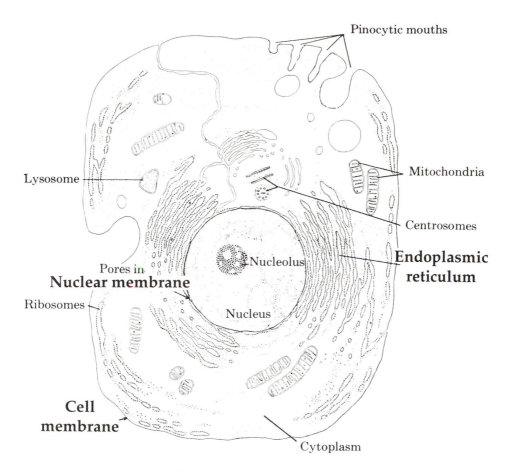

Figure 2:1 Typical Animal Cell. (Modified from Plate XI of Dorland's Illustrated Medical Dictionary, p. 236, 26th Edition — with permission of the W.B. Saunders Co.)

Charles Overton, in 1920, suggested that the cell membrane is composed of compound lipids such as fatty acids, sterols, and neutral fats. A few years later, in 1925, Gortel and Grendel speculated that the membrane lipids are arranged in bilayer fashion. Porter and Palade, in 1960, using an electron microscope, described the endoplasmic reticulum. The bilayered plasma cell membrane, they explained, had the tendency to extend itself inwardly when appropriate, forming a channel-like network allowing passage of nutrients, waste, and other molecules to and from the inner cell. This groundwork led Singer, in the 1970's, to describe the fluid mosaic model of membrane structure, which remains today our most widely accepted view of the cell membrane.[17] (Figure 2:2)

The fluid mosaic model demonstrates that the bilayered cell membrane is quite complex. Each layer consists of lecithin and other phospholipids with a mix of carbohydrate/fat combinations, fat/protein particles, and large molecules of integral protein. The membrane selectively serves as sentry to the inner cell. In performing this function it is constantly in motion, literally doing backward somersaults. Its flip-flop action influences selective permeability through changes in position of its membrane lipids. By this authority the cell membrane protects the cell and serves as "social director," mediating its interaction with all other cells and the environment.[18]

Certain membrane proteins serve as recognition sites for antigens— identity tags that prevent the body's surveillance mechanism from destroying the cell as it would any foreign body.[19] Sugar proteins and sugar lipids, together, form a communication system which recognizes neighboring cells. Through this system the cell membrane can signal its own cell nucleus for constraint of cell growth. In addition, the cell membrane synthesizes special protein receptors, as needed, or it provides the platform for cell-synthesized receptors to manifest, thereby encouraging attachment of chemical messengers from neighboring cells, glands, and organs. Through this action, cell membranes provide a sophisticated means of communication to synchronize body activities. The number and availability of receptor sites for these messengers may change as the bilayer flip-flops, or according to the rate of their biosynthesis.

Cholesterol is also a major component here, common to the cell membranes of all animals as well as humans. Because of this, cell membranes are similar in makeup to lipoproteins (while lacking triglycerides) that must carry cholesterol and the fat soluble nutrients to and from these cells. Being similar, lipoproteins and cell membranes actively exchange membrane components with one another. It is the membrane structure and its functional nature that allows this to happen, being two-dimensional, viscous, and fluid-oriented. Many of these same features can be found in the lipoprotein particle, which when compared structurally and functionally, could just as easily be construed as a circulating plasma membrane. In particular, the cell membrane must be compatible with both an outer watery environment and its inner cell constituents. When operating normally the cell membrane can then perform (at the very least) six basic functions. (Figure 2:3)

The characteristic which allows the cell membrane to carry out its normal function is membrane fluidity. In fact, as will be discussed in the next few paragraphs, membrane fluidity is the one major feature that separates healthy cells from stressed, malfunctioning cells. It may also be an important determinant of the level of serum cholesterol, significant now only to the extent that one can more easily see how solving heavy metal toxicity relates to the previously-stated, ultimate goal of attainment of optimal health while preventing heart disease.

Cell Membrane Fluidity

Cell membrane fluidity is perhaps the best known indicator of the state of cell health. Indirectly, it is a measure of lipid peroxidation—an indicator of the rate of free radical oxidation that is a constant threat to the health of cells. In health, fluidity allows cell diffusion to occur without interruption, while allowing a smooth molecular flow within the cell in spite of the extreme pressure exerted by circulating blood, lymph, and interstitial fluid. Fluidity also is important for the cell to be selectively permeable to constituents that satisfy its own needs. As membrane fluidity decreases, or increases (either may occur but the loss of membrane fluidity seems to be a more significant determinant of disease), the cell membrane loses part or all of this discriminating

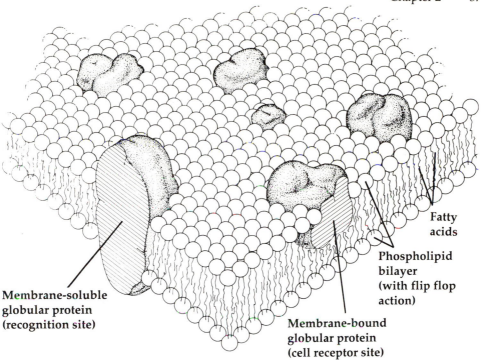

Figure 2:2   Fluid Mosaic Model of Plasma Cell Membrane: Modified from *Science* 175:72, 1972. Courtesy of S.J. Singer, Ph.D., Professor of Biology, University of California, San Diego, La Jolla, California.

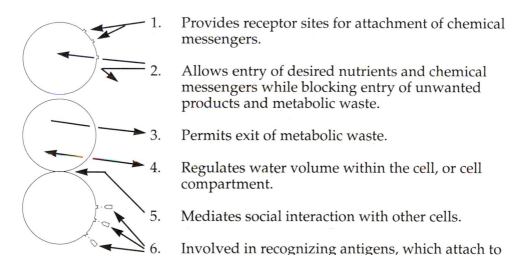

1. Provides receptor sites for attachment of chemical messengers.

2. Allows entry of desired nutrients and chemical messengers while blocking entry of unwanted products and metabolic waste.

3. Permits exit of metabolic waste.

4. Regulates water volume within the cell, or cell compartment.

5. Mediates social interaction with other cells.

6. Involved in recognizing antigens, which attach to glycoproteins.

Figure 2:3   Six primary functions of plasma cell membranes: Cadmium, lead, and mercury may interfere with normal function in any one of several ways, by attachment to membrane, sulfhydryl proteins, for instance, which may then promote oxidation of membrane constituents.

function. The loss of selective permeability also causes the cell to lose resistance to drastic changes that may occur in its watery outer environment, which results in a dysfunctional stressed cell. The consequence goes beyond lost permeability, however. Reduced membrane fluidity causes cell stress, which may interrupt all normally occurring functions of the cell membrane. This produces cell fatigue, ultimately causing the cell to dysfunction. (Figure 2:4)

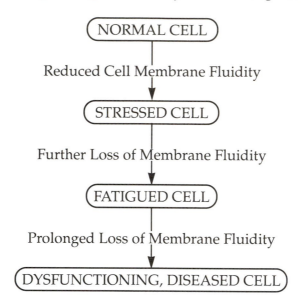

Figure 2:4

A reduction of membrane fluidity can result from many causes. Drs. Bauer and First[20] report that mercury and other heavy metals—which are easily taken up by cell membranes—represent one of the more significant ones. Ionic mercury reaches the cell membranes attached to circulating blood proteins, particularly the water-soluble, protein component of lipoproteins. Here, its affinity is strongest for the sulfhydryl proteins: methionine, cysteine, glutathione, and cystine. It is this feature, in fact, that allows ionic mercury to exchange freely between lipoproteins and the macromolecules (of ligands) of cell membranes, including red blood cells (RBC's). The hemoglobin portion of RBC's are particularly rich in sulfhydryl proteins, similar to lipoproteins, which further explains how ionic mercury reaches the various cell membranes via blood.

"This lipotropic relationship," explain Drs. Bauer and First, "facilitates a change in membrane permeability, in which mercuric ions bind to ligands and change transmembrane potentials." The change is believed to contribute to the symptoms of fatigue so often expressed by patients with chronic mercury toxicity. Ironically, however, the affinity of mercury for lipoproteins provides the basis by which mercury is most easily exited from the body, through the intestines as a component of bile.

Sulfhydryl proteins are characterized by the highly active thiol (SH) group that serves as an antioxidant, or reducing agent. The most important of these is glutathione (GSH). Like other cell membrane protectors (vitamins E, A, and C), GSH and other sulfhydryl proteins are destroyed by oxidative processes, and must thereby be regenerated daily to protect the cell. When mercury attaches to sulfhydryl proteins of cell membranes, the cell is subjected abnormally to oxidative processes and there is greater need for these nutrients. Because of the high content of sulfhydryl proteins in the normal lens of the eye, for instance, and the low content in the lens of patients with cataract, it is possible that chronic mercury toxicity is a contributing factor in the cataractous process. In fact, the accumulation of mercury in the eye of some people is known to express itself as band keratopathy, which affects the cornea and causes ocular rigidity and impairment of the visual field.

Galin and Obstbaum,[21] in studying this problem, learned that mercury may damage by acting as a denaturant of ocular protein. Attachment of mercury to the sulfhydryl proteins that are abundant in the eye occurs first, followed by altered cell membrane permeability (highlighted by a negative change in fluidity). This allows mercury to denature the cell's membrane proteins, thereby causing the deposition of calcium salts. Ironically, just as the affinity of mercury for lipoproteins provides a basis for its removal from the body, its strong affinity for sulfhydryl proteins does likewise, resulting in the recommendation of a diet high in both fat and sulfhydryl proteins.

Vitamin C offers some protection to the eye. As Varma[22] has noted, the healthy cornea has the third highest tissue concentration of vitamin C (the adrenals and the liver have higher levels). He also noted that structures of the neural retina undergo severe degeneration in scurvy. Based on this, his subsequent research confirmed that vitamin C and the cataractous process were directly related. Lohmann,[23] however, found that the relationship was due not to a deficiency of ascorbic acid, but to the rapid oxidation of ascorbic acid which is characteristic of chronic mercury toxicity.

Vitamin E, according to Welsh,[24] is an important antioxidant that provides the cell membrane with protection against mercury-induced oxygen radicals. When cells are deficient of this—and other protective agents such as vitamin C—both organic and inorganic mercury compounds promote oxidative damage to cell membranes.[25] Niki, who researched this relationship further,[26] revealed that vitamins E and C serve as antioxidants, or scavengers of oxygen radicals. In addition, vitamin C serves to regenerate membrane vitamin E—by converting the oxidized form of vitamin E back to its active, reduced form. Yet when vitamin E and/or vitamin C is deficient, (or when the demand for either is increased due to increased oxidation, as is characteristic of chronic mercury toxicity) the disease process begins as previously discussed, through interference with the selective uptake of nutrients by the cell membrane. It then disrupts the orderly discharge of cell waste, causing cell stress, leading to cell fatigue. This ultimately causes dysfunction and/or death for critical cells in the organ or cell group—a characteristic of almost all diseases, including the cataractous process and arterial disease.

As the process of disease progresses from the normal cell to the stressed cell, it becomes clear that each proceeding stage is most likely to develop when a combination of stresses are at work, and least likely to develop when the total number of stresses are held to a minimum. In this manner one can understand why people (some more than others) are vulnerable to heavy metals. "Theoretically," says Dr. Elhassani, "those who have the poorest diet and lifestyle are the most vulnerable, but we can't really know this for certain until a double blind study is performed." The concept that a poor diet and lifestyle predisposes one to disease in general, also emphasizes the role that continued heavy metal exposure might play in an individual whose cells are already stressed or fatigued from this or other causes. In these people the smallest additional burden of a heavy metal, particularly mercury, has the potential for causing disease, especially since mercury makes so many additional demands on one's nutritional status, and is so slowly removed—again remembering that methylmercury has a half life of 70 days in most tissues, and 240 days in the brain.

Researchers at Osaka City University Medical School, Osaka, Japan,[27] demonstrated that once mercury and other heavy metals pass through the cell membrane barrier, there is an immediate and varying effect upon the cell. As determined by Galin and Obstbaum, calcium deposits may occur, and/or the cell's enzyme system may be altered, resulting in either inhibition of enzyme activity or cell death. Mercury has a special affinity for enzymes, in addition to lipoidal cells, because sulphur-bearing amino acids are primary constituents of most enzymes.

This becomes significant when it is noted that specific enzymes are required to catalyze almost all major chemical reactions within cells. Therefore it is not surprising that mercury tends to accumulate mainly within organs that contain the most enzymes, sulfhydryl proteins, and fat. The liver, which is known to contain at least a thousand different enzymes, is a prime site. (In spite of this, liver function seems to be altered less severely than that of the brain or kidneys, most likely due to the liver's role in detoxifying toxins and metabolites.) The brain and CNS are the most sensitive targets, partially because mercury vapor readily oxidizes in brain and nervous tissue to its ionic form, where ionic mercury freely binds with sulfhydryl groups of cell membranes, protein, and brain enzymes; thereby having the potential to cause a wide variety of sensory, motor, and mental disturbances.

Since antibodies are normally synthesized from methionine, cysteine, and cystine—the major sulfhydryl proteins—mercury also tends to be incorporated as a constituent of new antibodies. This, and the demonstration by Hirokawa and Hayashi that mercury causes atrophy of the immune-producing thymic cortex of mice,[28] suggests that chronic mercury toxicity could be the co-factor in humans responsible for the progression from infection to illness due to bacteria or viruses.

The onset of Acquired Immune Deficiency Syndrome (AIDS) is a good example. According to the U. S. Public Health Service, as of February 1987 anywhere from one to one-and-a-half million people in the U. S. are infected with the human immunodeficiency virus (HIV). Yet it is expected over the next five years only 20 to 30 percent of them will develop AIDS. If the co-infection hypothesis—that the disease process of AIDS doesn't manifest until the patient's immune system is taxed by a co-existing infection—is correct, as many researchers now believe it is, it is important to those who _are_ infected with the virus, but who are free of symptoms, to avoid other viral infections that would allow the dormant HIV to develop into AIDS.

Because of the preferential binding of mercury with sulphur-containing amino acids, and because its transport hinges on proteins and lipoproteins, the effect of mercury becomes most apparent in particular organs and systems, as we have just demonstrated. Mercury tends to concentrate in brain and nerve tissue, where lipoidal tissue is dominant, and in the liver, kidney, spleen, lungs, intestinal wall, and smooth and skeletal muscles, where sulfhydryl proteins dominate. The same principle applies to any of the heavy metals, each having an affinity for specific tissues.

Referring again to Table 2:1, mercury has a special affinity for the kidneys. While kidney problems are slow to surface as a consequence of mercury intoxication, unhealthy changes in cell membrane fluidity are noted earlier. In acute mercurialism, for instance, the primary damage to the kidneys is caused by an increase in the permeability of the tubular epithelium. The subtle changes at first cause transient polyuria, due to the failure of tubular reabsorption. As the plasma membranes of the affected cells compensate, the symptom of polyuria reverses, sometimes correcting itself to the opposite extreme, causing anuria.

Anuria reflects total reabsorption of tubular fluid—a feature that parallels onset of the nephrotic syndrome, or nephrosis.* Mercury is, in fact, known to cause the nephrotic syndrome through just such a scenario. Although anuria is not a feature of the mercurial nephrotic syndrome, the presence of anuria in those people who are susceptible to nephrosis, or who formerly had nephrosis, raises suspicion that chronic mercury toxicity may be a contributing cause, in some people, of the irreversible degenerative changes which lead to endstage renal disease (as referred to earlier by Wedeen). Thus, since the nephrotic syndrome—and nearly every disease, including endstage renal disease—involves changes in cell membrane fluidity (which often accompanies chronic mercury toxicity), restoring membrane fluidity before these irreversible changes can occur (through purging the body of heavy metals) is believed to be an important first step in preventing disease and attaining optimal health.

Noticeable changes in a diseased cell membrane are: an alteration in the content of membrane cholesterol (usually reduced); a corresponding alteration in membrane fluidity (likewise, usually reduced); and an altered total serum cholesterol (usually elevated, but this is not a strict condition). It is this combination of features that may characterize cell stress due to any cause, and which has prompted the concept of disease held throughout this book and to be held in future books in the lifestyle series. Again, disease proceeds from a normal, healthy cell ultimately to cell dysfunction. The process may or may not be reversible, depending upon the extent of damage and whether or not the contributing causes can be identified and removed. The deciding factor rests with whether or not membrane fluidity can be restored to the cell group.

Because heavy metals are absorbed more easily than excreted, the intake of heavy metals usually exceeds output. The body can handle acute poisoning over time, but in any chronic exposure there is a net accumulation. Chisolm explains that the residence time for lead in soft tissues is 35 to 40 days, after which it may rest in bone tissue for 25 to 30 years. A similar problem exists with mercury and cadmium. A chronic exposure, particularly to lead, cadmium, and/or mercury, may cause a reduction in the translational property of integral protein, hindering the cell membrane's ability to communicate with other cells, as well as its own cell nucleus. The cell membrane is less able to exchange components with lipoproteins; it thereby becomes deficient of fat-soluble nutrients, such as vitamins E and A; and it becomes noticeably rigid, or stressed, when compared to normal. The health consequences of this may not be seen for 20, 30, or even 40 years, but may eventually surface as a problem that becomes diagnosed relative to the way it manifests. In these cases there is a

* According to the findings of Kantarjian,[29] these same changes underlie the clinical syndrome of amyotrophic lateral sclerosis (ALS). ALS was documented in eleven individuals in Iraq who had mistakenly eaten bread prepared from seed grain treated with a mercurial fungicide. This raises a question regarding the potential role of mercury in all such cases of ALS in which kidney disease is also present.

risk that the treatment regimen will address only the symptoms and not the cause.

For example: A patient with emphysema may be accumulating cadmium from a variety of sources; from cigarettes, from the air that he breathes normally, or from house dust. He is treated for the emphysema and advised to give up cigarettes, but the house dust and air supply at home or work may be the greater contributor of cadmium, so the lung condition continues.

A patient with cancer is treated for the cancer without knowing that years of nickel accumulation are the underlying cause. How is the doctor to know? It is close to impossible to determine whether or not nickel is contributing to the problem.

A patient with high blood pressure may be treated without the doctor knowing that he is highly sensitive to lead and has been over-exposed for many years. Perhaps this same patient has likewise been exposed to cadmium for many years. Now, suddenly, he also finds himself exposed to dental mercury.

A doctor administers medication to a patient for abnormal heart rhythm, all the while not understanding that mercury could be at the root of the problem. Moving further into the area of speculation, it is an equally good bet that a patient with mental depression who is mercury-sensitive and chronically exposed to mercury will likely be treated without the doctor ever having considered a heavy metal.

It is unlikely that the doctor will suspect the synergistic effect of heavy metals without the information in this book. Heavy metal poisoning has so many faces that it is seldom recognized. Hopefully, the information here will help the doctor realize that those important first steps in lifestyle counseling—helping patients rid themselves of heavy metal excess—are of much greater importance than has generally been assumed. By addressing the potential for heavy metal toxicity first, the doctor automatically enhances his chance of gaining positive results during the treatment program, whether when dealing with heart disease, periodontal disease, cancer, kidney disease, mental disturbances, or any other of a wide range of ailments. In fact, chronic heavy metal toxicity—a disease endemic to all peoples—is likely to play a factor in the onset and progression of all diseases that commonly afflict man.

PREVENTION AND TREATMENT OF HEAVY METAL POISONING: UNDERSTANDING THE NUTRITIONAL INTERACTION

To summarize so far: The danger of heavy metals is that they are absorbed easily and excreted with great difficulty. Prevention by removing the patient from further exposure is therefore a vital part of the treatment plan. In lieu of being excreted, each of the heavy metals attaches to cell membranes which are most sensitive to the toxin, making selectively permeable membranes tougher and less supple. This creates interference with selective uptake and excretion of nutrients, steroids and other chemical messengers and metabolites, and interferes with release of cellular waste in the affected tissues, as well as with other normal cellular functions, hence manifesting symptoms of chronic heavy metal toxicity. The procedures for treatment and prevention differ considerably, each demanding special nutritional considerations, as well as removal of the source of contamination. We will discuss these nutritional considerations, and then summarize them in a three-step program for ridding the body of heavy metals.

Lead

Recognition of the lead poisoning syndrome began in 1931 in Baltimore—a consequence of burning discarded battery casings in home cook stoves to retrieve the lead for resale. That incidence has led to our present understanding of how lead causes disease. The metal enters into the same respective metabolic pathways as zinc and calcium: the three compete for absorption. When dietary zinc and calcium are adequate, lead is not easily absorbed. Drs. Ashraf and Fosmire of Pennsylvania State University, in the March 1985 *Journal of Nutrition*, report that zinc deficiency favors absorption of lead. Consequently, an excess of lead inhibits zinc from performing its normal role of preventing high blood pressure.[30] "Provision of an adequate level of zinc in the diet would seem to lessen the danger of lead exposure," says Fosmire. That's not to say high doses of zinc will stave off lead poisoning, he notes. Excess zinc doesn't add further protection, and in large doses may have adverse effects, such as causing arthritic-like symptoms.

Lead competes with calcium in the intestine for attachment to calcium-binding protein (CBP),[31] a substance that is synthesized in the intestine, when needed, to aid in absorbing calcium. When dietary calcium is adequate, unwanted lead is rejected and excreted without entering the bloodstream, as CBP has a stronger affinity for calcium than lead. Conversely, insufficient calcium intake encourages CBP to attach to lead, thereby permitting absorption of lead.[32]

One of the net results of low calcium intake, according to interpretation of findings of the Center for Health Statistics, National Health and Nutrition Examination Survey I (NHANES 1),[33] may be high blood pressure. Excess vitamin D is also involved. Since vitamin D is known to stimulate production of calcium binding protein (CBP) with or without adequate calcium intake, excessive ingestion of vitamin D with insufficient dietary calcium may likewise promote absorption of lead. The danger of this is greatest when the diet contains an excess of red meat. Meat, while contributing to dietary vitamin D, also has the tendency to promote excretion of urinary calcium and the synthesis of CBP.* (There will be more on this topic in our discussion of kidney stones, Chapter 5). It becomes clear that an adequate intake of calcium with a limited intake of dietary vitamin D provides a major, shielding defense against dietary sources of toxic lead.

Once lead is absorbed, there are several important considerations. As Chisolm pointed out, bone has a special attraction for lead, just as it has for calcium. Levander explains that lead may contribute to red blood cell (RBC) fragility when vitamin E is deficient.[34] It may then interfere with heme synthesis, causing anemia and fatigue. One method of reducing the effect of lead is to provide an adequate supply of calcium, either through the diet or through supplementation. A diet high in phosphorous is also commonly used, along with lactates and citrates. This promotes the storage of lead in bone tissue. The problem with this approach is obvious. At some future time when dietary calcium is insufficient, especially when dietary phosphorous is excessive, the body begins quite naturally to draw upon bone tissue for its calcium requirements, thereby releasing the stored lead.

---

* Appendix D further explains how an excess of dietary vitamin D increases one's risk to heart disease, indicating that a variety of health dangers may loom from excessive vitamin D intake. In the volumes that follow in the lifestyle series this topic will be expanded upon further.

As stated previously, RBC's are particularly sensitive to lead accumulation, causing early RBC destruction followed by anemia. This occurs because cell membranes deficient of vitamin E and other protective factors are more susceptible to the intrusion of lead and other heavy metals, causing RBC's to rupture. For this reason it is common to supplement with iron and vitamin E when lead poisoning is suspected. This knowledge led to the standard porphyrin-based fingerprick test to screen children for high lead levels. It is also common practice to evaluate the extent of lead intoxication by observing RBC stippling through the microscope, which may be visually apparent in the lead-toxic patient.

When lead reaches such a level in the body as to cause general poisoning, or should the doctor and patient decide upon a more aggressive program for reducing the likelihood of lead intoxication, it is common practice to administer a chelating agent. One drug that is sometimes considered is D-Penicillamine, given orally. However it cannot be given when lead is present in the intestine, and is contraindicated when there is a history of penicillin sensitivity. Calcium Disodium Edetate (EDTA), the drug of choice, is given by intravenous infusion, while a second alternative, Dimercaprol (better known as BAL), is given intramuscularly. EDTA, given separately but concurrently with BAL, serves by exchanging its calcium for lead ions and thereby enhancing the urinary excretion of lead.

IV-EDTA is administered in a concentration of less than three percent diluted with isotonic saline or glucose. About 98 percent of the drug is recovered in the urine unchanged within 6 hours of its injection, thus accounting for its lack of unwanted side effects. There <u>are</u> two side effects that may occur, however. The first is tetany caused by too rapid or too frequent administration, a result of the strong affinity of EDTA for ionized blood calcium.* The second occurs when mercury and lead toxicity coexist in the same patient, in which case EDTA may cause nephrotoxicity.[35,36] Thus, it is recommended that EDTA not be administered to a patient with chronic mercury toxicity, since it is not always known whether or not the patient is afflicted concurrently with lead intoxication. If the same patient is suspected of being lead-toxic, it is recommended that one address chronic mercury toxicity first, using IV-C, followed by EDTA. (see Appendix H for this and alternative therapies.)

Cadmium

Cadmium sulfide is a byproduct of zinc refining. Mainly it is used in industry for electroplating—to rustproof tools. It is used also in welding and in the manufacture of paints, plastics, metallurgical fungicides, and superphosphate fertilizers. The workers in these types of operations are at a higher risk, as are the people who live downstream or downwind from the factories. Emitted dust settles in homes and on vegetation intended for animal and human consumption, and cadmium-rich fertilizer (made from industrial sewage sludge)

---

* This same potential threat to health is a feature that has made it popular among doctors offering alternative health care, who believe its use may reduce the calcium in diseased arterial tissues, thereby reducing one's risk to heart attack. Because of this and other potential health benefits from EDTA that go beyond its uses for lead poisoning, it has become a common but controversial practice among doctors to resort to EDTA as a regimen for treating almost all degenerative diseases. While this volume serves neither to condone nor to pass judgement on this practice, the reader may obtain additional information by contacting the American College of Advancement in Medicine and the American Heart Association. (Refer to Appendix E)

is used on many vegetable farms, where cadmium tends to "load" in particular plants, especially lettuce. Slowly, it enters the food chain (directly and indirectly) and concentrates in organ meats.

Waterborne pollution, on the other hand, enters the food chain primarily via rice and shellfish. Rice, the food grown most often in a river-fed bog, readily extracts its cadmium from water. Bottom-feeding shellfish become intoxicated when cadmium settles to the river's bed. Other fish are at risk also, but to a lesser extent. Regardless of its route of entry, however, cadmium does not cross the placental barrier, so whatever amount a patient now has within his system has been acquired since birth.

Beyond the acute episode, which causes abdominal pain with vomiting and diarrhea, cadmium sulfide is known to cause low back pain, painful bones, and restriction of spinal movement. The result is an affected patient who walks with a gait that resembles a duck's waddle. Calcium sulfide is also known to replace and antagonize zinc in some zinc-dependent enzyme systems. Through this mechanism Drs. Engvall and Perk of Oskarshamns, Sweden, believe that chronic exposure to cadmium may be an important cause of high blood pressure.[37] Among smokers, who acquire cadmium through contaminated tobacco, it may also be a cause of emphysema.[38] Cadmium absorption is prevented by an adequate intake of zinc and calcium. In addition, dietary iron and ascorbic acid, ingested together, serve to interfere with cadmium absorption[39] through an unknown mechanism.

Within the body, cadmium attaches to cell membranes (the kidneys a primary target) and becomes a source of exceptional stress. Rats intoxicated with cadmium demonstrate an exaggerated startle response. They tend to freeze in their tracks when a loud noise is heard, and (as revealed in the *Science News* report), express various other anxiety responses. Additionally, and perhaps important where some alcoholic patients are concerned, the researchers found that cadmium-intoxicated rats tend to prefer alcohol to water when presented with a choice. While these findings may or may not relate to humans, it is tempting to speculate that perhaps some alcoholics have chronic cadmium toxicity (just as some people have chronic mercury toxicity) as an underlying cause of their drinking problems. If so, then the **IV-C Mercury Tox Program**—which includes measures to deal with cadmium toxicity—would be doubly helpful for these people, especially since a report presented recently at the Third Conference on Vitamin C disclosed that megadose vitamin C protects against acute and chronic alcohol intoxication, making it an important antidote for the alcoholic patient.[40]

In addition to anxiety and stress, cadmium intoxication contributes to decreased resistance to infection. Dr. Ronald R. Watson[41] and Dr. Adria Rothman Sherman[42] separately reported that particular nutrients should be given consideration in bolstering the immune system. Included among these are vitamins A, E, C, B_6, B_{12}, and folic acid, as well as zinc and essential fatty acids (EFA), taking care to limit EFA and the total intake of polyunsaturated fatty acids to less than ten percent of total calories. Care should also be taken to limit vitamin E intake to less than 800 IU's, if megadose supplements are employed. In addition, to counter a depressed immune system,[43] adequate amounts of dietary protein are required. Special care should be taken to avoid excesses of protein, particularly from meats, as cadmium-induced stones may develop in the kidneys. Additionally, as explained in our discussion of lead, an excess of animal protein may be counterproductive by promoting excretion of calcium in the urine.

Zinc is also involved. In adequate amounts, zinc serves to stimulate an enzyme that neutralizes the toxic effects not only of cadmium, but also of lead, by promoting urinary excretion of the same.[44] Ultimately, however, the primary effect of cadmium intoxication is iron deficiency anemia. Iron supplementation, along with foods rich in iron, are needed to restore hemoglobin.[45] Copper and ascorbic acid (vitamin C) must be supplemented,[46] because the use of iron in hemoglobin formation is dependent upon an adequate intake of copper, while ascorbic acid improves the utilization of iron.*

Mercury

Chronic mercury toxicity offers a special challenge in its treatment. The first order of business is to remove the patient from further exposure. As we have already discussed, the source of exposure (without regard to the chemical species of mercury) may be the workplace, contaminated fish or seed grain, or mercury-based products. The patient may acquire the toxin as mercury vapor, through direct contact with the skin, or by eating contaminated food. Should the decision be made to replace the patient's dental fillings, it is probably best to treat the patient for chronic mercury toxicity first. If the fillings are indeed a source of chronic mercury toxicity, then replacement before treatment may only exacerbate the symptoms, since the patient risks becoming contaminated further during the replacement process.

When considering treatment, it is important to consider that mercury is excreted through every body fluid including perspiration, saliva, nasal discharge, vaginal and seminal fluids, urine, and feces. These latter two are the most important routes of exit. Elemental mercury may be exhaled also, via the lungs, but the significance of this is very low because tissues prefer to oxidize elemental mercury to mercuric mercury and most of the reduced mercury is reoxidized. The route of exit (depending on the chemical species, extent, and route of exposure) accounts for some of the early signs of acute poisoning, i.e. diarrhea, polyuria, excessive salivation, a nose that runs constantly, and a tendency to perspire profusely. It is therefore important to design a plan that encourages the discharge and replacement of these fluids, i.e. regular and sustained physical exertion, followed immediately by a shower.

A similar benefit might be derived from the regular use of a sauna. Putman and Madden, in their report for *National Geographic*,[47] described a treatment given to exposed miners of the Almaden mines in Spain. They alternated between a lamp-studded hot box and "the beach"—a room bathed in ultraviolet light. However, particular patients with heart problems and an electrolyte imbalance might not be well suited to this type of treatment. For those allowed access to a sauna, it is necessary to alternate the sauna with a cool shower every ten minutes; repeating the cycle three times per session. As an added precaution, the patient should have no more than three sessions daily, with each session preceded or followed by the consumption of an

---

* A unique twist to the use of iron supplements has to do with bioavailability, and the manner in which cadmium binds to RBC plasma membranes: Ferrous iron works, while ferric iron does nothing to correct the anemia. The ferrous forms of iron, such as ferrous sulfate and ferrous gluconate, replace cadmium in hemoglobin formation, whereas ferric iron (ferric citrate, ferric pyrophosphate, and ferric oxide) cannot. A more complete explanation can be found in the 1975 National Academy of Sciences source book.

electrolyte replacement beverage.

In regard to diet and the potential for chronic mercury toxicity from dental amalgam, preventing its absorption would seem to be an important defense. Many cooperating factors are, however, required. The inorganic, non-ionic mercury normally present in amalgam is least likely to be absorbed, but can be breathed as mercury vapor and converted in the brain and lungs into ionic mercury. As dental amalgam ages, there is risk of small pieces being swallowed.

In addition, as discussed earlier, inorganic mercury from amalgamated fillings can be converted (in the mouth and intestines) by normally occurring bacteria to its most toxic form—organic methylmercury. While the normal intestinal flora also have the capacity to degrade methylmercury, there is risk that such action is slow to occur when the organisms are deficient (a common event in chronic mercury toxicity, since the mercury tends to destroy the normal intestinal flora). Additionally, mercury-toxic patients have a tendency to consume too little fiber, which thereby promotes the reabsorption of mercury. (Methylmercury, however, may be the least significant source of amalgam-derived mercury, unless the patient has already been intoxicated from other sources of methylmercury.) This indicates the need for a dietary program designed not only to impede the intestinal absorption of mercury, but also to aid the body in excreting and detoxifying elemental and ionized mercury efficiently. To satisfy this need, individual aspects of the program are next discussed separately, although no one aspect of the program is more important than another. To maximize effectiveness, the program must be applied in its entirety.

Digestive Enzymes. Further complicating the role that the healthy gastrointestinal (G.I.) tract plays in preventing absorption, the findings of McNab[48] indicate that mercury may interfere with the activity of normally occurring digestive enzymes, impeding nutritional absorption and perhaps allowing absorption of poorly digested proteins. His findings also suggest that naturally-occurring food enzymes may be nearly as important in the digestive process as the body's own digestive enzymes. For this reason it may be wise to include high-enzyme foods, such as papaya, in the diet. Freshly sprouted seeds are also an excellent source. The work of Northcote[49] demonstrates that the enzyme activity of germinating seeds may increase several hundred times beyond that found in the nongerminating seed.

Manganese. Foods high in the trace mineral, manganese, may be of benefit to enzyme function. This is especially true in the synthesis of mucopolysaccharides—the intermediate forms of proteins that comprise the cell membranes of connective tissues. Because manganese is involved in many enzyme systems, and because mercury has an affinity for the sulfhydryl groups of enzymes, requiring a more rapid replacement of enzymes, larger quantities than normal are likely needed for those suffering from chronic mercury toxicity—well beyond the 2.5 to 5 mg per day that is otherwise adequate. Manganese is especially concentrated in the brain, therefore the coexistence of mercury poisoning with an insufficient amount of body manganese may be partially responsible for the associated neuromuscular and neurological symptoms. The affected patient should be instructed to add to his diet foods that are high in manganese. In some cases a food supplement may be desirable.

Cultured Dairy Products. Methylated mercury tends to destroy the normal intestinal flora, promoting the overgrowth of yeast just as would be expected during any long-term antibiotic therapy. This action requires replacement of these organisms through consumption of cultured milk products, containing any one or a combination of the following live, non-pathogenic cultures:

- Lactobacillus acidophilus
- Lactobacillus bulgaricus
- Lactobacillus bifidus
  (L. bifidus is known also as Bifidobacterium bifidum)

- Streptococcus faecium
- Streptococcus lactis
- Streptococcus thermophilus

Adequately supplied, these live bacteria serve by incorporating mercury into their enzyme systems, after which the mercury is excreted along with the remnants of the organism.* A diet that provides these organisms would include buttermilk, yogurt, cottage cheese, sour cream, and soft cheeses. Modulating the protein intake would encourage their growth. A key point to remember, however, is that hard cheeses and many brands of yogurt do not suffice, as the cultures used in their making have been prekilled. Observe labels carefully. If the live culture has been retained it will usually say so on the container. If not, then the dairy product will not serve to restore normal intestinal flora. Hence, when adequately supplied, milk cultures will block mercury absorption, aid in nutrient absorption, and prevent systemic yeast infections.

Those few people who offer resistance to the above therapy through allergies to milk products, are usually sufferers of lactose intolerance. This is due to a reduction of the lactase enzyme. Live dairy cultures are an important source of lactase. Thus, people who complain they are "allergic" to milk will generally find that they can tolerate cultured dairy products quite well. If not, then the doctor and patient might consider replacing the organisms through a nondairy, supplementary source.†

Sulfur and Selenium. Sulfur and selenium naturally provide fish with protection from the harmful effects of mercury.[50] This is important because the seas already contain 70 million tons of accumulated mercury, and industry is producing an additional 10,000 tons annually which ultimately finds its way to the sea. While the amount contributed by industry seems trivial in comparison to the total, it is significant because the dumping is not uniform. The discharge of waste causes particular areas of the ocean to become hazardous pockets of mercury pollution. Fortunately, some of the mercury pollutant combines with sulfur before reaching the sea, forming inactive mercury sulfide (HgS). Inactive HgS is a dominant factor in decreasing the availability of mercury for methylation. Without this action the organomercurial wastes are consumed and methylated by fish.

The fish which live the longest and grow to the largest size ultimately contain the most mercury. Relatively large tuna contain 0.5 ppm, while the larger swordfish and pacific blue marlin average 1.0 and 5 to 14 ppm respectively. The secret to the health of the fish, and perhaps to the health of

---

* These same organisms, according to preliminary data from animal research of Dr. S. E. Gilliland at Oklahoma State University, may also benefit those who are concerned with their blood cholesterol level. His findings—yet to be published—suggest that cultured milk products may have the ability to assimilate cholesterol from bile salts and thereby promote its removal.

† Two such distributors of a suitable product are Klaire Laboratories and the Neo-Life Company of America. (See Appendix E for addresses).

people who consume those fish, is dependent upon the ratio of selenium to mercury. The lower the ratio the greater the chance for acquiring chronic mercury toxicity.

When fish from unpolluted waters are eaten, having a high protective ratio of selenium to mercury, there is normally sufficient selenium to escort the mercury through the human gastrointestinal tract. If the fish source of mercury is methylated, selenium serves—in a manner that will soon be explained—to block its attachment to body proteins of cell membranes, bringing about its excretion beforehand. (Here again, normal intestinal flora are important in limiting mercury absorption.) It is only fish from polluted waters that present a health risk, because fish caught in the open sea have sufficient selenium to negate the toxic effect. Otherwise, methylmercury is absorbed and reabsorbed with ease as a part of bile acid. Yet, because the consumer is likely to be eating fish that has not been properly assayed for mercury,* it is important that the mercury-toxic patient either eliminates fish altogether, or consumes his fish in the same meal with garlic, onion, some source of animal protein, or a dietary supplement of selenium and activated charcoal. Reasons for this will be given shortly.

How does selenium work? Selenium is a trace metal that is classed along with sulfur in chemical systems. In fact, selenium has the ability to replace sulfur in chemical bonding. Therefore, since selenium and sulfur are chemically interchangeable, it is not surprising that high-sulfur cysteine, an amino acid, often includes traces of selenium. While the implication of this in treating chronic mercury toxicity is obvious, the sulfur/selenium relationship in chemical systems may be harmful or beneficial. In cattle fed vegetation from soil where selenium is high, "alkali disease" or "blind staggers" is a common occurrence. Appreciable amounts of the mineral tend to deform hooves of affected animals by replacing their high concentrations of sulfur. Through a related mechanism in humans, large amounts may be either toxic or beneficial in preventing the absorption of mercury.

Fang,[51] speculating on the mechanism for the mineral's role as protector, believes that the benefit of selenium to the mercury-toxic patient may be due not only to its close resemblance to sulfur, but also to its ability to replace sulfur. From his own studies he concluded that selenium protects by breaking the carbon/mercury bond. When this occurs in the gastrointestinal tract, selenium escorts mercury out of the body. Within the body, the breaking of the carbon/mercury bond redistributes mercury to other tissue, or to recently ingested sulfur-bearing proteins.[52]

To confirm this reported benefit of selenium, Ganther, et al.,[53] studied chronic methylmercury toxicity in quail. They noted a significant decrease in the quails' symptoms of chronic mercurialism in response to selenium. Khayat

---

* An article that appeared in *USA Today*, by Dan Sperling (Nov 20, 1986), indicates that while the consumption of fish and taking of fish oil supplements is now being touted as an important measure for preventing heart disease, the inspection requirements for fish are presently much too lax. Mr. Sperling cites statistics from the Center for Disease Control, which indicates that 25 percent of food-related illness is caused by fish, and that only 13 percent of fish eaten in the USA is government-inspected. Thus, to obtain the beneficial effect of fish oils many consumers are turning to supplements. Since there is also a danger of consuming toxins from fish oil supplements, it is important that your patient seek a reliable, safe source. The two safest sources to our knowledge are the MaxEPA supplement made by the R.R. Scherer Corporation, and the Salmon Oil Capsules made by the Neo Life Company of America.

and Dencker[54] attempted to explain the mechanism of selenium's protective action. They showed that selenium assists animals exposed to elemental mercury vapor (without promoting excretion of mercury) by distributing the mercury evenly among the tissues. This occurs through a process of <u>competitive equilibrium</u> in which an excess of selenium, relative to mercury, promotes displacement of mercury from its binding sites. The researchers thereby credited the reduction of symptoms to the redistribution of mercury; from highly susceptible mercury-sensitive tissues and organs, to tissue sites that were less crucial to total health.

While the mechanism just shown for selenium is helpful in detoxifying certain tissues, it still does not rid the body of mercury. To do so requires the simultaneous inclusion of a diet high in fiber and fat, because mercury has an affinity for lipoproteins required to transport fat and to synthesize bile. Hence, when the point of competitive equilibrium (selenium vs. mercury) is reached, the mercury displaced is then free to be transported to the liver via fat-stimulated lipoproteins, and excreted along with bile.

Selenium minimizes the toxic action of mercury attached to cell membranes, which otherwise promotes free radical oxidation and is a cause of cell membrane stress. In performing this role, selenium functions as a cofactor in the enzyme activity of GSH. Each molecule of the enzyme contains 4 selenium atoms. A sufficient supply of selenium is critical to its protective function. In fact, the specific affinity of sulfhydryl groups for mercury is particularly due to this enzyme. Through cooperation with vitamin E and other antioxidants (vitamins A and C included), GSH inhibits peroxidation of membrane lipids and fatty acids, thus protecting the cell from aging and destruction by free radicals. Supplemental and dietary selenium promote a marked increase in the biosynthesis of additional GSH, and protect the cells throughout the body.

The net effect of selenium is protection of nearly all cell membranes while redistributing the mercury so that its negative effect is reduced in any one part of the body. Ahlrot-Westerlund, et al.,[55] in support of this statement, reported that the higher the ratio of mercury to selenium, the more likely the patient will manifest symptoms of chronic mercury toxicity. In some people, therefore, in whom there is a deficiency of selenium, even the slightest amount of mercury may cause obvious health problems. Conversely, an increase in dietary selenium would decrease the mercury: selenium ratio—bringing the patient closer to the critical point of competitive equilibrium—and thereby exert a protective role.

As convenient as the use of selenium sounds for reducing the toxic effect of mercury, the concept presents an additional problem: The amount of selenium needed to accomplish the beneficial goal of redistribution, or competitive equilibrium, has not been established. An effective treatment plan for chronic mercury toxicity may require a toxic level for selenium.

Animal studies by Levander, et al.,[56] indicate that 0.1 µg selenium per gram of total dietary intake (or 50 µg per day for humans) prevents deficiency. Yet, in more direct studies with humans, Levander's group demonstrated that the daily need for selenium is 70 µg, which assumes about 80 percent absorption of food selenium (not controlling for vitamin E intake, which modulates the amount of selenium absorbed). Thus, a range of 50 to 200 µg per day has become the generally accepted RDA for selenium (assuming a vitamin E intake of 100 IU's per day). Selenium toxicity, on the other hand, is widely suspected to occur in humans, but has not been demonstrated, as it has in animals when the diet exceeds 3 µg per gram of diet—equivalent to about 200 to 300 times the RDA for humans. Using this criteria, it should be safe to supplement with up to 1000 µg of selenium daily, especially if megadose vitamin E (200 to 400 IU) and vitamin C (which serves to negate the toxic effect of megadose selenium) are simultaneously administered.

Dr. C. H. Hill, of the North Carolina State Poultry Science Department,[57] formulated a set of truisms from studying chicks that can perhaps be applied to human nutrition. Of great significance, Dr. Hill learned that supplemental vitamin C prevented the risk of intoxication from selenium—important in animal health because selenium is added to the chick's diet as an adjunct therapy for mercury poisoning. If we may apply these findings to human nutrition, then the equivalent of 3 grams per day of oral vitamin C may be sufficient to prevent selenium intoxication during the initial phase of treatment, assuming a treatment dosage of 400 to 1000 µg daily.

Onion and Garlic. These two are also excellent food sources of the sulfhydryl groups: either may serve to chelate mercury. Robert A. Good, M. D., Ph. D., has recently published an excellent report on the biological and nutritional benefits of the chemical compounds found in garlic.[58] Dr. Good explains that garlic contains a number of allyl-based sulfur compounds. An oxide of diallyl disulfide, called allicin, is built up from the sulfur-containing amino acid cysteine. Two additional ingredients are allyl sulfide and methyl trisulfide. Together, these ingredients of whole garlic offer an excellent source of a sulfhydryl chelating agent for escorting mercury out of the intestinal tract. "Onion, too, which contains a variant form of allicin that is structurally similar to the allicin found in garlic, may serve this purpose. With the help of allinase," explains Dr. Good, "the onion form of allicin creates the eye-irritant that produces tears." By ridding the body of harmful agents, such as mercury, the benefit of sulfhydryl proteins may be one of the ways in which garlic and onion are reported to reduce the risk of heart attack and cancer.

Sulfur-Bearing Amino Acids. Beyond the protection offered by normal intestinal flora and a high-fiber diet, there are other means by which mercury absorption is prevented; these are best explained by reexamining the manner through which mercury most often attaches to cell membranes. Again, mercury has a special affinity for sulfhydryl groups found in most integral membrane proteins.[59] This feature is accounted for by the predominance (in these proteins) of one or more of the sulfur-bearing amino acids: methionine, cystine, glutathione, taurine, or cysteine.

To reach the point of competitive equilibrium (sulphur vs. mercury) through diet, it is important to prescribe foods that are rich in sulfur-bearing amino acids. Animal protein (eggs, cultured dairy products, poultry and red meat) has a far greater concentration of sulfur-bearing amino acids than plant protein sources. (A couple of days before IV-C is administered, however, it may be important in certain patients at risk to stone development to minimize their intake of animal protein. [See Chapter 6.])

Some patients who are vegetarians, will need to understand the necessity of foregoing a strict vegetarian diet during the mercury treatment program. Ovolactovegetarians will have an easier time making the transition, as they will probably already be eating whole eggs and cultured milk products. Ovolactovegetarianism, in fact, may be an alternative for those patients who are following a vegetarian diet due to religious reasons.

In addition, it will be wise to supplement with vitamin B$_6$ or include foods that are a rich source of the vitamin* (Chapter 5). For patients known to be mercury-sensitive or mercury-toxic, it is also wise to eliminate fish from their diets. While fish is a good source of selenium, known to offer natural protection, it is hard to know for certain if the fish were caught in pure or contaminated waters, in which case the excess mercury would override the normal protection offered by selenium.

Butter. Butter, since it is high in fat, proves an advantage when removing mercury from the blood. While one might argue that mercury is not fat soluble, that ionic mercury is more soluble in water than lipids, and that it's nearly always attached to <u>any</u> of the sulfhydryl groups in circulating blood, one must keep in mind the fundamental (dual) property of lipoproteins. They are both hydrophilic and lipophilic, which allows them to transport water-soluble proteins and water-insoluble fats (including cholesterol) at the same time. Ionic mercury, while technically insoluble in fat and soluble only in water (blood), is transported by lipoproteins as a part of the sulfhydryl protein segment of the particle. Ultimately, it is deposited in the liver's catabolic pool to be excreted along with bile. In addition, fat is required to stimulate the flow of bile, so fat, therefore, is required to reduce the body burden of mercury. Assisting in this action, butter is known to stimulate the enzyme LCAT, which is necessary to transport both mercury and cholesterol out of the body. Butter is especially helpful as a replacement for fat from animal protein sources a few days before IV-C is administered—a period when the risk of kidney stones is greatest, and when animal protein must be reduced in favor of selenium supplementation. One-eighth to one-quarter pound of butter per day is recommended.

Thiol Resins and/or Activated Charcoal. Norseth and Clarkson report that methylmercury tends to reabsorb from bile,[60] making it essential that a way be found to block this tendency and promote the total excretion of bile. To explain: Bile acids enter the small intestine via the bile duct, along with reduced metabolites of cholesterol and methylated mercury. Fat absorption is facilitated in the process, first and foremost in the ilium and to a lesser degree in all levels of the intestine. Thereafter, much of the bile is reabsorbed, returning to the liver via the portal vein. Mercury is reabsorbed also as a part of bile, after which the liver returns the bile and its constituents to the intestine, completing the enterohepatic circulation. The cycle may be repeated 2 to 3 times during a fatty meal, averaging 6 to 10 times daily.[61]

Unless the diet contains adequate fiber, and the colon is evacuated regularly, the expanded enterohepatic circulation may be a cause of persistent chronic mercury toxicity and hypercholesterolemia. This, and the fact that methylmercury has a strong affinity for sulfur, prompted Clarkson, Small, and Norseth,[62] and then Bakir, et al.,[63] to study the efficacy of a thiol resin that would prevent the reabsorption of mercury from bile. The thiol resins, which contained a fixed sulfhydryl group that was nonabsorbable, effectively increased the excretion rate of methylmercury from bile by 50 percent. These

---

* A few years ago, Dr. Kilmer McCully, former professor of pathology at the Harvard medical school, advanced the concept that vitamin B_6 (pyridoxine hydrochloride) served as a coenzyme that facilitated the enzymatic conversion of toxic homocysteine (a metabolite of methionine) to nontoxic cystathionine. This is important, he believes, because unconverted homocysteine may promote arterial disease by causing the initial break in the arterial wall that leads to plaque formation. Thus, while consuming a diet that is high in animal protein, particularly the amino acid methionine, vitamin B_6 is required in amounts that surpass the RDA.

are today in common use for the treatment of acute mercurialism, and believed to be of equal value in the treatment of the mercury-toxic patient. Ideally, it is recommended that the thiol resin be administered with, or shortly following, meals.

Activated charcoal, unlike thiol resin, has the ability to adsorb a wide variety of drugs and toxic agents. It has become popular in the past ten years as an antidote for all types of poisoning, including food poisoning. Its popularity has grown to the point that charcoal hemoperfusion is now the treatment of choice for the emergency management of drug intoxication, especially when the intoxicant is unknown. This application, its ease of administration, and lack of serious side effects, has prompted Pertti Neuvonen[64] of Helsinki to suggest its use in the management of patients with chronic heavy metal toxicity—either in addition to the thiol resin or as an alternative to it.

The recognized value of administering activated charcoal to uremic patients has aided in our understanding of how it works. Friedman, et al,[65] observed that 35 grams per day administered to 6 patients with renal insufficiency and hyperlipidemia had the very good effect of significantly lowering both serum cholesterol and triglycerides. These findings prompted the Finnish team of Kuusisto and Neuvonen, et al,[66] to study more intensely the lipid-lowering effect of activated charcoal. They administered 8 grams of activated charcoal three times daily for four weeks to 7 patients with hypercholesterolemia. Plasma total cholesterol and LDL decreased 25% and 41% respectively, while high density lipoprotein (HDL) or "good" cholesterol increased 8 percent. The researchers reasoned that the observed benefit was due to the ability of activated charcoal to bind bile acids.

This being the case, it is perhaps reasonable to administer activated charcoal in conjunction with the thiol resin, but in a much smaller dose than what was used in the Finnish study (1.5 g vs. 35 g/day). In health food stores within the U. S., activated charcoal is available in 260 mg capsules. The general recommendation is 2 capsules taken with water after each meal, a regimen that is usually continued for at least 30 days. Do inform your patient that his stool will have a black color when taking charcoal. Other side effects are few, when used as intended. Neuvonen informs that the rapid ingestion of higher doses may cause vomiting, constipation, or diarrhea but this isn't likely to be a problem when the recommended dosage (1/2 gram following meals) for chronic mercury toxicity is followed closely.

Vitamin C. According to protocol, once the preliminary dietary requirements have been followed for a minimum of 36 hours, the patient is ready to begin oral vitamin C. The beginning dosage before administering IV-C, and the duration of such dosage, depends on the patient. Cameron and Pauling,[67] for instance, caution that when vitamin C is administered too rapidly to patients with widespread metastasis, extensive necrosis and hemorrhage may occur. The cancer patient, being the exception, should be given at first a smaller dosage (1 to 2 g per day), increased slowly over a two- to three-week period before IV-C is administered. The mercury-toxic patient who is free of cancer can begin the program with 3 grams per day, mostly to prepare the body for handling a much larger dosage. After following the prescribed diet, lifestyle, and supplement program for a week or two, the next step is to titrate dosage to suit the patient's need according to one of four acceptable methods for determining the correct dosage of oral vitamin C.

The Silver Nitrate Urine Test: This first test[68] was proposed and developed by the late Frederick R. Klenner, who is credited with having pioneered the use of megadose vitamin C in the general practice of medicine. Dr. Klenner claimed to have administered megadose vitamin C to over 30,000 patients. "The objective," he once explained, "is to administer vitamin C until it reaches a level in the urine that indicates acceptable saturation." To do this requires testing every fourth hour as the patient steadily increases his vitamin C intake at the rate of 4 grams per hour. The Silver Nitrate Urine Test employs 10 drops of 5% silver nitrate and 10 drops of urine placed in a test tube. Read in two minutes, it gives a color pattern relative to the amount of vitamin C excreted, showing white, beige, smoke gray or charcoal.

Correct, initial vitamin C dosage is reached when the test shows a fine charcoal-like precipitation with a clear supernatant liquid. Thereafter, the objective is to maintain a dosage that retains the Silver Nitrate Urine Test at or just below this degree of saturation. While effective in arriving at a dosage of vitamin C that satisfies the patient's bodily demand, the technique requires considerable attention. For this reason Dr. Robert Cathcart, a medical practitioner from Los Altos, California, has developed another method:[69]

Titrating to Bowel Tolerance: "Titrating to bowel tolerance," says Cathcart, "is based upon the premise that disease and bodily stresses substantially increase a patient's requirement for vitamin C." Derived from 18 years of experience of administering megadose vitamin C to 16,000 patients, Cathcart's formula is also based on the premise that each cell and cell group may individually suffer from what he terms acute induced scurvy, a consequence of the stresses placed upon them by the agents and processes that cause disease. When properly applied, the theory lays waste the conventional definition of scurvy, as scurvy is usually indicated by correlating outward physical symptoms with a plasma deficiency of ascorbic acid. Acute induced scurvy, he contends, occurs in every disease condition, requiring a different treatment dosage of supplemental vitamin C for each.

To further explain his concept, Cathcart refers to previous studies that have shown that the body of the average well-nourished person contains 5 grams of vitamin C. Stress and disease may significantly reduce this amount, which can cause what others before have referred to as subclinical scurvy. In addition, he believes that stress and disease cause the body to utilize vitamin C at a faster rate. To determine a patient's precise need, he began to administer oral vitamin C at an increasingly greater dosage, until the patient developed diarrhea. People who were stressed and diseased, he found, could handle a great deal more oral vitamin C before developing diarrhea than could well-nourished persons. He summarized further that the dose required was directly related to the toxicity or cell stress of the patient's disease, which he thus termed bowel tolerance.

Cathcart's preferred source of oral vitamin C for titrating to bowel tolerance is ascorbic acid—either tablets or powder.* While he has experimented with sodium ascorbate and a mixture of ascorbic acid and ascorbate salts (sodium, potassium, and calcium ascorbate), it is his experience that when titrating to bowel tolerance patients prefer ascorbic acid, and their conditions improve best on ascorbic acid. He has also found that magnesium ascorbate may actually be a cause of diarrhea in some people, sodium ascorbate may unhealthfully add to the total body burden of sodium in others, and the

* Both the powder and tablets of ascorbic acid can be obtained from Bronson Pharmaceuticals. See Appendix E.

additional calcium from calcium ascorbate is not a good idea over a lengthy treatment period.   There are exceptions of course.

For those patients who have an ulcer, esophagitis, or colitis—or related intestinal problems—Cathcart may administer an ascorbate salt in the beginning, but then shifts to 100 percent ascorbic acid as soon as possible. For other patients having a problem with straight ascorbic acid, he instructs them to take a little sodium bicarbonate, again switching to straight ascorbic acid as soon as possible. When asked about his experience with sodium ascorbate, he responded, "Both Irwin Stone and Dr. Frederick Klenner used sodium ascorbate and both died of heart problems. I don't know whether there is any relationship, but I have had patients come in with high blood pressure who were taking sodium ascorbate, who had their pressure go to normal on ascorbic acid. I have also had ladies complain of edema with sodium ascorbate orally. Nevertheless, I use sodium ascorbate exclusively—intravenously—and have never had trouble with it." So, after experimenting with the various sources and combinations of sources of oral vitamin C, Dr. Cathcart's first choice remains ascorbic acid.

Titrating to bowel tolerance requires the patient's total cooperation. The patient must learn to titrate between that amount which makes him feel better and that amount which almost—but not quite—causes diarrhea. Cathcart contends that patients who are less sick will require significantly less vitamin C to reach this point than those who are seriously ill. He has found, for instance, that 80 percent of adult patients will tolerate 10 to 15 grams of powdered vitamin C in one-half cup of water, divided into 4 doses per 24 hours, without having diarrhea. Those who present with more serious symptoms, however, will tolerate a much larger dosage, ranging up to 50 or 100 grams per day.

The doctor will want to encourage diarrhea when the patient first starts, however, regardless of the dosage required. This is because vitamin C serves as a natural cathartic for clearing the channel through which mercury and other toxins must exit. At or below the bowel tolerance dosage the intestines readily absorb whatever amount of vitamin C is presented, which to Dr. Cathcart is an indication of the dosage required to correct the patient's condition. "Clinical effectiveness," he contends, "is reached when a critical threshold is reached, as indicated by bowel intolerance to ascorbic acid in the form of diarrhea. It occurs both because megadose vitamin C can act as a non-rate-limited, antioxidant free radical scavenger (which will be explained in Chapter 4) and because acute induced scurvy is avoided." A dosage that exceeds bowel tolerance, therefore, is in excess of the body's immediate requirement. When this occurs the excess of vitamin C creates a hypertonic, or hyperosmolar, situation in the rectum, causing a benign and rapid diarrhea much like a water enema. In this manner vitamin C exerts its cathartic action.

Interestingly, during an interview, Cathcart informed me that IV-C raises the bowel tolerance threshold rather than lowering it, partially because IV-C cannot and does not enter the lower colon and rectum. Diarrhea due to vitamin C does not occur, therefore, while IV-C is being administered. Thus, he instructs the patient to continue taking oral vitamin C during the IV-C infusion. The combination of IV-C and oral vitamin C maximizes the amount of ascorbic acid a patient can take without producing diarrhea, since IV-C independently does not contribute to diarrhea. On the other hand, the patient's bowel tolerance dosage normally falls just before the IV-C is completed, so he instructs his nurse-therapist to discontinue oral vitamin C during the final 100 ml of the IV-

C infusion. Afterward, the bowel tolerance must be reassessed to prevent diarrhea. On the positive side, this change in bowel tolerance is one of the indicators used to assess the patient's improvement. A reduction in the dosage required to reach bowel tolerance following IV-C is believed to be an indication of reduced cellular stress. If so, and if the definition for disease given in the earlier part of the chapter is correct, then the patient's risk for disease should be lessened proportionately.

Titrating to Body Tolerance: This is a variation of the bowel tolerance method, developed by Jonathan V. Wright, M. D., who has been treating patients with megadose vitamin C since about 1972. Dr. Wright, whose specialty is nutritional medicine, is the author of two books on the topic,[70,71] and a medical columnist for Let's Live magazine. Wright has very little argument with Cathcart's method. He recommends only that the doctor instruct patients to take as much vitamin C daily as possible (regardless of source) without getting diarrhea or gas. By considering either the onset of gas or diarrhea as the end point, his approach is slightly more conservative in the dosage of vitamin C and equally acceptable for the purpose of treating chronic mercury toxicity.

The Vitamin C Flush: This also is a variation of the bowel tolerance method, first proposed by Dr. Hal Huggins of Colorado Springs. While the procedure has not been published, it is preferred by Dr. Huggins in treating the mercury-toxic patient. His method involves instructing the patient to drink 4 grams of powdered vitamin C* in 2 to 3 ounces of water every 30 minutes until diarrhea occurs. The dosage required for the average patient ranges from 16 grams to 20 grams, while people who are highly toxic may require from 32 grams to 40 grams, or more. Once diarrhea occurs, the average patient who is mercury-toxic is maintained on 3 grams daily before, during, and following the IV-C, or 5 grams daily if the person is severely toxic.

The rationale for the use of megadose vitamin C, particularly IV-C, in treating chronic mercury toxicity is presented in Chapter 4. Before administering IV-C, however, it is necessary to consider further the previously mentioned steps for ridding the body of the major heavy metals and preventing heavy metal toxicity.

A THREE-STEP PROGRAM FOR RIDDING THE BODY OF HEAVY METALS, PARTICULARLY LEAD, CADMIUM AND MERCURY

To restate a point made earlier in this chapter: The method for prevention and the procedure for treatment differ considerably. The doctor must decide how aggressive the treatment program should be, and, more importantly, initiate steps for prevention or for treatment. In every case, one or the other program should be implemented.

Step 1: Consider Chronic Lead Toxicity

Chronic lead poisoning is the most common of all forms of metallic poisoning, and at the same time one of the most insidious. The earliest and most common symptoms include irritability and nervousness, often with slight anemia. Subclinical poisoning (chronic lead toxicity) may also show high blood pressure. The symptoms proceed with loss of appetite, followed by nausea, constipation, and wasting. The symptoms may also include a metallic taste in

*Dr. Huggins instructs his patients to use sodium ascorbate powder, as he feels ascorbic acid is too acidic if used in this way.

the mouth.   Except for the constipation, these early symptoms are strikingly similar to those of chronic mercury toxicity.   Symptoms of gouty arthritis, however, which appear with the usual blood and urine picture of patients with gout due to other causes (hyperuricemia and hyperuricosuria, discussed in Chapter 6), are unique only to lead.   Because the characteristics of gout might increase the risk of kidney stones during IV-C therapy, it may prove necessary to have the patient with an identifying medical history, whose blood picture fails to respond appropriately to the usual therapy for gout, undergo the program outlined in Step 1 prior to IV-C.

If chronic lead toxicity appears to be evident, the following program should be adhered to for at least two weeks, depending entirely upon the doctors' assessment:*

- **Calcium**: Include at least 2 servings per day of a cultured milk product or supplement with 600 mg daily.
  CAUTION: This recommendation is for general prevention of further contamination.   Dr. Warren M. Levin, who instructs candidates for board certification in Chelation Therapy (See Appendixes E and H for further information), informs that calcium supplements would be restricted shortly before, during, and for 24 hours following EDTA therapy, after which replacement therapy is resumed.

- **Zinc**: Include 2 eggs per day with 2 tablespoons raw sunflower seeds or supplement with 15 mg daily.

- **Iron**: Include a daily serving of raisins and serve liver twice per week. Include also a daily serving of parsley, watercress, spinach or beans or supplement with two tablespoons daily of blackstrap molasses or supplement with 18 mg ferrous sulfate or ferrous gluconate per day for men and non-pregnant females. For pregnant and lactating women the recommended dosage is 30-60 mg daily.
  CAUTION: The addition of iron to the diet may mask the symptom of fatigue which is characteristic of mercury poisoning.

- **Vitamin E**: Include whole grains and unprocessed vegetable oils daily or supplement with 200 IU to 400 IU d-alpha tocopherol a day.

- **Vitamin D**: Restrict all foods supplemented with vitamin D.   Use cultured milk only. Obtain vitamin D requirements from sunshine. If calcium supplements are taken, purchase only those that do not contain vitamin D.

- **Protein**: Maintain a quality protein intake at about 50 g daily, taking care to limit red meat. Ideal protein intake, according to a 1975 report from the National Research Council, is about 700 mg/kg body weight.

* Dr. Wright cautions that this program assumes patient digestion and assimilation to be normal, and food allergies are not evident. Yet there is a 40 percent chance that this is not the case, and much greater odds when chronic mercury toxicity is involved. He recommends that the doctor investigate beforehand the absence or presence of food allergies, and perform at the very least gastric analysis and pancreatic enzyme studies—to be followed by replacement, or supportive therapy where indicated.

Step 2: Consider Chronic Cadmium Toxicity

Acute poisoning, while rarely encountered, is usually characterized by acute gastro-enteritis with pronounced vomiting. A headache and dry throat may be evident, along with diarrhea, brown urine, and renal failure. The treatment would include an emetic or gastric lavage with milk or albumin, saline catharsis, hydration, and respiratory support. BAL is not indicated, as explained in Chapter 4. Chelation may be indicated using EDTA, similarly to lead. An attempt should be made to maximize the immune system through the nutritional considerations listed earlier in this chapter.

Chronic cadmium toxicity may result in unexplained high blood pressure, similar to that of high blood pressure from lead. Likewise, a smoker's cough may be a sign of chronic, small-dose exposures. The patient may demonstrate signs of emphysema. If this is indeed a part of the patient's medical history, chronic cadmium toxicity should be suspected. Step 2 should therefore be followed before administering IV-C, as cadmium intoxication may place the patient at risk for developing kidney stones (Chapter 6). This being the case, the patient should be instructed to adhere to the following preventive regimen:

- Follow Step 1 for at least one week—preferably 6 weeks if lead exposure is also suspected.

- While continuing Step 1, begin the second week (or seventh week if lead exposure is initially suspected), with a consideration for dietary copper. Copper supplements should not be taken. There is too great a risk of surpassing the RDA (2 to 3 mg per day). Rather, it is more important to pay attention to dietary sources such as 1 serving daily of either 1/4 cup cashews, 1/2 cup raw mushrooms, 1/2 cup whole wheat flour, or 4 oz of dark meat chicken.

- Supplement daily with 3 g vitamin C, but only after the patient's risk category has been considered as outlined in Chapter 6. Make whatever lifestyle corrections are necessary beforehand.

- If the patient smokes, enter him in a STOP SMOKING program.

Continue Step 2 for three weeks, longer if necessary. If chronic mercury toxicity is also suspected, you might begin Step 3 during the second week of Step 2.

Step 3: Consider Chronic Mercury Toxicity

Chapter 3 will give a profile of the patient most likely to be in need of this step. Chapter 4 touches upon the standard treatment for acute poisoning, as well as the rationale for the use of IV-C in chronic mercury toxicity. Symptoms of chronic exposure, which may include abnormal heart rhythm, mental disturbances, a depressed immune system, muscular incoordination, irritability, nervousness, collagen disease, and a tingling sensation in the extremities, along with the sudden onset of allergies and frequent urination with nocturia, are of greatest concern. If the patient has any of these symptoms or if the patient fits the profile presented in Chapter 3, then the following additional lifestyle practices should be employed:

- Follow Steps 1 and 2 (including 3 g daily of vitamin C), with two exceptions:
  1. Discontinue any iron supplements, and restrict foods that contain iron. (Refer to Chapter 4)
  2. Discontinue all calcium supplements. Rely only on cultured milk products (2 to 3 servings daily) for calcium sources.

- Emphasize animal protein as opposed to vegetable protein, increasing to, but not exceeding, 100 g daily. Do not use fish as a source of protein unless combined with onion or garlic. Whole eggs should be included in the daily animal protein intake.

- If possible, on alternating days include a raw egg cocktail blended with fruit juice and 3 large scoops of fresh papaya. The combination of papaya and raw eggs will serve a dual purpose. Raw egg protein is easier to digest and papaya will serve to replace some of the digestive enzymes lost to mercury poisoning. When blended, the enzymes form a liposomal arrangement with free proteins, thereby allowing some enzymes to be absorbed unaltered.

- Prescribe a broad-spectrum, digestive enzyme supplement, to be taken in the same meal as the animal protein, or included in the whole egg meal, but not to be included in more than two meals daily. During the third meal it may prove beneficial to include a liberal serving of freshly grown sprouts, such as bean and alfalfa sprouts, which supply a wide assortment of enzymes.

- Include garlic cloves daily with at least two of the three meals. These can be added to recipes, and may be whole or crushed, but the patient should ingest at least two daily.

- Supplement with 6 capsules daily of the oil of garlic (2 per meal). These are best tolerated when taken about halfway into the meal.

- Include onion in as many meals as possible. Similarly to garlic, onion can be added to many recipes in various forms, but the patient should have the equivalent of 1 whole onion each day.

- Add butter to the diet, replacing margarine—1/8 to 1/4 lb daily. The objective is to stimulate lipoprotein production, necessary to transport mercury out of the body. Butter not only provides the saturated fat needed for this action, it also acts to maximally stimulate the LCAT enzyme required to load cholesterol aboard the HDL (high density lipoprotein, or good cholesterol) carriers. Mercury may then exit the body along with cholesterol via bile and the intestines.

- Supplement with selenium, using a minimum of 200 µg daily. In more serious cases, reaching the desired therapeutic point of competitive equilibrium (selenium vs mercury) may require supplementing up to 400 to 1000 µg daily.

- Include a daily serving of one of the foods high in manganese. Food sources include whole oats, oatmeal, rye, wheat, and brown rice. Peas, bananas, and beans are also excellent sources. In some cases a food supplement may be desirable. Manganese supplements should provide 5 mg daily.

- Prescribe a thiol resin, 1 capsule to be taken with each meal.

- Instruct the patient to purchase from his health food store a two month's supply of activated charcoal; and take two 260 mg capsules following each meal, or as you otherwise direct.

- A few days to a week before IV-C is to be administered have the patient titrate vitamin C dosage to bowel tolerance, or to body tolerance, and maintain this dosage during and following the IV-C, or until instructed otherwise. Alternatively, two days immediately preceding the IV-C instruct the patient to perform a vitamin C flush. Afterwards, instruct the patient to consume 3 g or 5 g per day before, during, and following IV-C, according to his degree of toxicity.

CAUTION: There are other lifestyle considerations that should be studied, especially as they relate to the individual. Additionally, there are hormonal and other factors that may alter body chemistry, thereby making it more or less difficult to rid the body of mercury and its toxic effect. This volume does not address the many possible exceptions, which only a doctor can determine. The objective here is to highlight the basic requirements, guide the doctor and staff into formulating a rational program for better health, and encourage the doctor to address the possible negative role that mercury might play in patients' current health problems. The intent, should the patient be mercury-toxic or mercury-sensitive, is to assist the doctor in ridding the patient's body of mercury even before amalgam fillings are replaced. Otherwise, the sudden additional load of body mercury that may result during amalgam replacement could very well cause a worsening of the patient's condition. As a precaution before administering IV-C, Chapter 5 examines additional lifestyle considerations. Again, only the doctor can fully judge what lifestyle regimen should ultimately be followed for any particular patient.

LITERATURE CITED

[1] R.P. Wedeen, "Lead, Mercury and Cadmium Nephropathy," *Neuro Toxicol*, 4 (3): 134-46, 1983.

[2] S.S. Jensensen and M. Willems, "The Hazards of Leadshot in Soil," *Science News*, 131 (15): 233, April 11, 1987.

[3] J. Raloff, "U.S. River Quality: Not All Signs are Good," *Science News*, 131 (14): 214, April 4, 1987.

[4] B. Bower, "High-Cadmium Diet: Recipe for Stress?" *Science News*, 132: 101, August 15, 1987.

[5] "Maximum Allowable Concentrations of Mercury Compounds.," *Arch Environ Health*, 19: 891, 1969.

[6] A. Grollman and E.F. Grollman, *Pharmacology and Therapeutics*, Lea & Febiger, Sixth Edition, Philadelphia, 1965.

[7] J.A. Clark, et al., "Mercury Poisoning from Merbromin (Mercurochrome) Therapy of Omphalocele," *Clin Pediatrics*, 21 (7): 445-7, July 1982.

[8] "Report of an International Committee: Maximum Allowable Concentrations of Mercury Compounds," *Arch Environ Health*, 19: 891-905, 1969.

[9] I.M. Trakhtenberg, *Chronic Effects of Mercury on Organisms*, Translated from the Russian language and reproduced in limited quantities by the Geographic Health Studies Program, U.S. Department of Health, Education, and Welfare, DHEW Publication No. (NIH) 74-473, 1974.

[10] R.J. Williams, *Nutrition Against Disease*, Pitman Publishing Corporation, 6 East 43rd Street, New York, NY 10017, 1971.

[11] T. Takeuchi, "Pathology of Minamata Disease," *Acta Pathol Jpn*, 32 (Suppl. 1): 73-99, 1982.

[12] A.M. Gotto and J. Ross, Jr., (Moderators), "Symposium: Cholesterol Consensus," American Heart Association's 59th Scientific Sessions, Dallas Convention Center, Dallas Tx, November 17-20, 1986.

[13] H. E. Morgan and B. Packard (Chairmen), "Symposium: New Guidelines for Treatment of High Blood Cholesterol," American Heart Association's 60th Scientific Sessions, Anaheim Convention Center, Anaheim, CA, November 16-19, 1987.

14 A.G. Shaper, "Cardiovascular Diseases and Trace Metals," *Proc R Soc Land B*, 205: 135-43, 1979.

15 H.M. Perry and M.W. Erlanger, "Metal-Induced Hypertension Following Chronic Feeding of Low Doses of Cadmium and Mercury," *J Lab Clin Med*, 83: 541-7, 1974.

16 H.L. Queen, "The Scientific Sessions Issue," *HEART TALK*, (ISSN:0882-1836), 5 (l): l-8, January 1987.

17 S.J. Singer and G.L. Nicolson, "The Fluid Mosaic Model of the Structure of Cell Membranes," *Science*, 175:72, 31, 1972.

18 C. K. Chow, "Nutritional Influence on Cellular Antioxidant Defense Systems," *Am J Clin Nutr*, 32:1066-81, May 1979.

19 L. Bolis, ed., *Membranes and Disease*, Raven Press, New York, N.Y. 1976.

20 J. G. Bauer and H. A. First, "The Toxicity of Mercury in Dental Amalgam," *Calif Dental Asso J*, June 1982.

21 M.A. Galin and S.A. Obstbaum, "Band Keratopathy in Mercury Exposure," *Annals of Ophthalmology*, 1257-61, December 1974.

22 S. Varma, "Ascorbic Acid and the Eye with Special Reference to the Lens," *Ann NY Acad Sci*, 498: 280-306, 1987.

23 W. Lohmann, "Ascorbic Acid and Cataract," *Ann NY Acad Sci*, 498: 307-11, 1987.

24 S.O. Welsh, "The Protective Effect of Vitamin E and N, N'-di-phenyl-phenylenediamine (DPPD) against Methyl Mercury Toxicity in the Rat," *J Nutr*, 109: 1673-81, 1979.

25 Editorial, *Medical Hypothesis*, December 1979.

26 E. Niki, "Interaction of Ascorbate and alpha-Tocopherol," *Ann NY Acad Sci*, 498: 186-99, 1987.

27 K. Kageyama, et al., "Effects of Methyl Mercuric Chloride and Sulfhydryl Inhibitors on Phospholipid Synthetic Activity of Lymphocytes," *J Applied Tox*, 6 (l): 49-53, 1986.

28 K. Hirokawa and Y. Hayashi, "Acute Methylmercury Intoxication in Mice—Effect on the Immune System," *Acta Pathol Japan*, 30 (l): 23-32, 1980.

29 A.D. Kantarjian, "A Syndrome Clinically Resembling Amyotrophic Lateral Sclerosis Following Chronic Mercurialism," *Neurology*, ll: 639-44, 1961.

[30] W.R. Harlan, et al., "Blood Lead and Blood Pressure," *JAMA*, 253(4): 530-534, January 25, 1985.

[31] J.J. Chisolm, Jr., "Poisoning from Heavy Metals (Mercury, Lead, and Cadmium)," *Pediatric Annals*, 9:458-68, December 12, 1980.

[32] V.N. Finelli, et al., Biochem Biophy Res Commun, 65: 303, 1975.

[33] D.A. McCarron, et al., "Blood Pressure and Nutrient Intake in the United States," *Science*, 224: 1392-1398, June 29, 1984.

[34] O.A. Levander, "Nutritional Factors in Relation to Heavy Metal Toxicants," *Federation Proceedings*, 36(5):1683-1687, April 1977.

[35] J. Glomme and K.H. Gustavson, "Treatment of Experimental Acute Mercury Poisoning by Chelating Agents BAL and EDTA," *Acta Med Scand*, 164: 175-82, 1959.

[36] M.E. Datyner and P.A. Cox, "Inorganic Mercurial Poisoning," *Anesth Intens Care*, 9:266-70, 1981.

[37] J. Engvall and J. Perk, "Prevalence of Hypertension among Cadmium-Exposed Workers," *Archives of Environmental Health*, 40(3): 185-190, May/June 1985.

[38] Bower, op. cit.

[39] Levander, op. cit. pp. 1683-87.

[40] V.G. Zannoni, et al., "Ascorbic Acid, Alcohol, and Environmental Chemicals," *Ann NY Acad Sci*, 498: 364-88, 1987.

[41] R.R. Watson, ed., *Nutrition, Disease Resistance, and Immune Function*, New York: Marcel Dekker, 1984.

[42] A.R. Sherman, "Alterations in Immunity Related to Nutritional Status," *Nutrition Today*, 7-13, July/August 1986.

[43] I.P. Gontzea, et al., *Arch Sci Physiol*, 18: 211, 1964.

[44] V.N. Finelli, et al., op. cit.

[45] D.L. Hamilton and L.S. Valberg, *Am J Physiol*, 227: 1033, 1974.

[46] G.W. Evans, et al., *Bioinorg Chem*, 3: 115, 1974.

[47] J.J. Putman and R.W. Madden, "Quicksilver and Slow Death," *National Geographic*, 142(4): 506-27, October 1972.

[48] J.M. McNab, "Factors Affecting the Digestibility of Nutrients," *Proc Nutr Soc*, 34 (1): 5-11, May 1975.

[49] D.H. Northcote, "The Induction of Enzyme Activity in the Endosperm of Germinating Castor-Bean Seeds," *Biochem J*, 152 (1): 65-70, October 1975.

[50] L. Magos, "Mercury and Mercurials," *Br Med Bull*, 31 (3): 241-45, 1975.

[51] S.C. Fang, *Res Commun Chem Pathol Pharmacol*, 9: 579, 1979.

[52] J. Parizek, et al., *Newer Trace Elements in Nutrition*, eds. W. Mertz and W.E. Cornatzer, New York Dekker, p. 85, 1971.

[53] H.E. Ganther, et al., *Science*, 175: 1122, 1972.

[54] A. Khayat and L. Dencker, "Whole Body and Liver Distribution of Inhaled Mercury Vapor in the Mouse: Influence of Ethanol and Aminothiazole Pretreatment," *J Applied Tox*, 3: 66-74, 1983.

[55] B. Ahlrot-Westerlund, et al., "Altered Distribution Patterns of Macro- and Trace Elements in Human Tissues of Patients with Decreased Levels of Blood Selenium," *Nutrition Research Suppl*, I: 442-450, 1985.

[56] A.O. Levander, et al., *Am J Clin Nutr*, 34: 2662, 1981.

[57] C.H. Hill, "Interactions of Vitamin C with Lead and Mercury," *NY Acad Science*, 355: 262-266, 1980.

[58] R.A. Good, *Journal USA*, l(3):l-12, September 1986. Published by the United Sciences of America Research Foundation, Inc. (now defunct), formerly of Dallas, TX.

[59] R.F. Burk, et al., *Proc Soc Exp Biol Med*, 145: 782, 1974.

[60] T. Norseth and T.W. Clarkson, "Methylmercury," *Arch Environ Health*, 22: 568-77, 1971.

[61] B. Borgstrom, et al., "Studies on Intestinal Digestion and Absorption in the Human," *J Clin Invest*, 36: 1521-36, 1957.

[62] T.W. Clarkson, H. Small, and T. Norseth, "Excretion and Absorption of Methylmercury after Polythiol Resin Treatment," *Arch Environ Health*, 26: 173-6, 1973.

[63] F. Bakir, et al., "The Employment of a Thiol Resin in Mercury Poisoning," *Science*, 181: 230-41, 1973.

[64] P.J. Neuvonen, "Clinical Pharmacokinetics of Oral Activated Charcoal in

Acute Intoxications," *Clin Pharmacokin*, 7: 465-89, 1982.

65 E.I. Friedman, et al., "Charcoal-Induced Lipid Reduction in Uremia," *Int Soc Nephrol*, 13 (Suppl 8): S-170-S-176, 1978.

66 P. Kuusisto, et al., "Effect of Activated Charcoal on Hypercholesterolemia," *The Lancet*, 16 (2): 366-7, August 16, 1986.

67 E. Cameron and L. Pauling, "Supplemental Ascorbate in the Supportive Treatment of Cancer: Prolongation of Survival Times in Terminal Human Cancer," *Proc Natl Acad Sci USA*, 73: 3685-89, 1976.

68 F.R. Klenner, "Observations on the Dose and Administration of Ascorbic Acid when Employed Beyond the Range of a Vitamin in Human Pathology," *J Applied Nutr*, 23: 61-88, 1971.

69 R.F. Cathcart, "Vitamin C, Titrating to Bowel Tolerance, Anascorbemia, and Acute Induced Scurvy," *Med Hypothesis*, 7: 1359-76, 1981.

70 J.V. Wright, *Dr. Wright's Book of Nutritional Therapy*, Rodale Press, Inc., Emmaus, PA, 1979.

71 J.V. Wright, *Dr. Wright's Guide To Healing With Nutrition*, Rodale Press, Inc., Emmaus, PA, 1984.

CHAPTER 3

Identifying the
Mercury-Toxic Patient

*"A sick man may wear a wrong diagnosis around his neck like a mill-
stone, and the doctor's task may be first to un_diagnose him so recovery can
begin."*

~John L. McClenahan [1915-   ]

Chronic mercury toxicity, because it is an endemic disease that's seldom
recognized, may unknowingly be an underlying factor in—or contributor to—
nearly any disease or condition that the doctor is treating; whether it be heart
disease, cancer, or toothache. This may occur especially when only the symptoms of a disease are being addressed, and when an underlying cause for the
condition is not sought. Mercury may also exacerbate symptoms, or make any
treatment program more difficult to manage. It is this feature of chronic mercury toxicity—which makes it difficult to recognize and a roadblock to
health—that necessitates the message of this chapter.

In making a diagnosis it is necessary first to rule out mercurial poisoning, as opposed to chronic mercury toxicity. IV-C is not indicated in the initial
treatment phase of mercurial poisoning. As a general rule, visible symptoms
and elevated blood and urine values characterize mercury poisoning. Characteristic of chronic mercury toxicity are symptoms that are difficult to recognize,
as well as borderline, normal, and below-normal blood and urine values. Even
so, reliance upon blood, urine, and laboratory testing are of only secondary importance to diagnosis. Until more specific tests become available, the primary
diagnosis must be made from the medical history and from the patient's symptoms.

A CASE HISTORY

To assist the doctor in his diagnosis, this chapter begins with the story
of an actual mercury-toxic patient. His experience took him from one doctor's
office to another without ever being correctly diagnosed and treated. The purpose of this account is certainly not to lay blame, but rather to help the doctor
identify similar patients and to emphasize the widespread failure among dentists and physicians to recognize not just chronic mercury toxicity, but acute
mercurialism as well.

A 25-year-old male medical laboratory technologist appeared in the
office of an M.D. The patient, known to the doctor as being energetic, productive, and generally outspoken, exhibited a variety of symptoms that were uncharacteristic for him. He was lethargic and complained of mild depression,
increasing episodes of forgetfulness, and short periods of amnesia. This was serious enough in itself, but the patient at the time was concerned mainly with
periods of general muscular weakness coinciding also with periods of abnormal
heart rhythm. In fact, it was the bothersome change in heart rhythm that
first prompted him to seek his doctor's help.

During the interview, the doctor noted that the patient was having personal and financial problems, and was daily growing more dissatisfied with his job in a major university-affiliated hospital where he was employed as evening and night supervisor of the blood bank and clinical laboratory. He also worked a full day each week in the blood chemistry section of the same hospital laboratory where he performed bicarbonate (plasma alkali reserve) determinations on the Van Slyke apparatus.*

In addition to his primary symptoms, the patient complained casually of increased urinary frequency and daily diarrhea that had been with him for several months. Without hesitation, the doctor concluded that the cause of the abnormal heart rhythm was life stresses, and that all of his patient's other problems were due to a reactionary neurosis that followed. The doctor's prescription was to "go home, rest, and have a little fun...change jobs if you must, but don't take life so seriously." Chronic mercury toxicity was not suspected.

As it turned out, the medical technologist did benefit from his doctor's advice. He not only changed jobs, but also professions, attaining a modest degree of success during the next few years as a pharmaceutical salesman. Gradually, his previously described symptoms subsided to a tolerable level, but none of the original complaints ever entirely cleared up.

Three years after his first break from health, the technologist-turned-salesman had three amalgam fillings placed by his dentist. Six months later, he reported to another medical doctor (this one specializing in internal medicine) with complaints of repeated outbreaks of mouth sores due to herpes simplex.

This doctor's interrogation revealed that the patient had been experiencing periodic episodes of mental depression—an on-again, off-again condition that had been with the patient for the entire time. In recent months the frequency and duration of these episodes had been increasing. During these periods the otherwise successful salesman was nearly nonproductive and had no spirit to do the tasks demanded of him. The doctor, believing the patient was experiencing burnout and no longer felt challenged by the sales position, suggested—just as the first doctor had—that the patient consider a professional change.   By doing so, the doctor believed the stress experienced would markedly subside. Again, mercury was not suspected.

Once again, the patient followed his doctor's advice and changed jobs, but this time without improvement. During the next three or four years the patient went "doctor hopping," seeing one specialist and then another. His

* To perform tests on the Van Slyke apparatus, approximately 250 ml to 300 ml of liquid mercury were required in a closed system, forming a vacuum. The system, however, wasn't always closed. There were two rotating stopcocks that allowed the technologist to bring acid in contact with a patient's serum, thereby releasing CO_2. The gas was measured by observing the volume of mercury displaced. The problem here was that the stopcocks periodically popped out, breaking the vacuum seal and spilling the mercury on the counter top. It was then necessary to pick up the mercury in the best manner possible and place it into a beaker for reuse. It was also necessary to periodically clean the mercury, requiring the technologist to empty the contents of the apparatus into a beaker, add an alcohol-based cleaner, and, using gauze, wipe away the protein residue. In the process the technologist breathed the vapors and at times actually had his hands in the liquid mercury while cleaning it. (OSHA standards were at that time not in force, and the dangers of mercury in the workplace, while known, were generally overlooked.) For the technologist-turned-patient, and for all others who regularly operated the apparatus, this represented a significant daily exposure to mercury.

stops included the offices of an allergist (for treatment of recurring contact dermatitis), a urologist (for recurring prostate infections), a second internist (for bothersome heart rhythm), and a dentist (for tending to his ever-increasing rate of tooth decay). The dentist placed an upper partial denture that was comprised primarily of a nonprecious metal. Within 24 hours the clasp that anchored the hardware turned black and broke, which more than suggested (retrospectively) that the patient was experiencing exceptional oral corrosion due to strong galvanic action.

Ultimately, the patient was referred to a a psychiatrist. It is important, perhaps, to point out here that nearly all mercury-toxic or mercury-sensitive people who are exposed daily to mercury—if not diagnosed and treated appropriately—will eventually be referred to a psychiatrist. This psychiatrist performed extensive testing and concluded that the patient was now suffering from progressive deterioration of the brain stem with altered brain chemistry. He was placed on a treatment regimen consisting of psychotropic drugs and psychotherapy. The patient was informed during one of his office visits that this was how things would be for the duration of his life. Without the treatment, he was told, he would soon die or end up in an institution.

This is how many people with chronic mercury toxicity end up: in a mental institution with neither the doctor nor the patient ever realizing what caused the steady deterioration of health. Fortunately, however, this particular story has a happy ending. The patient, having the faculty for discovery by accident, suddenly reached the conclusion that since none of his doctors had answers, he would elect to do things his own way. If he were going to die, he reasoned, he at least was not going to do so without a fight, and while heavily sedated at that. Thus, he discarded all medication, cancelled all further appointments with his psychiatrist, and opted for a total health program.

That was fifteen years ago. The once "condemned" patient today is in far better health than the average person of comparable age. He exercises regularly, has a positive outlook toward life, approaches every day with energy and vigor, and is again making a useful contribution to society. The only unusual aspect of his own case, he believes, is that he was lucky enough to have stumbled upon a solution before a solution was knowingly available. Only later did he associate former health problems with his earlier exposure to mercury in the clinical laboratory. He has since learned that he is highly mercury-sensitive, and has had his amalgam fillings replaced, resulting again in positive health results.

In retrospect, he can see that each reoccurrence of his former health problems was associated with a visit to his dentist. He had become sensitive to additional exposure to mercury. Consequently, he has had to become keenly aware of the various possible sources of further mercury exposure. He has since become interested in the many facets of lifestyle practices and learned how daily habits influence health and disease. Thus, for him and others like him, who have learned that sensitivity to mercury may be acquired from a previous significant exposure, attainment of health is an ongoing process.

I can attest to the fact that the above case is true, because I am the patient involved.

From this case there are several points to be discussed:

- Doctors of every specialty are disinclined to suspect chronic mercury toxicity, or mercury poisoning for that matter, and are generally unaware of the symptoms of either stage of intoxication.

- Doctors are unfamiliar with the nature of mercury intoxication and are equally uncertain as to what tests should be performed to study its effect.

- It may be that the potential for poorer health from dental amalgam fillings is much greater in those patients previously exposed to mercury.

- Some of the classic symptoms of acute mercurialism, as well as chronic mercury toxicity, were evident in the above case. The doctor may have made the link if he had perhaps asked a few more questions, or if additional information had been volunteered. For instance, I had a noticeable metallic taste with partial numbness of the lips and mouth, and I often experienced dizziness. My speech was slurred somewhat and I stuttered more than usual, but did not believe this to be important enough to mention, nor did the doctor observe this or include a question that pertained to such when my medical history was taken.

- If chronic mercury toxicity was indeed the underlying cause of the symptoms, then one could reasonably argue that symptoms of subacute, chronic mercurialism* may include: brain dysfunction with mental depression, irritability, amnesia and forgetfulness with a progressively destructive effect on the brain stem; a depression of the immune system, causing an increased tendency toward repeated viral infections; enhancement of the natural allergic response, as evidenced by repeated contact dermatitis; interruption in normal cardiac rhythm; and interruption of normal muscular contraction and nerve transmission, leading to unnatural fatigue, dizziness, muscular weakness, and incoordination. Many of these symptoms are the same as those of acute mercurialism.

- If the first doctor had suspected acute mercurialism, what tests could have been performed to verify his suspicion? Likely, he would have chosen (correctly) blood and urine mercury determinations. If the second, third, fourth, or fifth doctors visited had suspected chronic mercury toxicity, or a hypersensitivity to mercury, what tests would they have run to determine this? This has always been a difficult question to answer, mostly because the chronic stage of the disease seldom can be confirmed with blood, urine, and hair analysis. Even more

---

* The toxicology of methylmercury is different from any other mercurial, and the cardinal signs of methylmercury intoxication are not produced by mercury vapor or inorganic mercury salts. Yet there was a great overlap of symptoms in my case, which is probably a common occurrence. Several explanations are possible, but I personally feel that the reduction in my general state of health caused initially by inorganic mercury and mercury vapors greatly increased my susceptibility to the toxic effects of otherwise "acceptable levels" of other chemical species of mercury that generally pervade our environment. It is equally plausible that the galvanic current generated by my dental fillings perpetually disrupted normal brain waves, thereby exaggerating my psychological, neurological, and neuromuscular symptoms.

difficult is the task of deciding what to do about the problem. At that time—and until this book—there was no effective treatment for chronic mercury toxicity, only acute mercurialism, for which the doctor would include intramuscular injections of BAL (discussed shortly), or oral administration of penicillamine. Even if the therapy had been effective for acute symptoms, unwanted side effects would have plagued any attempt at long-term therapy, without which the mercury-toxic patient could never have expected to be entirely free of the effects of mercury. This is another reason for the renewed interest in IV-C, as IV-C has the effect of addressing a wide range of health adversities while simultaneously addressing the symptoms of chronic mercury toxicity.

- Finally, if doctors are not skilled in identifying the symptoms of acute mercurial poisoning, then how can these same health professionals expect to recognize the subtle symptoms of chronic mercury toxicity, particularly if previously unsuspected dental amalgam has become a contributing factor? The answer is that they can, but it probably won't happen without a greater level awareness.

THE PATIENT PROFILE

In an attempt to answer the question of what a doctor should look for in identifying the patient with chronic mercury toxicity, an interview was conducted with Dr. Hal A. Huggins.

Dr. Huggins is a dentist who no longer practices dentistry, but who in recent years has transformed his regular dental practice into treatment of what he regards as dentistry-induced, mercury-related health problems. Most importantly, he believes, he has assumed the task of informing other dentists and medical doctors as well. For the reader's interest, his approach and use of proprietary diagnostic testing is controversial, to say the least. He has written books for the lay public, his latest entitled *It's All In Your Head*,[1] and has published some of his clinical observations in scientific literature. However some groups of researchers and dental authorities charge that he does not provide them with enough data to back up his research. They claim that an exchange of data would improve his credibility and help solve the controversy that surrounds the long-standing use of dental amalgam. Dr. Huggins replies that he is offended by this charge, as he lectures regularly and spends much time on the phone with interested parties. "At the ADA meeting...I was requested four times to present only clinical observations—not scientific data. Some medical journals have called articles well-done, but potentially too much panic could be developed should this truth be explored." He believes that health authorities are trying to discredit him to avoid widespread litigation of their own.

Whether he prefers to retain his proprietary rights for the benefit of his own patients, or whether he fears that others may discredit his findings for the reasons just given, Dr. Huggins' comments on this topic, as one who has over fifteen years clinical experience, are nevertheless regarded as valuable:

Q: Dr. Huggins, what percentage of the population would you venture to say, right now, is walking around with dental amalgam?

Dr. Huggins: There are various figures on this...I'm not sure who to believe. The figures go from as low as 70 to as high as 85 percent of the population. We are talking about many millions of people.

Q: What percentage of the people with amalgams are showing some kind of symptoms that are related to their dental amalgams?

Dr. Huggins: If you will allow me to cite the results of biocompatibility testing developed in our own laboratory: the figure that has most often been used in the past—20 percent—is probably inaccurate today. By subjecting the blood of our staff and patients to mercury and measuring their reaction in a number of ways, all based upon established methodology, we found that the figure greatly exceeds that. We have over 1000 test subjects, 68 percent of that population record immune reactivity to low levels of mercury.

Q: You are indicating that the prevalence is equivalent to a general epidemic, a problem that may be affecting 35 to 45 percent, or more, of the American population—assuming, as you say, that 70 to 85 percent of the population now have amalgam fillings in their teeth. If these figures are accurate, as you believe, then this brings up a most important concern for doctors of every specialty. Can you describe the patient from your own clinical experience and help these doctors understand what they should be looking for?

Dr. Huggins: The reason that chronic mercury toxicity is difficult to diagnose is that it takes so many forms. For better understanding we have subdivided the condition into 5 different forms; neurologic, cardiovascular, collagenic, immunologic, and allergic, plus an all-encompassing form that we call miscellaneous. Because we all have our own genetic weak link, we are all susceptible to environmental challenges according to what our genetic code dictates (Chapter 2). Our weak link, therefore, will determine our degree of susceptibility to mercury and other dental toxic metals.

      The problem as we see it, is that initially the effectiveness of the immune system will be reduced in susceptible people. Once the immune system is compromised anything can happen, because the body's defenses are down, and we're talking about more than just bacterial and viral infections. For instance, we probably see more neurological problems in our practice than anything else. But one of the big keys is if a patient has been to six or eight or even fifteen doctors, and nobody's really come up with a positive diagnosis...more than likely this is another case of chronic mercury toxicity. There is no one test for this, but there are a large number of symptoms that are related to it. What is most often seen is a combination of symptoms such as unexplained fatigue, metallic taste in the mouth, emotional swings for no particular reason, numbness and tingling of the fingers and the toes...this would be, I think, about 58 percent of the patients we see. Other common symptoms include unidentified chest pains, and allergies. These serve to trigger the more serious symptoms of the five major forms and, initially, give an indication of where to look. This is how we determine our testing program.

Q: Relative to the testing, Dr. Huggins, if an allergist, or any other medical doctor called you and asked "how do I determine if mercury is a problem in my patient?" How would you respond to his question?

Dr. Huggins: We teach doctors of all specialties to diagnose from 23 potential parameters. As a basic screen we start out looking for changes in the blood chemistries; we look for changes in the complete blood count (CBC); we look for changes in the urine; and we look at the hair analysis for toxic metals. This is going to be used on all patients. The testing then becomes more sophisticated. Based upon the symptoms we look at, the hormone balance—or imbalance if they have an endocrine problem—we will probably look at biocompatibility testing results; we will look at lymphocyte reactions; we may involve retinal photography, or the use of results from an electroencephalogram, or electrocardiogram. There are many areas that change as a result of mercurialism, micromercurialism, or of mercury being placed in the body. It all depends on the patient, so we try to match the test with the patient's problem. For instance, if the patient has a sore toe you don't ask a cooperating facility to do an electroencephalogram on them, you try to match the test to what the patient's symptoms are. To diagnose I would suggest that the doctor learn all of these parameters to better evaluate his treatment program and to improve the odds for a successful outcome.

As our interview revealed, chronic mercury toxicity may take on any one, or a combination, of five basic forms, plus a sixth (miscellaneous), which is really the equivalent of saying that mercury has the capacity to contribute to the onset, severity, and progression of all diseases. This is not surprising, however, since findings[2] of the major Iraqi outbreak of mercury poisoning indicate a clear difference in variation in individual sensitivity. The same can be said for chronic, low-level exposure to mercury. It is therefore necessary to become familiar with each class of symptoms that may result from chronic mercury toxicity.

Neurologic Symptoms
    The Japanese and Iraqi experiences indicate that neurological involvement is a feature of severe methylmercury intoxication. Likewise, chronic methylmercury toxicity (accumulated from a combination of sources) may be indicated with all patients who complain of unexplained sensory symptoms, including pain, numbness, or burning sensations. Rustam and Hamdi found that symptoms of severe intoxication may include unexplained muscular weakness, tremor of the hands and feet, ataxia, speech and visual impairment, as well as deafness; suggesting that some degree of chronic methylmercury toxicity should be suspected in all patients with similar symptoms.
    Elhassani,[3] in summarizing the Japanese and Iraqi experiences, explained that methylmercury inhibits choline acetyltransferase, thereby blocking synthesis of acetylcholine and resulting in neuromuscular symptoms. Rustam[4] determined, in a second study, that these symptoms seem to respond positively to the drug neostigmine. The work of Cavanagh and Chen[5] revealed that the most affected part of the CNS, when dealing with chronic mercury toxicity, is the spinal ganglia, which causes impairment of amino acid incorporation, followed by nerve/fiber degeneration. In addition, some of the patients in the 1973 Iraqi outbreak had myoneural transmission failure resembling Myasthenia gravis, which again responded to neostigmine. Still others developed a condition resembling amyotrophic lateral sclerosis (ALS).[6] Through these mechanisms and reported symptoms there is suspicion that methylmercury poisoning may also mimic or exacerbate multiple sclerosis. Thus, as before, it may be important to the recovery of particular patients to suspect some degree of chronic mercury toxicity in any patient suffering from these symptoms and diseases.

Mental and Emotional Symptoms
    Dr. Tadao Takeuchi,[7] reporting autopsy findings on patients with

Minamata disease, determined a difference in brain pathology between patients who died of acute poisoning (death occurring within 100 days of onset of disease) and those who died of chronic mercury toxicity (death occurring after one year). The acutely-poisoned patients suffered quick, cytotoxic brain damage as well as hypoxemic and anoxemic damage; whereas patients with chronic mercury toxicity exhibited a slow, neurotoxic effect on brain neurons.

There were other marked differences. Brain atrophy with up to 49 percent reduction in brain size was noted for those who died of chronic mercury toxicity; very little atrophy or reduction in brain size was noted in acute poisoning. Death came quickly in acute poisoning; whereas the scenario of chronic mercury toxicity developed slowly—symptoms progressing from mental depression to apathy, withdrawal, psychoses, and organic brain disorders. It was the neurotoxic effect in the latter that was responsible for causing the wider variety of symptoms. The difference, Takeuchi believed, could be attributed to the period of time over which exposure occurred, and to the half life of methylmercury—which, again, is 70 days in the body as a whole, but 240 days in the brain. Acute poisoning generally distributed the least amount of mercury to the brain. Repeated, low-level exposure to mercury resulted in a greater accumulation of brain mercury.

An M. D., Ph. D. from Sweden, Dr. Patrick Störtebecker,[8] wrote an excellent book on this topic, *The Effect of Mercury On The Brain*, giving special emphasis to dental mercury. The possibilities of subclinical effects are so broad, he believes (elemental mercury and mercury vapor, he found, were equally as damaging to the brain as methylmercury), that the doctors who must deal with this category, particularly neurologists and psychiatrists, might do well to routinely address the issue of mercury and other heavy metal intoxication in each of their patients.

To describe the psychic and behavioral characteristics that are so often a part of the mercury profile, the term "erethism" is often used. Erethism consists of subtle or dramatic changes in behavior and personality, such as depression, irritability, despondency, fearfulness, irascibility, restlessness, indecision, timidity, and a tendency toward easy embarrassment. Companion symptoms are drowsiness, headache, fatigue, dizziness, and insomnia, with an exaggerated response to stimulation. These are the neurotoxic symptoms of chronic brain involvement for which the electroencephalogram, along with other tests, may prove useful in confirming the diagnosis. In treating these patients I strongly recommend a companion book (one which played a part in my own recovery) that's consistent with the principles of this book. The title is *Psychodietetics*, by Drs. E. Cheraskin and W.M. Ringsdorf, Jr., with Arline Brecher.

Cardiovascular

The cardiovascular area of symptoms might include any patient with abnormal heart rhythm. A Russian scientist, Dr. A. O. Saytanov,[9] learned from studying rabbits exposed to mercury vapor that abnormal changes were observed in the electrocardiogram (EKG), as characterized by a lowering and broadening of the P-waves. He believed this was a consequence of cardiac sulfhydryl enzyme inactivation by mercury, causing an interruption in the energy/contraction cycle of the heart muscle. Damluji,[10] who studied the cardiovascular effects of the 1970 outbreak in Iraq, noted that methyl mercury caused abnormal changes in the S-T segment of the EKG. Chronic mercury toxicity, therefore, should be considered in any patient suspected of having been exposed to mercury, and who has similar findings on EKG.

The works of Shaper,[11] and of Perry and Erlanger,[12] respectively, demonstrate that mercury may be a contributing factor in arterial disease, as well as a wide assortment of maladies affecting the heart and arteries. It interferes with the normal processing of nutrients that feed the arterial intima and the cells of arterial smooth muscle, causing proliferation and rigidity of the inner arterial wall.

The works of Brown and Goldstein[13,14] explained how mercury may contribute to the problem of Type II Hyperlipoproteinemia—a genetic defect in which those affected have difficulty processing cholesterol from their arterial cell walls. Type II people tend to overproduce liver cholesterol, and show exceptional difficulty in depositing cholesterol in the liver's catabolic pool for removal from the body. Brown and Goldstein's revelation that sulfhydryl proteins are key links to the correct protein sequencing of receptors for LDL cholesterol may be interpreted to indicate that mercury has the capacity to interfere with the availability of receptors for LDL cholesterol, thereby contributing to the lethal characteristic of Type II Hyperlipoproteinemia. For this reason, and because mercury has the capacity to initiate arterial disease, chronic mercury toxicity could be suspected in any Type II patient.

In support of mercury's demonstrated involvement in arterial disease, researchers at Osaka City University Medical School demonstrated the detrimental effect that mercury has on fat-removing enzymes like LCAT and ACAT.[15] When the researchers compared the effects of methylmercury and other sulfhydryl inhibitors which affect enzymes in phospholipid systems, such as exist in the fat-removing LCAT and ACAT enzymes, methylmercury was the only inhibitor that actually killed the cells being studied. Through a closely related mechanism, it is believed that by interfering with fat-removing enzymes, mercury may be contributing to the high total serum cholesterol that is characteristic of these people, and to many other people at risk to arterial disease. Considering this possibility, chronic mercury toxicity should be suspected in those people who have an unexplained, elevated cholesterol, and who also show some evidence of mercury exposure. The following suggests that these people are at risk to manifesting violent, emotional behavior, as well as neuromuscular and neurological dysfunction when placed on the contemporary, cholesterol-lowering drug and diet regimen.

The Threat Of Chronic Mercury Toxicity Presents An Unforeseen Health Risk From A Sudden Drop In Cholesterol. The U. S. Government's now-famous, $150 million study into the relationship of cholesterol and heart disease, termed the LRC-CPPT Study,[16,17] was interpreted as proof that cholesterol-lowering through the use of diet or drugs, or a combination of these, would prevent the premature death and disability of those whose cholesterol was elevated. **HEART TALK**[18,19] has strongly challenged this interpretation of results, labeling it "The Government's $150 Million Dollar Fallacy."*

In order to arrive at their conclusion, it was argued, the interpreters of the study wrongly omitted from the analysis of the test group several deaths due to violence (murder, suicide, and auto fatalities). While the deaths should not have been excluded from the final tally, the authors believed the violent deaths were unrelated to the diet and drug being studied, and that no plausible explanation had been offered to make them believe otherwise. The evidence that has since surfaced, however, leads one to believe there is now sufficient

* Refer to Appendix I for information and address for **HEART TALK**.

reason to regard <u>chronic mercury toxicity</u> as a very sound reason for the un-counted deaths within the study group. In fact, the evidence suggests that a similar fate awaits many other people who are now mercury-toxic, undiag-nosed, and will soon be placed on a cholesterol-lowering diet combined with one of the newer, cholesterol-lowering drugs.

Dr. Matti Virkkunen[20] of the Psychiatric Clinic of Helsinki University compared the personality inventory of patients with varying levels of blood cholesterol. He found a significant connection between low cholesterol levels, or sudden drops in cholesterol, and a tendency toward impulsive homicidal and suicidal behavior. Although an explanation for his findings was never pro-posed, Virkkunen's observation gave reason to suspect (as we shall soon see) that chronic mercury toxicity is in some way involved.

Tamashiro, et al.,[21] in a study of leading causes of death among the people of Minamata Bay, likewise noted a higher than normal incidence of ac-cidents, poisonings, and suicides, which they credited indirectly to Minamata disease. The people who became prone to accidents and suicide did so, they be-lieved, as a consequence of ataxia and blindness. Although Tamashiro's group did not compare cholesterol levels, these facts and the characteristics of mer-cury disclosed in Chapter 2 strongly suggest that a more than casual link exists between the sudden lowering of blood cholesterol, violent emotional behavior, and chronic mercury toxicity.

Chapter 2 explained that methylmercury is transported to and from cells with the aid of lipoproteins. In fact, mercury's affinity for the protein segment of lipoproteins accounts (at least in part) for its strong attraction to the lipoidal tissues, such as brain and nerve cells. The process for mercury's release from binding sites requires administering sufficient selenium and sulfhydryl proteins to reach or surpass the point of competitive equilibrium. Once accom-plished, the mercury is then free to take either of two pathways: (1) it can re-distribute from affected tissue sites to sites that are less affected, or (2) it can exit the body.

Getting mercury to exit the body, however, isn't an easy task. Suffi-cient dietary fat is required to stimulate synthesis of the lipoproteins and cholesterol necessary for transporting cholesterol and mercury (attached to the sulfhydryl protein component of lipoproteins) to the liver for excretion along with bile. A low-fat, low-cholesterol diet, if recommended for the mercury-toxic patient, would be counterproductive.* The reduced intake of animal pro-tein from such a diet would limit the availability of sulfhydryl protein needed to compete with mercury for its binding sites. The low fat intake would inhibit the transport of mercury, and it would encourage retention rather than excretion of mercury. Furthermore, it would encourage accumulation of mercury in sensi-tive cells and tissue types, such as lipoidal tissues comprising nerve and brain cells. This would then cause symptoms of chronic mercury toxicity, such as erethism, neurological and neuromuscular disorders, and suppression of the immune system, to manifest. A review of my own experience offers a case in point.

At several times during my rehabilitation, when I was feeling my best, I noted that my total serum cholesterol ranged from 180 to 215. Not until I reduced my consumption of fat and had over-trained for a 10 mile run did my TSC drop into the range of 155 to 165, at which time symptoms of irritability and mental depression reappeared. Suddenly, I found myself crying for no

---

* For this reason, the **IV-C Mercury Tox Program** requires a diet high in fat.

apparent reason, and discovered that other symptoms, such as prostatitis, had also returned. Fortunately for me, however, I had by that time sufficient experience with the problem to be suspicious of the sudden change in TSC. Upon changing my diet and exercise habits in such a way as to raise TSC levels to "normal," the symptoms subsided. Since that experience I've heard similar reports from others and—as I've been told by those who are most affected—it didn't seem to matter from what point they had started; whether their TSC went down from 200 to 165 or whether it fell from 305 to 265, the symptoms of irritability and depression recurred.

The question immediately comes to mind: If fat and cholesterol are necessary to transport mercury through and out of the body, is it not logical to assume that symptoms of chronic mercury toxicity are least likely to manifest in people who are overweight, and most likely to manifest in people who are underweight? If one again examines the Minamata experience, the answer would seem to be a resounding "Yes". Being underweight and having little appetite is a feature of Minamata disease (in the most severely affected),* so the connection <u>does</u> make sense. Speculating further, it is tempting to ask: Are overweight, mercury-toxic people least likely to get themselves involved in violent acts? While the answer remains obscure, an important clue was provided by a coroner's report from New Mexico.

Dr. Kenneth Warner, while serving as county coroner in Albuquerque, New Mexico, made an analysis of body types of people who were brought to him for autopsy following violent death due to suicide, murder, or auto accident. In private correspondence he reported that normal weight individuals were twice as likely to die violently than overweight and obese people. While the report remains in rough draft form and unavailable for distribution at this time, his preliminary data supports the suspicion that the threshold of manifestation of symptoms of chronic mercury toxicity is linked to body fat and cholesterol.

In conclusion, the evidence indicates a possible coexistence of chronic mercury toxicity and Type II Hyperlipoproteinemia in certain participants of the LRC Study who died of violent death. I suggest the findings also offer a plausible explanation for their actions. Because mercury has an affinity for lipoproteins and lipoidal tissues, any sudden lowering of cholesterol without a reduction in the body burden of mercury would encourage the transfer of previously circulating mercury to the lipoidal tissues of nerve and brain cells. This possible behavioral reaction, I believe, <u>should require a warning on the package insert of the powerful new drugs being developed for cholesterol-lowering</u>. The enzyme inhibitor drugs, for instance, are said to be capable of reducing TSC by 25 to 30 percent; and by 40 to 50 percent when combined with a bile acid sequesterant. While not every recipient of these drugs will be mercury-toxic, the evidence suggests that those who <u>are</u> can expect to manifest the variable symptoms of chronic mercury toxicity. The doctor's task, therefore, is to be aware of this possibility, in which case monitoring the patient's behavior would be advised for those already on a cholesterol-lowering regimen.

---

* The poorest of the fishermen in the Minamata experience, who were forced to depend upon their own catch for 3 meals per day, were underweight even before the Chisso factory began releasing mercury into the bay. In such cases the fishermen were more susceptible to the consequences of mercury. Thus, being underweight was not a direct cause of methylmercury poisoning in their situation, but a factor which predisposed them to the most serious consequences.

Otherwise, an attempt should be made to identify beforehand any high-risk patient who may qualify as a candidate for the **IV-C Mercury Tox Program.**

The Fish Recommendation. Doctors in Japan, who treated the people of Minamata Bay poisoned by methylmercury, reported that the people at greatest risk to Minamata disease were those who ate the most fish caught in the bay. The researchers considered it unlikely that the chronic mercury toxicity/fish consumption pattern was limited only to Japan's Minamata Bay, since mercury is a growing contaminant of man's environment. While methylmercury epidemics have not occurred elsewhere, and while epidemics are not likely to occur as a result of contamination in the open seas, milder effects of methylmercury will likely occur (and probably do occur) as the consumption pattern of fish increases. Thus, the current recommendation that everyone increase their fish consumption as a means of preventing heart attacks gives additional reason for doctors to screen cardiovascular patients. Beyond the recommended intake of fish (3 to 4 servings per week), a significant number of people who habitually follow the latest health advice will surely reason that if a little is good, more is better...and better yet, they will figure, to supplement their diet with fish oil capsules.

While the concept of fish oil supplementation and the practice of consuming more fish appears valid, there is growing concern among scientists that the likelihood of excess may result in stroke, excessive bleeding, and chronic mercury toxicity in some people. The findings of Tamashiro's team of researchers gave support to this concern. They were surprised to learn that heart attacks as the cause of death was low among those who died of Minamata disease—surprising because Shaper had reported earlier that poisoning due to elemental mercury caused a rise in incidence of heart attacks. Even more surprising was the significant and alarming rise in incidence of cerebral hemorrhage among the Minamata Bay residents.

Those who were poisoned with mercury drank the most alcohol and ate the most fish, and thereby consumed more of the omega-3 fatty acids than those who ate less fish. This is significant since omega-3 fats are credited not only with preventing heart attacks, but with prolonging bleeding time. Together with alcohol, this may have played an indirect role in the increase in death due to cerebral hemorrhage. While this is still to be researched, it would appear prudent to suspect chronic mercury toxicity in those cardiovascular patients who are lean, who react emotionally to cholesterol-lowering, who are heavy drinkers, who are exposed to mercury in their work or have silver amalgam fillings, and who depend upon fish as their primary source of protein.

Again, the possibilities for involvement of mercury in cardiovascular ailments are so broad that the doctors who must deal with this category, especially the internist, family practitioner, and cardiologist, might do well to routinely address the issue of chronic mercury toxicity (and other heavy metal toxicities) early in the patient's treatment program. In turn, it would allow the doctor to attain better results with whatever treatment is chosen for his cardiovascular patients, especially if that treatment involves a combination of the powerful, cholesterol-lowering drugs.

Collagenic

The Minamata experience indicated that chronic mercury toxicity can mimic many of the collagenic diseases. These symptoms may include a wide assortment of conditions, not the least of which are periodontal disease and malocclusion (Chapter 4), as well as lupus erythematosis, scleroderma, and other collagenic vascular diseases that affect the skin. Included in this category also are unexplained bleeding (especially of the gums), loosened teeth, poor wound healing of arteries, and congenital defects such as collagen-induced platelet aggregation. Low back pain and the many types of arthritis are perhaps the most common degenerative diseases in this grouping. Because vitamin C and anabolic enzymes are required in the synthesis, growth, and repair of collagen, and because all enzyme systems are a possible target of chronic mercury toxicity, the slightest suspicion of a history of exposure to mercury is reason enough to enter all patients with collagenic disease in the **IV-C Mercury Tox Program.**

Immunologic

In any condition in which there is a reduction in the immune system response, mercury could very well be contributing to the problem. Hirakawa and Hayashi's study[22] of mice poisoned with methylmercury revealed that methylmercury causes atrophy of the thymic cortex. When this occurs, mercury reduces the ability to fight infections mainly by reducing the body's ability to produce T-Lymphocytes (T-cells). T-cells are activated in the thymus gland and form the backbone of the cell-mediated arm of immunity. They guard against most viral and fungal infections (candida, for instance), as well as mycobacterial infections and cancer. So it would seem appropriate, in treating and preventing these conditions, to rid the body of whatever mercury might be available for attachment to the thymic cortex and to the membranes of T-cells.

Likewise, to bolster the immune response, it would seem prudent to rid the body of any possible mercury contaminants that affect B-Lymphocytes (B-cells) from bone marrow, since bone marrow is a rich source of sulfhydryl proteins and thereby attracts mercury. B-cells comprise the humoral arm of immunity, and protect us from most bacterial and some viral infections. The antibodies produced by B-cells also allow vaccinations to work, and are required to provide passive immunity passed to the fetus from the mother across the placenta or through breast milk. Thus, the possible role of mercury in contributing to lost immunity may be equally important to the obstetrician, pediatrician, and oncologist, as well as the doctor specializing in geriatrics who must always be concerned with the reduction in immunity that is a part of the aging process. To this end, with patients who are mercury-toxic, administering the **IV-C Mercury Tox Program** would likely improve the doctor's treatment outcome, and subsequently reduce the risk of recurrent infections.

Allergic

Chronic mercury toxicity may create a hypersensitivity reaction (allergic or idiosyncratic)—either immediate or delayed—which may be caused by, or acquired through, exposure to any number of allergens. Many people who work with organomercurials, for instance, become sensitized, causing severe dermatitis; and must be removed from further exposure for their therapy to be effective. Since allergens are mostly protein, and since mercury is known to inactivate all types of enzymes, including those required in protein digestion, the question must be raised as to whether mercury interferes with digestive enzymes. If so, then it is reasonable to assume that improperly digested proteins may be contributing to at least a portion of the reported sensitivities to mercury.

Exposure and re-exposure to mercury alters one's capacity to react. Thus, with patients with unexplained reactivity, the doctor may find that mercury is contributing to, or causing the problem. An unusually low urine mercury is often a distinguishing feature for this. (It is well documented that the hypersensitive state occurs without showing the traditional dose-response relationship. The mercury-related nephrotic syndrome, dermatitis, and the infantile syndrome, acrodynia, are good examples, making an analysis of body fluids of little value.) This recently was the case in Africa, where black natives developed symptoms of hypersensitivity from the use of skin lightening creams containing mercury, and in Argentina where babies reacted similarly to diapers washed in a mercury-based solution intended to prevent diaper rash. An understanding of this relationship can perhaps best be obtained by studying acrodynia (which will be done shortly).

Miscellaneous

General fatigue is included in this category—a symptom that nearly everyone has experienced at some time in his life. Fatigue, as most family doctors will agree, is perhaps the most common complaint among a majority of patients. While low levels of hemoglobin and iron are a major cause of fatigue, many of the people who are mercury-toxic are deficient of neither. Arguably, it is speculated that mercury-toxic patients suffer impairment in their oxygen delivery system, since hemoglobin is a rich source of sulfhydryl proteins. Mercury, it is reasoned, can easily attach to these and become a toxic ligand that interferes with the normal functioning of hemoglobin, contributing to the patient's fatigue even when iron is adequate. The antithesis, on the other hand, contends that mercury does not interfere with the oxygen-carrying capacity of hemoglobin—that it is equally possible that the binding of mercury to hemoglobin is part of the protective mechanism, which serves by protecting more vital binding sites. If the **IV-C Mercury Tox Program** does indeed improve the oxygen-carrying capacity of hemoglobin, the patient was likely either cadmium-toxic or lead-toxic in addition to mercury-toxic; and the benefit experienced by the patient was a result of correcting the former two conditions. Regardless of the correct explanation, any unexplained symptom of fatigue should be cause enough to suspect chronic mercury toxicity, especially in those patients who are suspected of having been exposed to mercury.

Kidney disease and a variety of liver afflictions may also be included here, as mercury is known to have a strong affinity for both organs. A patient's complaint of fatigue may reflect the total involvement of these systems.

Fetal and Neonatal Involvement. Clarkson, et al.,[23] determined that methylmercury (and all other chemical species of mercury) passes readily through the placenta, and that the fetus is several times more sensitive to mercury than the mother. Choi reports[24] that *in vitro* methylmercury particularly has an affinity for human fetal neurons and astrocytes that is several times greater than the affinity of methylmercury for adult human neurons. Thus, congenital health problems are possible, and likely outcomes of a mother's exposure to chronic, low levels of mercury before or during pregnancy. The Minamata experience vividly illustrates that congenital defects occurred even when the mother showed no outward signs of poisoning, or chronic methylmercury toxicity.

The affinity of mercury for fetal hemoglobin is especially strong, as it is for fetal neurons. Tejning,[25] for instance, determined the affinity factor to be 30 percent greater for fetal RBC's than for the mother's RBC's. To make matters worse, mercury passes through the mother's milk,[26] containing about 10 percent of her blood level of mercury. Tedeschi, who performed this study, cited a list of congenital outcomes of methylmercury poisoning that included cerebral palsy, cleft palate, microcephaly, and the nephrotic syndrome, with an average mortality rate of 7 percent. In addition, he cited the following other conditions which tended to surface from one to six months after birth:

- retardation in speech development
- intelligence disturbances
- pyramidal symptoms
- disturbed body growth
- anorexia
- dysarthria
- limb deformity
- weakness

- hands and feet red, swollen, and cold
- slight, persistent fever
- mental retardation
- primitive reflexes
- hyperkinesia
- irritability
- fretfulness

The key point to be made here is that fetuses and infants are much more susceptible to chronic, low-level exposure to mercury than adults. The mothers of affected children in Minamata Bay seldom showed any outward signs characteristic of mercury poisoning. The mother's condition, in fact, most often went undiagnosed until the infant developed problems. Yet the variety of disease conditions that surfaced in the infants demonstrated the subtle, but deadly, nature of congenital, chronic mercury toxicity. The consequence of prenatal exposure, in fact, was much more serious than if the exposure occurred after birth. These findings have very serious consequences, strongly suggesting the wisdom of assessing every would-be mother's history of exposure to mercury and, if need be, entering her in the **IV-C Mercury Tox Program** before she becomes pregnant. It also provides sufficient reason to suspect chronic mercury toxicity as a contributing factor in any of the infantile conditions just discussed. At the very least, the prospect should encourage the doctor to engage in some method of routine testing.

Finally, irritability and a tendency toward violent, irrational behavior may be included in the miscellaneous category. Although it is difficult to separate irritability from nerve involvement, one may become irritable from dysfunction of any body part, as well as brain neurons, again indicating the breadth of the role that mercury can play in disease.

TESTING FOR CHRONIC MERCURY TOXICITY

Analysis of Body Fluids

The concept of testing would seem simple enough. Urine, blood, and hair analysis for chronic mercury toxicity have been available for many years, with urine testing the most dependable of the three. Yet Jay M. Arena, the editor of *Poisoning*,[27] cautions that not even in acute poisoning should urine, blood or hair analyses be used as the primary diagnostic tool. The physical examination and history of exposure are much more reliable. On the other hand, some type of testing is desired if for no other reason than to confirm the doctor's diagnosis.

Urine mercury levels by x-ray spectrochemical analysis is the method suggested by Arena for reasons of speed and accuracy. The time required to complete this analysis is only a fraction of the time required by classic procedures, and he says that he can measure concentrations as low as 3 μg of mercury per 100 ml urine using this method. This is one-tenth the clinically maximum allowable concentration. Hair and salivary (parotid) mercury levels can also be measured. The former is an excellent indicator of exposure, the latter the better measure of the rate of excretion. There are problems with these tests, however; the validity is greater in acute poisoning, and less in chronic mercury toxicity.

The usual interpretation of blood and urine tests does not apply to the chronically ill, mercury-toxic patient. Acceptable levels of mercury in blood and urine, for instance, are generally considered to be the average level at which no recognizable symptoms (a normal dose/response curve) of toxicity are apparent. Lower readings assume the absence of intoxication. The reading required for the standard interpretation may, however, be much too high for the patient with chronic mercury toxicity who, according to his threshold of sensitivity, may fall into a category of his own. The usual interpretation, by not allowing for biochemical individuality, may regard as normal some patients who are truly mercury-toxic and react to unusually low levels of mercury.

The disappearance of mercury from blood and urine, as reflected in lower readings, does not necessarily mean a normal body burden of mercury, or that mercury has exited the body. It is possible that an exceptionally low urine mercury indicates that the body cells are retaining mercury rather than releasing it. An example of this is apparent in the common syndrome known as acrodynia—a form of subacute or chronic mercurialism seen in infants. Also called "pink disease" because of the color of the extremities, the infant with acrodynia has many of the symptoms of acute mercurialism, yet urinary mercury levels are frequently low, though not lower than 5 µg per 100 ml.[28] The urinary excretion of methylmercury is so low, however, that it can not be used as an index of body burden. Another way of explaining this, perhaps, is to take a closer look at the differences between the terms "toxicity" and "sensitivity," or biocompatibility.

Biocompatibility

The differences between toxicity, sensitivity, and biocompatibility are important to the diagnosis of chronic mercury toxicity, and to predicting the level of exposure at which any given patient could be expected to manifest symptoms. Toxicity implies a biochemical reaction capability—an interference in biological systems. Sensitivity is much more, as it involves all aspects of the body's natural immune response. This includes not just the antigen/antibody response, but also serological and other body responses that are not as well defined. Biocompatibility is often considered a better term than sensitivity, since it more accurately refers to the body's total reaction—or lack of reaction—to a particular material.

There is need for a scientifically-accepted procedure that can test the full spectrum of biocompatibility, and one that is also available for widespread use. Once operational, dentists would have a means of determining whether or not a particular dental material, such as dental amalgam fillings, was compatible with the intended recipient.* Of equal importance, the doctor would have a basis for recommending the replacement of dental amalgam fillings in patients who are not currently mercury-toxic, and could predict with some degree of certainty which replacement material would be best suited for a particular patient. For accomplishing this feat, perhaps the biocompatibility methods employed by Huggins noted in the interview are conceptually correct.

---

* Dr. Huggins reports that high copper amalgam has become state of the art, and that of his 1000 test subjects, copper reacts in 62 percent of those tested. Thus, even the newer amalgam materials present a potential health problem.

If so, then these methods should be tested and proven in research laboratories and made available for broader use.

The Porphyrin Fingerprint

In addition to biocompatibility, a more promising approach to detecting a patient's susceptibility to mercury is perhaps through establishing a porphyrin "fingerprint" for recent mercury exposure. The porphyrin fingerprint is an adaptation of the standard porphyrin-based fingerprick test used to screen children for high lead levels. The practicality for using the test similarly as a means of detecting chronic mercury toxicity was discussed recently at an international conference in Rye, New York.[29] Sponsored by the New York Academy of Sciences, the guest toxicologists explained porphyrinopathy as a means of determining the extent of functional impairment due to a toxin—like lead or mercury—without regard to the blood or urine level of that toxin.

Porphyrins are a constituent of every eukaryotic cell (a cell with an organized nucleus bounded by a membrane). Particularly, they are involved in the multi-step synthesis of heme—the iron-carrying component of hemoglobin. The synthesis of heme, however, occurs not just in hemapoietic tissues, such as spleen and bone marrow, but in essentially all tissues including liver, lung, and kidney. Bound to protein, heme plays the role of essential mediator in a range of metabolic functions, including cellular respiration, energy generation, and chemical oxidation. During heme synthesis—requiring the sequential synthesis of seven different porphyrin molecules—a number of important enzymes are likewise required to convert one porphyrin into the next, with heme as the final product of the cascade-like sequence.

Interruption in these enzyme processes, by mercury and other toxins, alter blood and urine levels of various porphyrin constituents. Uniquely, each toxin seems to interfere with a different enzyme of the heme biosynthetic pathway, causing some porphyrins to accumulate and others to decrease in body tissues, thereby creating a distinct pattern, or porphyrin fingerprint, for each toxin, toxic metal, and combination thereof. Generally, the pattern is detected by measuring the relative levels of porphyrins or their precursors aminolevulinic acid (ALA), uroporphyrin (UP), coproporphyrin (CP), in blood cells or urine.[30]

Lead, for instance, was reported by Dr. Sergio Piomelli and his colleagues at Columbia University to have some effect on all the porphyrin-metabolizing enzymes, but it characteristically blocks ferrochelatase, the final enzyme in the heme pathway. In so doing it competes with iron for attachment to the enzyme, displacing iron during heme biosynthesis. The pattern that results is quite different than for any other toxin.

The dioxins and polychlorobiphenyls similarly interfere with heme synthesis. They were found, by Dr. George H. Elder and co-workers, at the University of Wales College of Medicine, to modify a porphyrin-metabolizing enzyme known as uroporphyrinogen decarboxylase (UROD). In so doing, the resulting porphyrin fractions demonstrate a pattern distinctly their own. The team of Alfred M. Bernard, on the other hand, at the University of Louvain in Brussels, Belgium, showed in animal studies that mercury, as well as copper, silver, zinc and cadmium, can all interfere with the porphyrin enzyme, aminolevulinic acid dehydratase (ALAD), creating again a porphyrin fingerprint that differs from all others. The exact source (or sources) of interference, they believe, can then be differentiated by studying the biomarker in its entirety.

Janet Raloff of *Science News* reports that initial research into chronic mercury toxicity is promising. Work now being conducted at the Battelle Seattle Research Center and the University of Washington in Seattle, by Dr. James S. Woods, supports the premise that early signs of developing chronic mercury toxicity might be detected by measuring porphyrin profiles in either a single blood specimen or a 24-hour urine sample. Dr. Woods believes the test has several attractive features. It is inexpensive, easy to perform, and can serve to indicate recent exposure. Dr. Bruce Fowler, of the National Institute of Environmental Health Sciences, found that such measurements can actually reveal initial biochemical disturbances in the patient's metabolism. This, perhaps, is the test's greatest potential value—as a useful index of exposure to mercury. To this end it is hoped that whatever research is necessary to establish the porphyrin fingerprint as an index of chronic mercury toxicity will soon be completed.

While we await the concluding research that would give us a definitive means of determining the extent of functional impairment due to mercury exposure, however subtle that exposure or impairment, there are other avenues for testing available to us now. Addresses and further information on the companies and/or products that are discussed can be found in Appendix E.

Electrodiagnostic Studies

Kamla Iyer, et al.[31] studied a 53-year-old dentist who had also gone "doctor hopping" in search of an answer for his declining state of health. Upon arrival at the office of Dr. Iyer, a neurologist, the dentist complained of feeling like a senile old man, following years of emotional instability and depression. He reported having first seen an internist friend who found nothing wrong. He was then referred by the internist to a psychiatrist who placed him on drugs and psychotherapy for four months without benefit. His symptoms began to include a tingling and numbness of both feet, which was exaggerated by walking. This prompted him to consult a second internist. All laboratory findings were normal, but as so often is noted in senile patients (and mercury-toxic patients as well), he had difficulty distinguishing cold from hot water when bathing. He then saw a cardiologist, who found no evidence of peripheral vascular disease, but happened to note diminished-to-absent vibration and position sense in both legs, and was thus referred to Iyer's neurology clinic for evaluation.

While the neurological examination was normal, electrodiagnostic studies led to a diagnosis of sensory polyneuropathy on the basis of abnormal sensory nerve action potentials in the lower extremities, which suggested to the neurologist that the dentist was manifesting the effects of a toxic substance. "It was only after detailed persistent questioning" said Iyer, "that a history of handling mercury in the preparation of amalgam for fillings was revealed."

He concluded that elemental mercury can measurably alter conduction along the sensory nerve fibers due primarily to lesions of the central nervous system. The peripheral nerves in lower extremities are most sensitive, especially the superficial peroneal. He recommended that in suspected cases of chronic mercury toxicity, either organic or elemental, the superficial peroneal (sensory) and sural nerves be carefully examined electrophysiologically for evidence of neuropathy. Conversely, chronic mercury toxicity should be suspected in patients who demonstrate evidence of neuropathy from a cause of unknown origin.

Electrophysiological evidence may be equally important in more serious cases, like my own. Rustam and Hamdi, for instance, in collaboration with

Von Burg,[32] studied the victims in Iraq who had eaten seed grain contaminated with mercurial fungicide. Through this method, in patients with apathy, withdrawal, and depression, there was evidence of severe damage to the lower brain stem, similar to what I had experienced from exposure to elemental mercury and mercury vapors. Unfortunately, however, these people died a slow death. The **IV-C Mercury Tox Program** was not yet available.

Electroencephalogram

Brenner and Snyder[33] have clearly demonstrated a particular electroencephalographic pattern that ultimately develops following organic mercury poisoning. Because the delayed, neurological symptoms that are associated with this pattern are typical of chronic mercury toxicity, it may be wise for doctors to personally review Brenner and Snyder's interpretation when studying the electroencephalographic report of a suspected mercury-toxic patient.

Mercury Vapor Analyzer

The Arizona Instrument Corporation manufactures an instrument that can precisely measure mercury in the air at the touch of a button. It also measures oral mercury vapor through the use of an adaptor. While generally expensive, ranging in price from $4000 to $7000, the instrument can detect oral mercury vapor at concentrations as low as 0.001 mg/m3. The advantage of this test would be the confirmation or dismissal of the doctor's suspicion that a patient's dental amalgam fillings are contributing to his body burden of mercury. Interested doctors can often arrange to borrow a mercury vapor analyzer from their local dental society, or from their state toxicology laboratory. The data obtained can be most informative.

Mercury Patch Test

The patch test, in which a patch containing mercury is directly applied to the patient's skin, offers data that complements other forms of testing by examining patient sensitivity. Ammoniated mercury and mercurous chloride are the two materials most commonly used in patch tests. Dr. Levin adds "There's a sub-specialty in Dermatology, comprised of physicians who are particularly interested in diagnosis of skin sensitivity by patch testing, and who recommend ammoniated mercury over mercurous chloride. In my experience I use both, as some patients react to one and not the other, and vice versa. While there is always the risk that a particularly sensitive patient will experience a serious reaction, there is no simpler way (at this time) of demonstrating sensitivity, and since sensitivity is of critical importance in young people as to whether or not they need to be pushed into removing their amalgam fillings right away, I continue to use this test and find it very useful."

You would think that because the patch test is a reliable test for sensitivity, and because it's such an easy test to administer and interpret, such testing would become mandatory before the dentist places mercury-laden fillings in a patient's mouth, but it isn't. If the patient _were_ sensitive, it would be much better for the patient to react to the patch test than to the fillings. Mercurous chloride patches can be obtained from Toxsupply.

White Blood Cell Viability

Because mercury interferes with enzymes in cells, causing cellular dysfunction and cell death, the white blood cell viability test, subjecting the patient's whole blood to standard mercury concentrations, may be a sensibly-priced alternative. This would tell, without risking the patient's health, if he is mercury-sensitive at concentrations of mercury that are less than what is normally considered toxic.

Cytotoxic Testing
         The familiar cytotoxic testing, a form of biocompatibility testing in which mercury is combined with the patient's own cells in culture, may be of value. The concept of white blood cell viability was derived from this. It is a proven—but limited—method of determining the level of mercury or any other substance that is needed to totally rupture the cells being tested. The problems here are high cost, the short period of time allowed from the moment the sample is collected until the test is performed, and the need for exceptional and expensive equipment, all of which indicate that the test would not be practical on a national or international level.

         The widespread use of mercury in dentistry, and the extraordinary number of patients who manifest many of the symptoms of chronic mercury toxicity and have amalgam dental fillings, indicate that there is immediate need for doctors of every specialty to become more aware of the potential for micromercurialism underlying a wide assortment of health problems. Perhaps the simplest means of determining whether or not a patient will react to mercury is through testing before and after dental amalgam placement. Except for a lack of routine testing beforehand, this is the method currently used in dentistry. If reactive, the patient simply becomes ill and turns up in another doctor's office, where the doctor (who is, unfortunately, generally uninformed of the mercury issue) has difficulty determining the cause of the health problem and resorts again to treating symptoms rather than the cause. Most often, long-term treatment results are unsatisfactory, and the patient goes from doctor to doctor. Those few doctors who are informed are still faced with the problem of determining what regimen to follow in treating their mercury-toxic patient, as past treatment programs have generally not been successful. Thus, doctors and patients alike are sorely in need of the **IV-C Mercury Tox Program's** receiving an immediate evaluation.
         Other than the above suggestions, there is presently no acceptable protocol for determining whether or not a patient is mercury-toxic before treatment, or currently suffering from chronic mercury toxicity. Yet, the routine use of some of the above testing procedures would be of value to the doctor who suspects chronic mercury toxicity, and to the dentist who elects to continue placing dental amalgam restorations. In fact, with the potential for health risk to particular patients, it would seem only prudent to adopt some sort of testing procedure beforehand. It is likely only a matter of time before this is required in the U. S. and elsewhere.

LITERATURE CITED

[1] H.A. Huggins and S. A. Huggins, *It's All In Your Head*, Privately published. (See Appendix E for information.) 1985.

[2] H. Rustam and T. Hamdi, "Methyl Mercury Poisoning in Iraq," *Brain*, 97: 499-510, 1974.

[3] S.B. Elhassani, "The Many Faces of Methylmercury Poisoning," *J Toxicol: Clin Toxicol*, 19 (8): 875-906, 1983.

[4] H. Rustam, et al., "Evidence for a Neuromuscular Disorder in Methylmercury Poisoning," *Arch Environ Health*, 30: 190-195, 1975.

[5] J.B. Cavanagh and F.C.K. Chen, *Acta Neuropathol*, 19: 216-24, 1971.

[6] H. Rustam, et al., op. cit.

[7] T. Takeuchi, "Pathology of Minamata Disease," *Acta Pathol Jpn*, 32(Suppl l):73-99, 1982.

[8] P. Störtebecker, *The Effect of Mercury On The Brain*, A private publication. (See Appendix E for information.)

[9] A.O. Saytanov, as quoted by I.M. Trakhtenberg, *Chronic Effects of Mercury on Organisms*, trans. Geographic Health Studies Program, U.S. Dept of Health, Education, and Welfare, DHEW Publication No. (NIH) 74-473, p.200, 1974.

[10] S.F. Damluji, "The Clinical Committee on Mercury Poisoning: Intoxication Due to Alkylmercury-Treated Seed, the Clinical Aspects of the 1971-1972 Outbreak in Iraq," *Bull WHO*, 53 (Suppl.): 65, 1976.

[11] A.G. Shaper, "Cardiovascular Diseases and Trace Metals," *Proc R Soc Lond*, B-205: 135-43, 1979.

[12] H.M. Perry and M.W. Erlanger, "Metal-Induced Hypertension Following Chronic Feeding of Low Doses of Cadmium and Mercury," *J Lab Clin Med*, 83:541-7, 1974.

[13] A.M. Gotto and J. Ross, Jr., Moderators, *Symposium: Cholesterol Consensus*, American Heart Association's 59th Scientific Sessions, Dallas Convention Center, Dallas, TX, November 17-20, 1986.

[14] H.L. Queen, "The Scientific Sessions Issue," *HEART TALK*, (ISSN: 0882-1836), 5 (l):l-8, 1987.

[15] K. Kageyama, et al., "Effects of Methyl Mercuric Chloride and Sulfhydryl Inhibitors on Phospholipid Synthetic Activity of Lymphocytes," *J Applied Tox*, 6 (l): 49-53, 1986.

[16] "The Lipid Research Clinics Coronary Primary Prevention Trials Results. I. Reduction in Incidence of Coronary Heart Disease," *JAMA*, 251(3): 351-64, January 20, 1984.

[17] "The Lipid Research Clinics Coronary Primary Prevention Trial Results. II. The Relationship of Reduction in Incidence of Coronary Heart Disease to Cholesterol Lowering," *JAMA*, 251(3): 365-74, January 20, 1984.

[18] H.L. Queen, "The Scientific Sessions," *HEART TALK*, 3(l): 1-8, February 29, 1984.

[19] H.L. Queen, "Controversy and New Hypothesis: The LRC Study," *HEART TALK*, 3(2): 9-12, November 1984.

[20] M. Virkkunen, "Behavioral Changes Relating to Changes in Total Serum Cholesterol," *JAMA*, 253(5): February 1, 1985.

[21] H. Tamashiro, et al., "Methylmercury Exposure and Mortality in Southern Japan: a Close Look at Causes of Death," *J Epidemiol and Commu Health*, 40:181-5, 1986.

[22] K. Hirakawa and Y. Hayashi, "Acute Methylmercury Intoxication in Mice—Effect on the Immune System, *Acta Pathol Jpn*, 30(l): 23-32, 1980.

[23] T.W. Clarkson, et al., "The Transport of Elemental Mercury into Fetal Tissues," *Biol Neonate*, 21: 239-44, 1972.

[24] B. Choi, et. al., "Abnormal Neuronal Migration, Deranged Cerebral Cortical Organization, and Diffuse White Matter Astrocytosis of Human Fetal Brain: A Major Effect of Methylmercury Poisoning *in utero*," *J Neuropathol Exp Neurol*, 37:719-733, 1978.

[25] S. Tejning, "Mercury Levels in Blood Corpuscles and in Plasma in 'Normal' Mothers and their Newborn Children. A Report Of The Department of Occupational Medicine," *Lung Stencils*, 68:02:20, 1968.

[26] E. Fujita, "Experimental Studies of Organic Mercury Poisoning on the Behaviors of Minamata Disease Causal Agent in the Maternal Bodies and its Transference to their Infants via either Placenta or Breast Milk," *J Kumamoto Med Soc*, 43: 37-62, 1969.

[27] J.M. Arena, *Poisoning: Toxicology, Symptoms, Treatments,* Fifth Edition. Charles C. Thomas, Springfield, Illinois, p 202, 1986.

[28] R.E. Goselin, R.P. Smith, and H.C. Hodge, eds., *Clinical Toxicology of Commercial Products*, Williams & Wilkins, Baltimore/London, p.III-265, 1984.

[29] J. Raloff, "Embedded Sentinels of Toxicity: The Porphyrins," *Science News*, 131: 123-25, February 21, 1987.

[30] J.T. Hindmarsh, "The Porphyrias: Recent Advances," *Clin Chem*, 32(7): 1255-63, 1986.

[31] K. Iyer, et al., "Mercury Poisoning in a Dentist," *Arch Neurol* 33: 788-90, Nov. 1976.

[32] H. Rustam, and T. Hamdi, op. cit.

[33] R.P. Brenner and R.D. Snyder, "Late EEG Findings and Clinical Status after Organic Mercury Poisoning," *Arch Neurol*, 37: 282-84, 1980.

CHAPTER 4

The Rationale for the Use of Intravenous Vitamin C (IV-C) for Chronic Mercury Toxicity

"While it is to be insisted on that rationality is not the ultimate test of scientific truth, there is no reason to question the value of the rational process as an implement of research."

~Wilfred Trotter [1872-1939]

Acute mercurialism has long been treated successfully with a variety of agents. Of these, Penicillamine and BAL are the two most often used.[1] Unfortunately, following rescue from acute poisoning there has not been a totally effective therapy to counter the gradual disability, and eventuality of death, which are due to the effect of mercury on the central nervous system. Further, as reported by Elhassani,[2] patients with no more than a minor exposure to methylmercury, and with no apparent reason to see a doctor, may present years later with symptoms of seemingly unrelated diseases, for which a cause may never have been determined.

The growing popularity of the use of IV-C to treat chronic mercury toxicity arose, in part, from the need for a safe and effective therapy that would address all the diverse symptoms of chronic mercury toxicity. IV-C was rediscovered during this search, and has filled the need perfectly. It serves a useful purpose in nearly all disease processes, and complements other treatment regimens. In addition, it has been found that IV-C is not a new treatment for the mercury-toxic patient, having been used sparingly only a few years ago to counter the toxic effects of organomercurial therapeutics.

To explain this evolvement of discovery, it will be helpful to retrace the development and use of BAL and Penicillamine. BAL, an acronym for British Anti-Lewisite and chemically known as Dimercaprol, was first developed as a neutralizer of arsenic-based war gases. It was later found to be effective in treating the toxic effects of certain additional heavy metals, particularly gold, lead and mercury. Its value is questionable, however, in poisoning caused by some other heavy metals, such as antimony and bismuth.* The secret to its action in acute mercurial poisoning is the presence of unstable sulfhydryl groups attached to two of its three carbons.

Following intramuscular injection, BAL detoxifies by binding free mercury (Hg) to its two sulfhydryl (SH) groups. It does this by competing successfully with critical bindings sites for mercury on proteins and other cellular constituents, effectively keeping mercury away from them. The mercury bound to BAL can then be excreted, primarily via the kidneys and intestines. (See Figure 4:1)

Penicillamine, an amino acid (dimethylcysteine) derived from penicillin, works in a similar manner. Its unstable SH groups remove unbound,

---

* According to product information given by Hynson, Westcott & Dunning, original makers of BAL injectable, it should not be used in iron, cadmium, or selenium poisoning because the resulting metal complexes are extremely toxic to the kidneys.

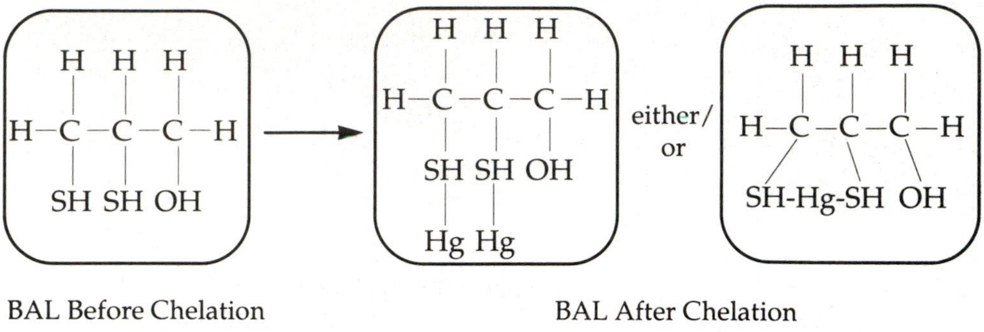

BAL Before Chelation   BAL After Chelation

Figure 4:1   Dimercaprol (BAL) and its two chelation products

absorbed mercury before it can attach to SH groups of cell membranes and cellular enzymes. It is then excreted by the kidneys.

In choosing between BAL and Penicillamine, it is important to consider that each exerts an opposite effect on the kidney and brain. In experiments with mice, BAL has been shown to increase the uptake of mercury in the brain,[3] while protecting the kidneys. Penicillamine has been found effective in removing brain mercury,[4] but tends to promote the accumulation of mercury in the kidneys. Thus, in acute poisoning one may be preferred over the other, according to the patient's condition; or both may be employed, delaying the use of Penicillamine until the first neurological symptoms appear.

The problem with both of these products is that neither is safe nor effective in the long run, and an extended treatment period is generally required to counter the effects of chronic mercury toxicity. Both may be fatal. For instance, reactions to Penicillamine, which occur in about one-third of patients, include fever, rash, leukopenia or thrombocytopenia. Penicillamine may also cause vitamin B_6, iron, and copper deficiency, so it is a self-defeating feature unless supplements are simultaneously administered. In addition, Penicillamine may precipitate Goodpasture's syndrome. BAL is contraindicated when kidney and liver function is insufficient. It also increases the risk of developing hypertension and an abnormal heart rhythm.

Thus, when the need first arose among doctors to counter the growing risk of subacute mercurialism due to the expanding presence of mercury in our environment, the growing consumption of fish, and the continued use of mercury in dental amalgam fillings, it was necessary to look beyond the standard methods of treatment. They discovered that megadose vitamin C met all three of their basic requirements. It was safe as well as effective—when used correctly—and had a very good history as an adjunct therapy for nearly all diseases, including oral diseases. Recognizing that there are those who question the wisdom of choosing vitamin C, let alone intravenous vitamin C, for such an important role, it is perhaps best to explain the choice by tracing the history of vitamin C and its use in health and medicine.

HISTORY OF THE USE OF VITAMIN C

"That experienced and brave admiral, Sir Charles Wager, once told me...his sailors were terribly afflicted with the Scurvy...Recollecting, from what he had often heard, how effectual these fruits (oranges and lemons) were in the cure of this distemper, he ordered a chest of each to be brought upon deck, and opened every day. The men, besides eating what they would, mixed the juice in their beer. It was also their constant diversion to pelt one another with the rinds; so that the deck was always strewed and wet with the fragrant liquor. The happy effect was, that he brought his sailors home in good health."

~Richard Mead [1673-1754][5]

Albert Szent-Gyorgyi, from 1928 to 1933,[6,7] was first to isolate the anti-scurvy factor, derived from adrenal cortex tissue. Since the term scorbutic pertains to scurvy, it was named ascorbic acid, and designated vitamin C. Only a very small amount (40 to 45 mg) of the vitamin was needed on a daily basis to prevent symptoms of scurvy in humans. It was thus assumed that larger amounts provided no additional benefit. "At that early point in time," Dr. Szent-Gyorgyi stated,[8] "the medical profession itself took a very narrow and wrong view: Lack of ascorbic acid caused scurvy, so if there was no scurvy there was no lack of ascorbic acid. Nothing could be clearer than this. The only trouble was that scurvy is not a first symptom of lack but a final collapse—a premortal syndrome—and there is a very wide gap between scurvy and full health." Henceforth, two camps emerged in the research community; one maintaining that our need for vitamin C should be restricted only to prevention of scurvy (40 to 45 mg per day); the other contending that attainment of optimal health may require many times this basic requirement. This latter view implies that the role of ascorbic acid in human health goes beyond its vitamin function.

Megadose Vitamin C

By 1940, shortly after its discovery, vitamin C researchers began to study the effect of massive doses of ascorbic acid on the treatment of human disease. They derived the megadose concept by applying a common principle of pharmacology: adjusting the dosage level to get the desired effect. At various levels it was found effective in inactivating the viruses that caused polio,[9] herpes,[10] rabies,[11] hoof-and-mouth disease,[12] and the tobacco mosaic disease, among other uses.[13] Researchers found that ascorbic acid not only bolstered the natural immune system while inactivating the viruses, but that it actually destroyed the viruses.

To attain this level of clinical success, the oral dosage of ascorbic acid ranged from 4.5 to 17.5 grams every two to four hours around the clock, or 27 to 210 grams daily.[14] This amount went far beyond what is generally prescribed today, but is probably the desired dosage for countering most diseases. The research findings, however, were subsequently faulted by scientists who worked with lesser quantities; who attempted similar studies using only 5 to 25 grams per day, and who reported that vitamin C was safe but ineffective.[15] While the results of high-dose/low-dose comparisons were totally unrelated, as Cathcart has since demonstrated in clinical practice,[16] the damage had long-lasting ramifications. Thereafter, the credibility of research using megadose vitamin C was severely blunted. Even the research that continues today using megadose vitamin C does so without the advantage of a wide audience of listening scientists, making it necessary to reexamine the reasons for use of megadose vitamin C, and to examine the mechanisms by which it works.

The use of megadose vitamin C evolved quite naturally following the discovery that many animals produce their own vitamin C according to the biosynthetic pathway depicted in Figure 4:2.

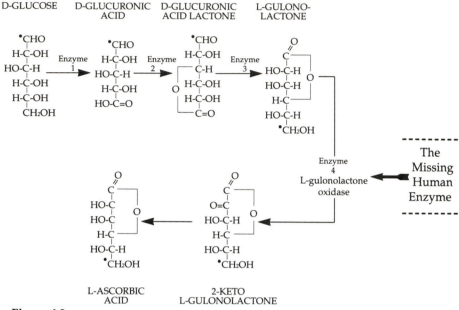

Figure 4:2

Figure 4:2. (Taken from Irwin Stone's book, *The Healing Factor: Vitamin C Against Disease.* Reprinted and modified with permission of Grosset & Dunlap, New York, 1972.) This scheme represents the pathway in the mammalian liver that leads to the biosynthesis of ascorbic acid. While the amount of ascorbic acid produced by this natural body process ranges from 5 g to 40 g per day,[17] the potential output is nearly endless. Stress from any cause stimulates its synthesis and release directly into the bloodstream.

Professor Robert Jenness, retired from the University of Minnesota College of Biological Sciences,[18] and now a visiting research professor at the Primate Research Institute of New Mexico State University, explains that several mammals and other animals are not able to produce their own vitamin C because they lack the critical enzyme, L-gulonolactone oxidase (GLO) which catalyzes the last step in the synthesis of L-ascorbic acid from D-glucose.*

Guinea pigs and anthropoid primates (monkeys, apes, and man) lack GLO. For humans, therefore, ascorbic acid is a vitamin—an essential nutrient that is obtainable only through the diet. However, reliance upon diet as our only source of vitamin C puts us (when under stress) at a distinct disadvantage to other mammals. Only select foods contain vitamin C; there is a limit to the

* See Appendix F for a further discussion of the topic of the production of vitamin C in animals.

quantity of vitamin C-rich foods that someone will willingly eat on a daily basis; and it is doubtful that any human diet would contain more than a gram of vitamin C per day without unusual effort. Yet, if other animals can be used as a model, there is evidence that when under stress the human body might benefit from supplemental vitamin C. To this end, Klenner believed it more relevant to think of vitamin C in terms of maximum daily requirement rather than minimum daily requirement.[19] His treatment objective of administering megadose vitamin C to every patient, was simply an effort to mimic what other animals do naturally during health as well as disease circumstances.

Dr. Cathcart is in agreement with this concept. He prefers to think of megadose vitamin C as "the missing stress hormone," a basic substance which almost all mammals utilize and produce when under stress. Under normal health conditions, he believes, the amount required by humans when experiencing normal stress is based on the average daily output of other mammals (5 to 15 grams per day),[20,21] also referred to as the "rat-no-stress" equivalent (the amount of vitamin C produced daily by a rat under no stress). Similarly, low-to-medium stress conditions require a range of 5 to 40 grams. Under moderate-to-severe stress conditions (due to emotional or physical trauma, or disease) the need for vitamin C increases proportionately. Cathcart contends that the reason the body requires additional vitamin C during these periods is due not to its antiscorbutic role but to its role as a nonrate-limited, antioxidant free radical scavenger.

While vitamin C is not the most potent of the antioxidants that protect cell membranes, it is certainly the most available. In this context Cathcart contends that vitamin C is the premier free radical scavenger. Its value is such that any unusual demand for its action, created particularly by illnesses that single out specific tissues, may cause a condition that he has termed "acute induced scurvy." In such cases, acute induced scurvy may occur even when the total body load of vitamin C is adequate (as judged by contemporary standards) or when the daily intake of vitamin C is purportedly being met. When this happens, vitamin C is required in amounts that go far beyond the minimum RDA. Cathcart has found that patients who are ill require a great deal more vitamin C to reach the bowel tolerance level discussed in Chapter 2. When given in lesser amounts the vitamin doesn't seem to work. "It's as if a threshold must be reached," Cathcart observes, "at which point the ascorbate becomes effective, and below which it has little therapeutic value."

The Reducing Redox Potential (Equilibrium) Determines Effectiveness. From his observations, Cathcart speculates that vitamin C's effectiveness has to do with the concentration of the vitamin required to healthfully influence its reducing redox potential (equilibrium); or, the balance of oxidation and reduction reactions that occurs continuously between ascorbic acid and dehydroascorbic acid (the reversibly oxidized form of ascorbic acid). The process occurs in the following manner:

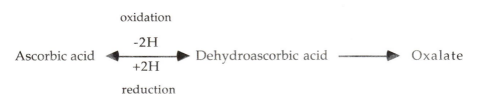

The principle is based on an equation* which relates the standard potential to the concentration of the species in equilibrium (ascorbic acid being the reactant, dehydroascorbic acid the product). In those people who are free of disease (free of stress and disease-causing free radicals, or other harmful oxidizing substances), and are consuming no more than the RDA for vitamin C, the ratio between ascorbic acid and dehydroascorbic acid is adequate to sustain health in that individual. Yet, during periods of increased cellular stress and disease in these people, the quantity of the reactant (ascorbic acid) is insufficient to provide the necessary electrons for reducing stress-causing agents. In these circumstances a higher tissue level of ascorbic acid (a ratio of ascorbic acid to dehydroascorbic acid favoring ascorbic acid) is required to reduce the disease-causing free radicals and other reactive oxidizing substances.

To obtain the desired change that is consistent with health (i.e., a change in equilibrium of the reducing redox potential), it is necessary to supplement megadose vitamin C periodically throughout the day. Megadose vitamin C becomes its own source of electrons required for its role as a non-rate limited, free radical scavenger to protect cell membranes. This need for protective action is most likely why many animals under stress synthesize throughout the day what appears, at first, to be an excess of ascorbic acid.

When the equilibrium of the reducing redox potential is shifted slightly towards the left (when the ratio of the reactant [ascorbic acid] and its product [dehydroascorbic acid] favors the reactant—and when the concentration of the ascorbate reactant is sufficient to satisfy its role as a free radical scavenger) the patient is better able to withstand any additional stresses (chronic mercury toxicity particularly). When the patient's vitamin C intake is marginal, however, or when only the minimum RDA for vitamin C is being provided during the stressful period, the equilibrium of the reducing redox potential shifts unhealthfully towards the center; a condition that slows the healing process and eventually allows disease to manifest.

This was recently supported by Dawson, et al.,[22] who found that the ratio of ascorbic acid to dehydroascorbic acid reflects one form of control on cell biosynthetic processes. Thus, to effectively treat an ill patient, Cathcart contends that the doctor must administer enough vitamin C so that it may satisfactorily perform its role as a non-rate limited, free radical scavenger, which depends on the availability of ascorbic acid and the rate at which free radicals are being produced. The more free radical reactants—increased normally during stress, fatigue, and disease—the more ascorbate that's required to reach that ratio.

The effect of this can be seen in the extremely large dosage that is required by sick people when titrating to bowel tolerance. For these people clinical effectiveness cannot be reached until the critical threshold is reached. The supplemental dosage must be kept high enough to encourage a shift in the equilibrium (reducing redox potential) from right to left. A smaller dosage that doesn't do this, and falls short of reaching the critical threshold, isn't likely to improve the patient's symptoms. Cathcart contends that this is the reason so many researchers fail to attain desired results when administering vitamin C. I believe it is also a major reason megadose vitamin C is desired for treating chronic mercury toxicity. The mercury-toxic patient most often presents with a

---

* The Nernst Equation, found in any textbook of physical chemistry, disentangles—through mathematics—the axiom that free energy is the fundamental driving force in nature, and that free energy in nature is always decreasing.

variety of disorders, each manifesting a variation of acute induced scurvy. Megadose vitamin C aids in improvement of this general condition, in addition to ridding the body of mercury.

Established Biochemical Effects of Vitamin C

In a recent, important review of vitamin C,[23] Mark Levine, M. D. (of the National Institute of Arthritis, Diabetes, and Digestive and Kidney Disease, National Institute of Health) highlighted several biochemical effects for vitamin C other than its role as antioxidant.

As an antiscorbutic, no more than 60 mg daily is the required therapy to restore the body pool of vitamin C to 1500 mg and correct the major symptoms of scurvy—best remembered through "the four H's": hemorrhagic signs, hyperkeratosis of hair follicles, hematologic abnormalities (mostly anemia due to errored folate metabolism and a reduction in iron absorption), and hypochondriasis.

Beyond its antiscorbutic function, vitamin C also serves as a hydroxylating agent. Specifically, ascorbic acid transfers electrons to enzymes that provide reducing equivalents in hydroxylation and amidation reactions. To this end, however, Levine informs that ascorbic acid is not essential, as the body can call on other reducing agents for this role. Yet vitamin C in adequate amounts is an important prerequisite if one hopes to maximize hydroxylation reactions. The biosynthesis of catecholamines (the conversion of dopamine to norepinephrine), is one example. When vitamin C is inadequately supplied, both the synthesis and release of norepinephrine is hindered.

Although Levine didn't state so directly, his report demonstrates that an adequate body pool of vitamin C (significantly greater than what's required to prevent scurvy) is needed to maximally optimize enzyme function—a fact that can't be overemphasized when one considers that reduced enzyme function is a feature of chronic mercury toxicity, as well as many other disease conditions.

Intravenous Vitamin C

Many attempts have been made, through supplementation of the diet, to offset the advantages of vitamin C synthesis held by other mammals. Titrating to bowel tolerance has narrowed the gap, but a threefold problem remains: 1) there are some people with certain health problems who for one reason or another cannot take oral medication; 2) there is a limit to the amount of vitamin C that the gastrointestinal tract will accept; and 3) there are situations, such as chronic mercury toxicity, where the amount of vitamin C required to be effective goes far beyond what is possible through titrating to bowel tolerance. Thus, there are limitations to oral vitamin C, and what is needed to rid the body of mercury goes far beyond what oral vitamin C can provide. Many doctors have thus turned to intravenous administration.

IV-C offers the maximum potential of quickly reaching the blood level that other mammals routinely experience when diseased or under stress. It also raises the bowel tolerance threshold, so that the combination of IV-C and oral vitamin C maximizes the amount of ascorbic acid a patient can take without producing diarrhea, since IV-C independently does not contribute to diarrhea. The resulting dosage possibilities, while not required in ridding the body of mercury, may be important in treatment of the patient whose primary problem is other than micromercurialism, or whose condition has become severely debilitating. These latter two instances are not at all uncommon. In fact, chronic mercury toxicity probably occurs just as often, if not more, as a secondary condition than as the primary problem. Thus it is important to the mercury-toxic patient that megadose oral vitamin C and IV-C have been used for many years to effectively treat nearly every disease.

Diseases Treated with Megadose Vitamin C

While Drs. Wright and Cathcart are perhaps the two most frequent prescribers of megadose oral vitamin C and IV-C in the U.S. today, Dr. Linus Pauling (the only winner of two Nobel Prizes: for Chemistry, in 1954, and for Peace, in 1962), has in recent years been the most visible proponent. Pauling and Cameron's work with cancer and the common cold has been widely publicized. What is not well known is that virtually every human disease has been treated safely and effectively by them—and by many other doctors before them—using megadose vitamin C, particularly IV-C. Some of those treated successfully, either with oral or intravenous vitamin C are:

- Periodontal disease[24]
- Connective tissue diseases[26]
- Arthritis[28]
- Poor eyesight[30]
- Glaucoma[32]
- Ocular hypertension[34]
- Physical stresses
  - heat[37]
  - cold[39]
  - bone fracture[41]
- Food allergy[25]
- Asthma[27]
- Hay fever[29]
- Bronchitis[31]
- Atherosclerosis[33]
- Anaphylactic shock[35]
- Ulcers[36]
- Mental disease[38]
- Multiple sclerosis[40]
- Cancer[42]

The fact that megadose vitamin C therapy has been used with varying levels of success in virtually every disease process, further substantiates its role as a basic substance in human health—a role which may carry its importance far beyond that of the antiscorbutic vitamin. Albert Szent-Gyorgyi, who eventually received the Nobel Prize for his work on vitamin C, and who originated the concept that popularized IV-C, refers to ascorbic acid as "a substance basic to all mammalian life, as a protector against disease."

Attempting to further explain its protective role beyond antioxidant, antiscorbutic, reducing and hydroxylating properties, Cameron[43] suggests that ascorbic acid exerts its biological function indirectly by incorporation into a glycosaminoglycan residue to form an inhibitor of hyaluronidase. Hyaluronidase is an enzyme that possesses the ability to hydrolyze and depolymerize the ground substance, glycosaminoglycans, causing erosion of many cell groups. An increase in hyaluronidase, therefore, is seen in scurvy as a consequence of cellular damage, and in almost every disease involving cellular proliferation. The list includes not only cancer, but atherosclerosis as well, in which there is significant proliferation of the intima of the inner arterial wall.

It is the inhibition of hyaluronidase by vitamin C—which aids in preventing cellular proliferation—that led Pauling,[44] Cameron,[45,46] and others[47,48,49] to boldly administer megadose vitamin C to patients with various cancers. While the validity of this concept is often disputed[50,51] it can be argued that the differences in outcome may be due only to differences in research design, rather than efficacy. It is all but impossible to compare results when the studies are conducted under varying conditions. Those who failed to duplicate Pauling and Cameron's results generally administered a lesser dosage over a shorter period. Drawing upon the protective effect of vitamin C on hyaluronidase and scurvy, those who were seeking a treatment adjunct for the mercury-toxic patient noted that megadose vitamin C had been used successfully in treating virtually every condition that associates with chronic mercury toxicity.

During a recent interview, Dr. Cathcart expressed confidence in the value of megadose vitamin C (and IV-C) in the practices of medicine and dentistry, stating that "...if it ever becomes widely used, it could very well bankrupt many hospitals." He believes it to be that effective. "While it isn't a panacea," Dr. Wright has been quick to admit, "I consider IV-C and megadose oral vitamin C to be a *sine qua non* for any nutritionally-oriented practitioner."

The Periodontal Disease Connection. In the book, *The Vitamin C Connection*,[52] Drs. Cheraskin, Ringsdorf, Jr., and Sisley cite statistics from NHANES 1, which revealed that one of every four adult Americans is missing at least half of his teeth. In older adults with teeth, about 64 percent are afflicted with one or more of the symptoms of periodontal disease: inflammation of the gums, periodontal pockets, and/or a lack of firmness in body sockets. (Many of these symptoms reflect underlying collagen disease—one of the many possible adversities of chronic mercury toxicity.) Researchers have since studied the effect of vitamin C on this widespread oral disease. In one such study of 78 people (average age 29), Cheraskin, et al., cited the work of Adrian Cowan of the Faculty of Dentistry, Royal College of Surgeons in Dublin, Ireland, who compared tooth roots of patients before and after vitamin C supplementation with those of patients receiving no supplementation. "In a significant number of patients treated with vitamin C", said Cowan, "there was noticeable improvement of outline as judged by x-ray in areas of irregularity in the (periodontal) membrane." The doctor noted that optimal improvement was obtained with a vitamin C dose of about 1 gram per day. These results were obtained regardless of whether chronic mercury toxicity was suspected or not. While many similar reports appear each year in the literature, there are additional uses of vitamin C in dentistry that go beyond periodontal disease.

Collagen Disease in Malocclusion. Drs. T. Graber and B. Swain, in their second edition of *Current Orthodontic Concepts and Techniques*,[53] go into much detail to explain the importance of collagen in the prevention and treatment of problems of malocclusion. They explain how a deficit of vitamin C may affect the therapeutic outcome and, since ascorbic acid plays a vital role in connective tissue growth, repair, and biosynthesis,[54] they further explain how vitamin C deficit may be the source of the problem.

Not only is ascorbic acid required to induce the synthesis of collagen but, as the work of Murad, et al.,[55] suggests, a shift in the equilibrium of the reducing redox potential to the left of midline is required if healing is to proceed at optimum efficiency. Whatever treatment regimen is chosen, therefore, for collagen disease, quite naturally will benefit from megadose vitamin C. How much vitamin C is needed depends upon the individual. In many cases, contend Cheraskin, Ringsdorf, Jr., and Sisley, a small daily dosage like 500 mg is simply not enough. Significant megadose vitamin C therapy is believed to be required to attain the desired therapeutic effect even in orthodontics. To what extent the toxic effects of mercury may be contributing to collagen disease in malocclusion has generally not been studied, but mercury's role in other collagen diseases does suggest that such involvement is possible and plausible.

Chronic and Acute Hepatitis, and Other Uses of Megadose Vitamin C. When referring to the books written by Wright, and the journal articles of Cathcart, it is clear that megadose oral vitamin C and IV-C perform nearly miraculous feats in certain disease conditions. During our interview Dr. Wright became quite enthusiastic as he related the quick and positive response to IV-C of patients with both chronic and acute hepatitis. "I would get patients who had just been prescribed Prednisone and who were told their only alternative was a liver transplant; but...soon after administering IV-C their yellow color began leaving and I discontinued the Prednisone. Their laboratory values returned to near-normal, and after a few weeks it became obvious to them, me, and everybody they were no longer a candidate for a liver transplant. To be precise," he continued, "it was quite common for the patient's color and laboratory results to improve within a couple of days following IV-C, and their fatigue lifted accordingly." To accomplish these results it sometimes requires an exceptionally large dose of oral vitamin C, and an average of five treatments using IV-C, with some improvement seen following each session.

Dr. Wright has treated many diseases other than hepatitis effectively with megadose vitamin C and IV-C. A few good examples include arthritis, acute infectious mononucleosis, and a large number of allergic conditions. In fact, allergies of all kinds seem to respond positively to megadose oral vitamin C and IV-C. He cautions, however, that there are other features to his treatment approach which must be considered equally.* Likewise, Dr. Cathcart has had a great many victories in treating difficult conditions with the assistance of megadose vitamin C and IV-C, a few of which include babies at high risk for sudden infant death syndrome, select patients with AIDS who responded by going into remission, drug dependencies, and a number of patients who recovered from various poisonings and toxic conditions.

Vitamin C in Poisonings and Chronic Intoxication

In early studies on the effect of ascorbic acid on human bacterial infections, vitamin C was shown to be an excellent bacteriostatic agent.[56,57] Its bacteriostatic action, it was learned, was actualized at the equivalent of 7 grams per day for a 154 lb person. Later, it was determined that the main beneficial action of ascorbic acid on bacteria was its power to neutralize a wide variety of bacterial toxins.[58,59,60] This led to the successful application of ascorbic acid in neutralizing the powerful toxins of organisms that cause botulism[61] and tetanus,[62] as well as the deadliest snakebite venoms [63,64] and the most powerful chemicals and drugs containing benzene[65] and strychnine.[66] Hence, vitamin C has long been established as a key remedy for dangerous toxins and poisons.

Of the many ways that the body has for engaging in biotransformation (detoxifying harmful poisons, toxins, and byproducts of metabolism), the liver is by far the most important site of such activity. The liver is therefore quite vulnerable to these same harmful agents. Perhaps that is why nature located the capability for making ascorbic acid within the liver: to provide a means by which it can protect itself while making the toxins harmless. "Vitamin C does this," Dr. Wright points out (referring to published research), "by speeding up the activity of microsomal enzymes within the liver, enabling these enzymes to do their natural job." Humans, however, are lacking in liver vitamin C, due to the absence of Enzyme 4 (See again Figure 4:2), except for that which is derived

---

* Dr. Wright conducts seminars on these topics for doctors interested in nutritional therapy. See Appendix E for a contact address.

from diet. Consequently, liver damage is quite common among humans exposed to toxic chemicals such as mercury and chronic alcohol intake, and who also suffer from acute induced scurvy.

Clinically, the protective action of ascorbic acid against liver damage was demonstrated first by Beyer in 1943,[67] and again in 1965 by Soliman, et al.[68] This action rendered harmless the many chemical agents produced by the body itself, performing in a manner simulating its role in detoxifying bacterial agents. Ascorbic acid has thus received much of the credit for the detoxifying property of the liver. It is this acclaim, and the fact that victims of Minamata disease quite often suffer serious liver disease, that has given scientists reason to study the effect of ascorbic acid in protecting us from harm, not only from mercury, but from other heavy metals as well.

Vitamin C in Drug Overdose and Drug Dependencies

The risk of drug overdose is a fact of life in the practices of medicine and dentistry. It is a problem for which a safe and effective remedy is often unavailable. In fact, the antidote can be just as dangerous. For these reasons, Dr. Wright relies on IV-C as an adjunct therapeutic in drug overdose. In one of his cases, a patient overdosed on digitalis and subsequently developed bigeminal heart rhythm, a potentially fatal condition. The overdose was neutralized with 25 grams of IV-C. On other occasions, IV-C was administered to patients with one or more drug dependencies, such as hashish, cocaine, and marijuana. In none of these instances was it necessary to send the patient to intensive care. Rather, Dr. Wright said, "the patients all recovered in the emergency room and were sent home." Again, the evidence indicates that megadose oral vitamin C and IV-C have a tremendous range of useful indications, further supporting its value in treating the wide range of symptoms and conditions that are commonly associated with chronic mercury toxicity.

Vitamin C and Diet: Protection from Mercury Poisoning

As long ago as 1840,[69] a London physician noted that symptoms of scurvy were more severe when they appeared in people who were taking mercury compounds either for syphilis or as an occasional purgative. Ninety years later, another scientist noted that a certain dose of mercuric chloride injected into guinea pigs normally killed 100 percent of the animals within an hour. If, however, the animals were given an amount of ascorbic acid beforehand (the equivalent of 35 g per day for a human weighing 154 lb), 40 percent survived.[70]* Thereafter, because mercury was a common component of diuretic drugs up until the 1950's and the 1960's (and which are still being used sparingly today), it became accepted medical practice to give ascorbic acid to heart patients who were taking organomercurial diuretics.[71] In these patients, ascorbic acid reduced the side effects due to mercury, and in some manner that is still incompletely understood, it increased the desired diuretic action by 50 percent. Its effectiveness was so pronounced that until the mid- to late-1960's, ascorbic acid was often given as the antidote of choice for poisonings caused by fatal doses of mercury.[72]

* These experiments described the effect of ascorbic acid on s.c. (subcutaneously) and i.m. (intramuscularly) injected mercuric chloride. Ascorbic acid in these circumstances does not exert a true therapeutic effect, but decreases the absorbed dose by converting mercuric mercury to insoluble mercurous mercury and elemental mercury (by reduction) at the injection site.[73]

During the 1970's, vitamin C began losing favor for a combination of reasons, some of them previously cited. One reason for its sudden decline was because it was being touted as a cure for the common cold. Doctors and patients were unable to duplicate the original results. There were various reasons, but mostly they failed to duplicate the schedule for dosage, the dosage frequency, and the duration of dosage used in the original research. Its use and misuse became so widespread among lay nutritionists that the medical profession became skeptical. Thus the serious use of megadose vitamin C lost favor among medical practitioners. In spite of this, vitamin C research continued, and in the mid-1970's two separate studies renewed the shadow of questionable efficacy, perhaps unjustifiably, this time on the use of vitamin C in chronic mercury toxicity.

Blackstone[74] and Chatterjee[75] concluded from animal research that megadose vitamin C in micromercurialism was neither effective nor appropriate, reporting that vitamin C megadoses promoted the accumulation of mercury in particular organs and tissues. These studies were countered by Murray and Hughes,[76] and Hill,[77] who reported—as older studies had indicated—that megadose vitamin C was an effective treatment for mercurial poisoning, with or without the excretion of mercury. Together, these studies found that ascorbic acid significantly reduced the concentration of mercury in guinea pig tissues, which resulted in a substantial decrease of symptoms.

With conflicting reports, who is one to believe? Arguably, there are several plausible explanations. The researchers did not fully take into consideration the role that fat and selenium play in detoxifying the mercury-toxic patient, nor did they have available to them other essential facts for removing mercury from the body, such as were presented in Chapter 2. Another credible explanation was arrived at by reviewing the work of Carroll, et al.,[78] and through later works of Chatterjee, et al.,[79] and Hill.[80]

Carroll had observed that the protection offered by ascorbic acid against mercury poisoning was a clinical phenomenon, but could not be demonstrated objectively. It <u>was</u> demonstrated, however, that the observed protection from what is now considered a low dosage schedule of vitamin C was not due to its causing the immediate excretion of mercury. These findings, though not surprising—since the dosage was far below what is now recommended—were followed a few years later by the second study of Chatterjee, et al., who had found by administering mercury to rats that the metal in some way interferes with the working of enzymes required in vitamin C biosynthesis.* The researchers learned that by administering vitamin C to these animals their capacity to produce ascorbic acid was restored, and the protection that vitamin C normally provides against mercury intoxication was returned.

Perhaps the best explanation for understanding the discrepancies was provided by Dr. C. H. Hill. From his research Dr. Hill formed a plan for successive steps that he believed should be taken to obtain the most desired results from administering ascorbic acid for heavy metal intoxication:

---

* This is not too surprising, since mercury is known to damage the working of all enzymes that it encounters. High level contamination of mercury in vitamin C-producing mammals causes a scurvy-like reaction by interfering with their normal process of vitamin C biosynthesis. This interruption in vitamin C biosynthesis would confuse the observer and cause a misinterpretation of results, making one believe that animals that should enjoy the normal protection from mercury by synthesizing their own vitamin C when needed, were no better protected than humans.

1. One must first address chronic lead toxicity. Ascorbic acid does not protect against lead,* while iron is protective, and calcium is likewise protective.

2. One must secondly address chronic cadmium toxicity. Ascorbic acid is protective against cadmium, but does not correct anemia. Likewise, iron in the form of ferrous iron is effective and, together with ascorbic acid, corrects anemia and makes the oxygen-carrying capacity of hemoglobin more efficient.

3. Addressing chronic mercury toxicity is the third step. While iron supplementation is ineffective in ridding the body of mercury (other than misleading the observer to believe that a correction of fatigue was indication of effectiveness), megadose vitamin C is highly effective in overcoming chronic mercury toxicity,† but selenium should be given first in combination with a high-fat/high animal-protein diet. Selenium and the sulfur-bearing amino acids of animal protein replace and compete with mercury for binding sites on cell membranes; the plenitude of fat (forming lipoproteins) allows mercury to be escorted to the liver for excretion as a component of bile; and ascorbic acid protects against symptoms of selenium toxicity, among its many other roles. Working together, this action negates and reverses the toxic symptoms of mercurial exposure—acting independently of iron.

In dealing with mercury, Hill concludes ascorbic acid is very important. Its effect on mercury poisoning is quite positive—the effect is not credited to improved iron metabolism, as might be expected.‡ In fact, iron depresses the effectiveness of ascorbic acid in overcoming growth inhibition in animals due to chronic mercury toxicity, which presupposes that one should not use iron in humans to correct the mercury problem. It may only mask an important symptom (fatigue) and lead one to believe the patient's condition has improved, or that the patient's condition was due to something other than mercury.

Additionally, in some undetermined way excess iron may interfere with the positive effects of ascorbic acid. Hill further confirmed that the use of selenium should precede the use of ascorbic acid, pushing the dosage to border on intoxication. This, referred to in Chapter 2 as competitive equilibrium, disperses concentrated areas of tissue-bound mercury and better prepares for the

* From his clinical experience, Dr. Wright disagrees. Citing the work of Klenner, he believes that ascorbate serves to chelate many metals, including lead and mercury. He believes it plausible that lead and mercury are excreted as lead and mercury ascorbate during and following administration of IV-C and megadose oral vitamin C. A study of vitamin C 's effectiveness in reducing lead toxicity in animals confirms Wright's observations, which showed vitamin C to be even more effective than EDTA.[81] In human studies the reports have been conflicting.[82,83,84,85]

† A study by Calabrese, et al,[86] typically demonstrates that the majority of research that has shown vitamin C to be ineffective in treating chronic mercury toxicity was flawed by design. In this study, for instance, healthy patients were chosen rather than mercury-toxic patients. Additionally, the test subjects had baseline levels of blood and hair mercury that were well below normal, and urine mercury was not determined, so the findings were of little use in establishing vitamin C's worth.

‡ In Chapter 2 we discussed how vitamin C enhances iron utilization in cadmium toxicity, and that improved oxygen delivery is a consequence of improved iron metabolism. General fatigue and weakness is a feature of chronic mercury toxicity, and iron might improve this one symptom even without detoxifying the mercury.

beneficial action of ascorbic acid, both oral and intravenous. In contrast, a selenium deficiency and a diet low in fat that may have existed before administration of ascorbic acid may partially account for the original negative results reported first by Blackstone, and then Chatterjee.

After reviewing the many studies which report on the clinical value of the use of ascorbic acid in mercury poisoning, the exact mechanism by which it works remains unanswered. One other possibility was suggested by Dr. Huggins during our interview (Chapter 3). Because vitamin C is a proven chelating agent of some metals, he suspects (as Wright does) that mercury is excreted in the urine as mercury ascorbate. While additional research is needed to prove or disprove this hypothesis, an immediately plausible explanation can be derived from the combined works of Murata and Uike;[87] of Bielski, Richter, and Benon; and of Chan.[88] Although the best known function of ascorbic acid is as an antioxidant, the researchers remind us that it also functions as a prooxidant—that is, a free radical intermediate which does not react with oxygen (as does the antioxidant form of vitamin C). Bielski referred to a concept which holds that ascorbic acid undergoes enzymatic oxidation to form a free radical intermediate before becoming dehydroascorbic acid, and before attaining its antioxidant configuration. (Figure 4:3)

Figure 4:3

Ascorbic Acid—▶ Enzymatic Oxidation

⬇

Ascorbic Acid Prooxidant Intermediate

⬇

Enzymatic Oxidation—▶ Ascorbic Acid Antioxident

Theoretically, if the functional life of vitamin C is long enough—that is, if its equilibrium of the reducing redox potential is shifted to the left of midline as Cathcart has suggested, characterized by a constant and high rate of metabolic degradation (which may depend upon its concentration and pH, among other factors)—the prooxidant intermediate of ascorbic acid could be produced rapidly enough and of such a concentration as to function to attack double bonds, such as those seen in aldehydes and sulfhydryl proteins.

Certainly, Murata and Uike indicated a similar mechanism at work in the inactivation of viruses by ascorbic acid. The prooxidant intermediate of ascorbic acid could do this directly or indirectly by reacting first with molecular oxygen to form singlet oxygen (O_1). Through further research, by learning more about the potential role of this mechanism, one might at the very least learn more about how megadose vitamin C serves as a detoxifying agent. If this is indeed another correct explanation for the mechanism by which vitamin C detoxifies mercury—and it certainly seems possible—then the mercury released from the double bond of the sulfhydryl protein could, in due time, be excreted through the intestines, in the urine, or both.

In a purely scientific sense, the rationale for the use of IV-C in treating the mercury-toxic patient is supported by its proven record of efficacy, by its long-standing use in both dentistry and medicine, and by mechanisms that have either been theorized or demonstrated, and which require concomitant support from other nutritional and lifestyle factors. The conclusion of this chapter from the human aspect, however, is much more exciting.

Regardless of the exactness of the mechanism by which megadose vitamin C improves the condition of the mercury-toxic patient, the fact that it works is undeniable. To my good fortune, I've had the privilege of witnessing improvement not only in myself, but in hundreds of others being treated by dentists and physicians alike. I believe this is sufficient reason to launch a cooperative, worldwide research effort into refining its use in the practices of dentistry and medicine. To aid in this effort, PARTS II and III of this book will examine the risks and suggest a protocol for its administration based on our current understanding. This approach will minimize risks to the patient, while maximizing the potential for benefit.

LITERATURE CITED

[1] R.H. Dreisbach, *Handbook of Poisoning: Diagnosis and Treatment*, 6th edition. Lange Medical Publications, Los Altos, CA, 1969.

[2] S.B. Elhassani, "The Many Faces of Methylmercury Poisoning," *J Toxicol: Clin Toxicol*, 19 (8): 875-906, 1983.

[3] M. Berlin and T. Lewander, "Increased Brain Uptake of Mercury Caused by 2,3-Dimercaptopropanol (BAL) in Mice Given Mercuric Chloride," *Acta Pharmacol Toxicol*, 22: 1-7, 1965.

[4] J. Aaseth, "Mobilization of Methylmercury *in vivo* and *in vitro* Using N-Acetyl-DL-Penicillamine and Other Complexing Agents," *Acta Pharmacol Toxicol*, 39: 289-301, 1976.

[5] M.B. Strauss, ed., *Familiar Medical Quotations*, Little, Brown and Company, Boston, 1968.

[6] A. Szent-Gyorgyi, *Biochem J*, 22: 1387, 1928.

[7] W.N. Haworth and A. Szent-Gyorgyi, *Nature*, 131: 24, 1933.

[8] I. Stone, *The Healing Factor: Vitamin C Against Disease*, Grosset & Dunlap, NY, 1972.

[9] C.W. Jungeblut, "Inactivation of Poliomyelitis Virus by Crystalline Vitamin C (Ascorbic Acid)," *J Exp Med*, 62: 517-521, 1935.

[10] M. Holden and R.J. Resnick, "*In vitro* Action of Synthetic Crystalline Vitamin C (Ascorbic Acid) on Herpes Virus," *J Immunol*, 31: 455-462, 1936.

[11] G. Amato, "Azione Dell'Acido Ascorbico sul Virus Fisso della Rabbia e Sulla Tossina Tetanica," *Giornali di Batteriologia, Virologia et Immunologia*, (Torino), 19: 843-849, 1937.

[12] W. Langenbusch and A. Enderling, "Einfluss der Vitaminine auf das Virus der Maul-und Klavenseuch," *Zentralblatt fur Bakteriologie*, 140: 112-115, 1937.

[13] M. Lojkin, "Contributions of the Boyce Thompson Institute," 8 (4): 1936, by Martin, LF, *Proceedings Third International Congress of Microbiology*, New York, p 281, 1940.

[14] F.R. Klenner, "The Treatment of Poliomyelitis and Other Virus Diseases with Vitamin C," *Southern Med & Surg*, III: 209-214, 1949.

[15] O. Gsell and F. Kalt, "Treatment of Epidemic Poliomyelitis with High Doses of Ascorbic Acid," *Schweizerische Med Wochenschrift*, 84: 661-666, 1954.

[16] R.F. Cathcart, "Vitamin C: The Nontoxic, Nonrate-Limited, Antioxidant Free Radical Scavenger," *Med Hypo*, 18: 61-77, 1985.

[17] I. Stone, *op.cit.*

[18] R. Jenness, private correspondence, April 6, 1976.

[19] F.R. Klenner, "Observations on the Dose and Administration of Ascorbic Acid when Employed Beyond the Range of a Vitamin in Human Pathology." *J Applied Nutr*, 23: 61-88, 1971.

[20] J.J. Burns, et al., *J Biol Chem*, 207: 679, 1954.

[21] A.H. Conney, et al., *NY Acad Sci*, 92: 115, 1961.

[22] E.B. Dawson, et al., "Effect Of Ascorbic Acid On Male Fertility," *Ann NY Acad Sci*, 498: 312-23, 1987.

[23] M. Levine, "New Concepts In The Biology and Biochemistry of Ascorbic Acid," Seminars in Medicine of the Beth Israel Hospital, Boston (J.S. Flier and L.H. Underhill, Ed.), *N Eng J Med*, 314(14): 892-902, April 3, 1987

[24] A. Cowan, "The Influence of Vitamin C on the Periodontal Membrane Space—A Radiographic Study," *Irish J Med Sci*, 145: 9, 273-284, September 1976.

[25] M. Walzer, "A Critical Review of the Recent Literature on Vitamin C in Relation to Hypersensitiveness," *J Allergy*, 10: 72-94, 1938.

[26] J.M. Rivers, "Ascorbic Acid in Metabolism of Connective Tissue," *NY State J Med*, 65: 1235-1238, 1965.

[27] N.B. Silbert, "Vitamin C. Critical Review," *Medical Times*, 79: 370-376, 1951.

[28] B.F. Massell, "Antirheumatic Activity of Ascorbic Acid in Large Doses," *N Eng J Med*, 242: 614-615, 1950.

[29] H.N. Holmes and W. Alexander, "Hay Fever and Vitamin C," *Science*, 96: 497-499, 1942.

[30] H. Heath, "Distribution and Possible Functions of Ascorbic Acid in the Eye," *Exp Eye Res*, 1: 362-367, 1962.

[31] W. Dawson and G.B. West, "Actions of Sodium Ascorbate on Smooth Muscle," *Brit J Phar and Chemo*, 31: 269-275, 1967.

[32] M. Virno, et al., "Sodium Ascorbate as an Osmotic Agent to Reduce Intracranial and Intraocular Pressures," *Policlinico Sezione Pratica* (Rome), 72: 1746-1752, 1965.

[33] G.C. Willis, "An Experimental Study of the Intimal Ground Substance in Atherosclerosis," *Canadian Med Asso J*, 69: 17-22, 1953.

[34] B.B. Bietti, "The Value of Osmotic Hypotonizing Means for the Treatment of Ocular Hypertension," *Trans Ophthalmol Soc*, United Kingdom 86: 247-254, 1966.

[35] S. Yokoyama, "On the Influence of Vitamin C on Anaphylactic Shock," *Kitasato Archives Exp Med*, 17: 17-37, 1940.

[36] R.L. Russell, et al., "Ascorbic Acid Levels in Leucocytes of Patients with Gastrointestinal Hemorrhage," *Lancet*, 2: 603-606, 1968.

[37] W.L. Weaver, "The Prevention of Heat Prostration by Use of Vitamin C," *Southern Med J*, 41: 479-481, 1948.

[38] A. Hoffer and H. Osmond, "Scurvy and Schizophrenia," *Diseases of the Nervous System*, 24: 273-285, 1963.

[39] L.P. Dugal, "Vitamin C in Relation to Cold Temperature Tolerance," *Annals NY Acad Science*, 92 (l): 307-317, 1961.

[40] E.Y. Williams, "Treatment of Multiple Sclerosis," *Medical Record*, 160: 661-663, 1947.

[41] M.F. Merezhinskii, "Preservation of Ascorbic Acid and Glutathione Resources in Tissues of Animals Suffering from Trauma and Supplied with Various Amounts of Vitamin C," *Chemical Abstracts*, 57 :15712-17713, 1965.

[42] L. Pauling and E. Cameron, *Cancer and Vitamin C*, The Linus Pauling Institute of Cancer and Medicine, 1979.

[43] E. Cameron, "Biological Function of Ascorbic Acid and the Pathogenesis of Scurvy: A Working Hypothesis," *Med Hypotheses*, 2(4): 154-63, July 1976.

[44] L. Pauling and E. Cameron, "Supplemental Ascorbate in the Supportive Treatment of Cancer: Prolongation of Survival Times in Terminal Human Cancer," *Proc Natl Acad Sci*, 78(10): 3685-89, October 1976.

[45] E. Cameron, et al., "Ascorbic Acid and Cancer: A Review," *Cancer Res*, 39: 663-81, March 1979.

[46] E. Cameron, et al., "The Orthomolecular Treatment of Cancer III. Reticulum Cell Sarcoma: Double Complete Regression Induced By High-Dose Ascorbic Acid Therapy," *Chem Biol Interactions*, 11: 387-93, 1975.

[47] H.J.R. Bussey, et al., "A Randomized Trial of Ascorbic Acid in Polyposis Coli," *Am Can Soc*, 50: 1434-39, October 1982.

[48] H.M. Anthony and C.J. Schorah, "Severe Hypovitaminosis C in Lung-Cancer Patients: The Utilization of Vitamin C in Surgical Repair and Lymphocyte-Related Host Resistance," *Br J Cancer*, 46: 354-67, 1982.

[49] M.F. McCarty, "An Antithrombotic Role for Nutritional Antioxidants: Implications for Tumor Metastasis and other Pathologies," *Med Hypotheses*, 19: 345-357, 1986.

[50] E.T. Creagan, et al., "Failure of High-Dose Vitamin C (Ascorbic Acid) Therapy to Benefit Patients with Advanced Cancer," *NEJM*, 301 (13): 687-90, September 27, 1979.

[51] C.G. Moertel, et al, "High-Dose Vitamin C versus Placebo in the Treatment of Patients with Advanced Cancer Who have had No Prior Chemotherapy," *NEJM*, 312 (3): 137-141, January 17, 1985.

[52] E. Cheraskin, W.M. Ringsdorf, Jr., and E. Sisley, *The Vitamin C Connection*, Harper & Row, Publishers, Inc., NY NY 10022, 1983.

[53] T. Graber and B. Swain, *Current Orthodontic Concepts and Techniques*, Second Edition, Volume 1, The W.B Saunders and Company, Philadelphia, 1981.

[54] M.J. Barnes, "Function of Ascorbic Acid in Collagen Metabolism," *Ann NY Acad Sci*, 258: 264-77, 1975.

[55] S. Murad, et al., "Collagen Synthesis in Cultured Human Skin Fibroblasts: Effect of Ascorbic Acid and Its Analogs," *J Invest Dermatol*, 81: 158-62, 1983.

[56] G.C. Gupta and B.C. Guha, "The Effect of Vitamin C and Certain Other Substances on the Growth of Microorganisms.," *Annals Biochem and Exp Med*, 1: 14-26, 1941.

[57] M. Sirsi, "Antimicrobial Action of Vitamin C on M. Tuberculosis and Some Other Pathogenic Organisms," *Indian J Med Sci*, (Bombay) 6: 252-255, 1952.

[58] C.W. Jungeblut, "Inactivation of Tetanus Toxin by Crystalline Vitamin C (Ascorbic Acid)," *J Immuno*, 33: 203-214, 1937.

59 C.W. Jungeblut and R.L. Swemer, "Inactivation of Diphtheria Toxin *in vivo* and *in vitro* by Crystalline Vitamin C (Ascorbic Acid)," *Proceedings Soc Exp Biol Med*, 32: 1229-1234, 1935.

60 T. Kodama and T. Kojima, "Studies of the Staphylococcal Toxin, Toxoid and Antitoxin; Effect of Ascorbic Acid on Staphylococcal Lysins and Organisms," *Kitasato Archives of Exp Med*, 16: 36-55, 1939.

61 A. Buller-Souto and C. Lima, "Action of Vitamin C on the Toxins of Gas Gangrene and Others," *Memorias do Institute Butantan*, 12: 265-296, 1938.

62 P.K. Dey, "Efficacy of Vitamin C in Counteracting Tetanus Toxin Toxicity," *Naturwissenschaften*, 53: 310, 1966.

63 I. Nitzesco, et al., "Antitoxic Powers of Vitamin C," *Bulletin Academie de Medicin de Roumanie*, 3: 781-782, 1938.

64 J.H. Perdomo, "Snake Venom and Vitamin C," *Revista de la Faculatad de Medicina*, (Bogata) 15: 769-772, 1947.

65 S. Forssman and K.O. Frykholm, "Benzene Poisoning II," *Acta Medica Scandinavia*, 128: 256-280, 1947.

66 P.K. Dey, "Protection Action of Ascorbic Acid and Its Precursors on the Convulsive and Lethal Actions of Strychnine," *Indian J Exp Biol*, 5: 110-112, 1967.

67 K.H. Beyer, "Protective Action of Vitamin C against Experimental Hepatic Damage," *Arch Int Med*, 71: 315-324, 1943.

68 M.A. Soliman, et al., "Vitamin C as Prophylactic Drug Against Experimental Hepatotoxicity," *J Egyptian Med Asso*, 48: 806-812, 1965.

69 R.E. Hughes, *Nutritional Interactions Between Vitamin C and Heavy Metals in Vitamin C*, Birch, G.C., and Parker, K., Eds: 68-77, John Wiley & Sons, Inc. NY, NY; 1974.

70 M. Vauthey, "Protective Effect of Vitamin C against Poisons," *Praxis*, (Bern) 40: 284-286, 1951.

71 D.W. Chapman, and C.F. Shaffer, "Mercurial Diuretics," *Arch Int Med*, 79: 449-456, 1947.

72 M. Mokranjac and C. Petrovic, "Vitamin C as an Antidote in Poisoning by Fatal Doses of Mercury," *Comptes Rendus Hebdomadaires des Seances de l'Academie des Sciences*, 258: 1341-1342, 1964.

73 L. Magos, "The Uptake and Retention of Mercury by Kidneys in Rats," In *Mercury, Mercurials and Mercaptans*, M. W. Miller and T.W. Clarkson, Charles C. Thomas, Springfield, 167-186, 1973.

[74] S. Blackstone, et al., *Food Cosmet Toxicol*, 12: 511, 1974.

[75] G.C. Chatterjee and D.R. Pal, "Metabolism of L-Ascorbic Acid in Rats Under *in vivo* Administration of Mercury: Effect of L-Ascorbic Acid Supplementation," *Int J Vit Nutr Res*, 45: 284, 1975.

[76] D.R. Murray and R.E. Hughes, "The Influence of Dietary Ascorbic Acid on the Concentration of Mercury in Guinea Pig Tissues," *Abstract: Proc Nutr Soc*, 35: 118-119, 1976.

[77] C.H. Hill, "Studies on the Ameliorating Effect of Ascorbic Acid on Mineral Toxicities in the Chick," *J Nutr*, 109 (l): 84-90, 1979.

[78] R. Carroll, et al., "Protection Against Mercuric Chloride Poisoning of the Rat Kidney," *Arzneim Forsch*, 15 (ll): 1361-1363, November 1965.

[79] G.C. Chatterjee and D.R. Pal, op. cit., 284-292.

[80] C.H. Hill, "Interactions of Vitamin C With Lead and Mercury," *NY Acad Science*, 355: 262-266, 1980.

[81] R.A. Goyer, and M.G. Cherian, "Ascorbic Acid and EDTA Treatment of Lead Toxicity in Rats," *Life Sci*, 24: 433-438, 1979.

[82] A. Sohler, "Blood Lead Levels in Psychiatric Outpatients Reduced by Zinc and Vitamin C," *J Othomol Psych*, 6 (3): 1-5, 1977.

[83] R. Lauwerys, et al., "The Influence of Orally-Administered Vitamin C on the Absorption of and Biological Response to Lead," *J Occup Med*, 25 (9): 668-78, 1983.

[84] H.N. Holmes, et al., "The Effect of Vitamin C on Lead Poisoning," *J Lab Clin Med*, 24: 1119-27, 1939.

[85] S.W. Marchmont-Robinson, "Effect of Vitamin C on Workers Exposed to Lead Dust," *J Lab Clin Med*, 26: 1478-81, 1940.

[86] E.J. Calabrese, et al., "The Effects Of Vitamin C Supplementation on Blood and Hair Levels of Cadmium, Lead, and Mercury," *Ann NY Acad Sci*, 498: 347-53, 1987.

[87] A. Murata and M. Uike, "Mechanism of Inactivation of Bacteriophage MS2 Containing Single-Stranded RNA by Ascorbic Acid," *J Nutr Sci Vitaminol*, 22: 347-54, 1976.

[88] H.J. Bielski, et al., "Some Properties of the Ascorbate Free Radical," *Annals New York Academy of Sciences*, 231-236, 1973.

PART II

IV-C Safety

CHAPTER 5

IV-C Safety:
Knowing the Risk

"Even in medicine, though it is easy to know what honey, wine and hellebore, cautery and surgery are, to know how and to whom and when to apply them so as to effect a cure is no less an undertaking than to be a physician."

~Aristotle [384-322 B.C.]

The evidence derived from the first fifty years of use of megadose vitamin C and IV-C, including evidence presented at the Third Conference on Vitamin C[1] sponsored by the New York Academy of Science, suggests that its potential for health benefits is many times greater than the risk. In fact, Dr. Cathcart has found from his experience that the margin of safety for megadose vitamin C is greater than for aspirin, diuretics, all pain medications, tranquilizers, sedatives, muscle relaxants, antibiotics, or antihistamines.[2] A similar safety record has been reported by all of the major users of megadose vitamin C, both past and present. In addition to Cathcart, several others have contributed to this record in their respective fields: Wright (general nutritional medicine),[3] Klenner (general medicine and surgery),[4] Cameron and Pauling (cancer research),[5] Hoffer and Osmond (psychiatry),[6] and Cheraskin and Ringsdorf (dentistry and nutritional medicine).[7]

The successes of these doctors speak loudly. Yet some very severe reactions have been reported by infrequent users of megadose vitamin C: four of which have terminated in death. Three of these occurred in people with pre-existing kidney dysfunctions. This lone fact seems to indicate that certain people are predictably at risk, requiring precautionary steps that must necessarily preclude successful treatment. Therefore, Part II of this book will be devoted to identifying those risks, and, where possible, to choosing the appropriate corrective steps. Chapter 5 will first review the danger signals the doctor must recognize in order to safely administer IV-C, listing the most common—and generally least dangerous—reactions first. Next the truly serious, life-threatening conditions will be addressed: those that (however rarely they occur) make administering IV-C hazardous.

Chapter 6 will cover factors that influence kidney stone formation, and will offer suggestions as to how the doctor might effectively minimize the patient's risk. When these steps are closely followed, the risk of kidney stones is greatly reduced.

Then, based on the information in these next two chapters, a patient questionnaire will be proposed. From this, a pre- and post-treatment diet and lifestyle will be outlined that will minimize or eliminate adverse reactions. The patient questionnaire will help the doctor predict which patients are most and least likely to benefit from IV-C. It will aid in identifying those who present an unacceptable risk, along with serving as a guide for counseling the patient as per his protective pre- and post-IV-C diet and lifestyle. Thereafter the patient will not only be prepared for the **IV-C Mercury Tox Program**, but ideally suited for continual lifestyle counseling sessions.

VITAMIN C IN THE DIET

With the exception of water, vitamin C derived from foods is the most benign constituent of the human diet. Synthetic vitamin C (crystalline ascorbic acid) is likewise safe and nontoxic when consumed in quantities that duplicate dietary expectations. This can be credited partly to its water-soluble property and partly to an efficient urinary excretion rate: It is detectable in urine within minutes following a substantial intake of oral vitamin C. For all but a rare few individuals, dietary and supplemental vitamin C in amounts that do not exceed the Recommended Daily Allowance (RDA)* are virtually innocuous, causing little or no reaction other than that which benefits the human body. For most people this same harmless effect remains constant even when the supplemental dosage reaches and exceeds one hundred times the RDA.

In 1971, following their first 35 years of evaluating the safety of vitamin C, the American Medical Association concluded, "there is no evidence that large doses of vitamin C are harmful."[8] Soon afterwards, the use and popularity of the vitamin became widespread among doctors and laymen alike, particularly due to Linus Pauling's books on vitamin C's connection with the common cold and flu. Vitamin C thereafter became a household word. Its widespread use had the valuable effect of allowing scientists to more thoroughly evaluate its safety. Consequently, four major reviews[9,10,11,12] and a myriad of other related findings have since revealed that the earlier AMA report was generally correct, but still too lenient for total assurance. Though rarely encountered, megadose vitamin C does have the potential for causing harm through a variety of pharmacological actions. When unwanted reactions occur they are generally related to dosage, increasing in duration and severity as the dosage exceeds the RDA. Conversely, reactions become predictably less severe and nonexistent with dose reduction.

On the positive side, this investigative report reveals that most of the unwanted reactions to vitamin C—even those that have terminated in death—are predictable and preventable. The reactions may be related to individual tolerance levels, the patient's lifestyle circumstances, or to predisposing factors that may flag the patient as a high risk candidate. Steps are given herein that will greatly minimize risk, either by alteration of the patient's lifestyle before and after IV-C, or by determination through the patient questionnaire and other means that the risk/benefit ratio is unacceptable. It is these considerations that make this report necessary and worthwhile to those who wish to administer IV-C.

LESS SEVERE REACTIONS AND CONCERNS

Gastrointestinal Upset

Gastrointestinal (G. I.) disturbance is the most commonly reported side effect of vitamin C intake. It is dose-related and dependent upon individual

---

* The RDA for adults of both sexes, as determined by the National Research council, is now 60 mg. On this intake, the average body reserve will generally remain at 1500 mg, sufficient to sustain an individual for 30 to 45 days. After this period symptoms of scurvy will appear. In comparison, the RDA for premature infants is 100 mg; for newborn infants 35 mg; for women 80 mg during pregnancy, and 100 mg during lactation. Larger daily amounts may be required by those people who smoke, and by those people who are under greater-than-average stress from toxins, infections, mental stress, disease, physical strain, or metabolic disorders.

tolerance. Particularly, it is limited to the oral route of administration and is not associated with IV-C.

The most common G. I. disturbance is a laxative-like reaction, purportedly caused by the action of ascorbic acid on the osmotic load or, as Cathcart believes, due to a hypertonic situation in the rectum where the action of excess vitamin C (any amount that exceeds bowel tolerance) causes a benign and rapid diarrhea. This is often welcomed, however, by those who suffer from varying grades of constipation. The dosage required is usually in excess of 3 grams per day, but G. I. disturbances may begin with as little as 200 mg. To remedy the situation, many doctors now prescribe sodium ascorbate rather than pure ascorbic acid. Ascorbate acts as a buffer and is less likely to promote diarrhea, just as it reduces the likelihood of many other reported side effects. Unique to those people who report diarrhea on lower doses of ascorbic acid, is a drying of the mouth and reduced semen production, as noted by Smith.[13] The dry mouth is generally correctable with the switch to sodium ascorbate, but the effect on semen production has not been thoroughly evaluated.

The Sodium In Sodium Ascorbate. Doesn't It Cause A Problem? The use of sodium ascorbate in place of ascorbic acid raises several questions that must be addressed. Most importantly, what about the additional sodium? What effect does sodium ascorbate have on a sodium-free diet? Cathcart, who admits to taking the safer road on this issue, prefers ascorbic acid as his oral megadose vitamin C source. He administers sodium ascorbate only as an intravenous source, and only to those few patients whose conditions warrant, as discussed in Chapter 2. In this way he minimizes the risk to the patient of excess sodium, except for whatever is contributed from the IV-C.

While Cathcart's method offers a prudent alternative, the evidence does not support the fear of risk. When questioned by the Food and Drug Administration (FDA) on this matter in the late 1960's, Klenner replied that he had personally taken 10 to 20 grams of sodium ascorbate daily for many years, all the while maintaining a normal blood sodium, and a urine pH at just above 6.0. The FDA cautioned otherwise, however, until startling new evidence was presented in the 1980's by Elliott[14] on the kinetics of vitamin C.

Elliott studied the effect, on blood and urine, of a 3 gram supplement of vitamin C (as taken in 1 gram increments, as sodium ascorbate, three times a day for 12 weeks). He reported that despite a small daily sodium load of approximately 15 meq/liter from sodium ascorbate, the serum sodium and chloride values decreased significantly after the 12th week in 19 of 26 subjects. For example, said Elliott, "the mean serum sodium during the ascorbate loading period decreased to 139.2 meq/liter from the baseline mean of 140.8," the drop per person ranging from 1 to 6 meq/liter. The change, he reported, was not due to chance, but was highly significant. A rise in total urine sodium excreted per 24 hours, from 3.6 to 77%, was reported in 13 of 16 subjects (the remaining 10 subjects elected not to contribute to this aspect of the study). The increase in excreted sodium, as a consequence of vitamin C loading, was greater than what could be accounted for in the sodium ascorbate source. According to Dr. Elliott, "this effect (of a reduction in total body sodium through enhanced urinary excretion) of ascorbate loading had not been previously reported."

In an attempt to explain the relationship between sodium ascorbate loading and a reduction in total body sodium, Elliott pointed to the earlier findings of Selkurt and Houck.[15] They had reported, in 1943, that hypertonic sodium and potassium chloride solutions impaired the reabsortive activity of the tubules for ascorbic acid. The mechanism served to inhibit reabsorption of the ascorbic acid form of vitamin C, while promoting its excretion. This same action, Elliott reasoned, should logically interfere with sodium reabsorption and promote its excretion along with ascorbic acid. He believes this scenario could be expected when administering sodium ascorbate, regardless of the route of administration.

To obtain his most recent viewpoint for this book, Dr. Elliott was contacted by letter. He replied that while, "I do think that some (additional) experimental evidence would have to be shown in support of my idea (the hypothesis that sodium ascorbate impairs the sodium reabsorbtive activity of the tubules), I do believe it remains a plausible explanation." The Elliott findings strongly suggest that sodium ascorbate does not, as suspected, present a health risk for people who are free of hypertension.

Confirmation of the Elliott hypothesis that sodium ascorbate may actually be supportive of the goals of a low-sodium diet, was provided only recently by Kurtz, et al.[16] at the University of California, San Francisco, General Clinical Research Center. In a study of five men with essential high blood pressure, the researchers showed that the anionic component of an orally administered sodium salt is the real determinant of the salt's capacity to increase blood pressure. Sodium chloride, they found, raised the men's blood pressure, while sodium citrate did not. The observed differences were related to the varying effect of the anionic component (chloride) on plasma volume. Sodium chloride increased plasma volume and thereby increased blood pressure, while sodium citrate given in an equal osmolar concentration had no effect. Kurtz's team concluded that today's prevalent view of sodium—that the capacity of sodium chloride to increase blood pressure depends only on its sodium component—just isn't correct. Additional support was added by the team's animal model studies, in which they found that an expanded plasma volume (with an increase in blood pressure) occurs only when sodium is administered as the chloride salt. Neither plasma volume nor blood pressure increase when sodium is administered as bicarbonate, phosphate, glutamate, glycinate, aspartate, or the ascorbate salt.[17,18]

Thus, based on the findings of Kurtz and Elliott, there is little-to-no risk of normal people developing high blood pressure from sodium ascorbate administered orally or intravenously (in sterile water) as the megadose source of vitamin C. Whatever risk that does occur would be evident only if IV-C were administered in a high-chloride parenteral fluid, such as normal saline. (Parenteral fluids will be discussed in Chapter 9.) As for people with active hypertension, the results (while speculative) more than suggest that megadose sodium ascorbate may actually support the goals of a low-sodium diet.

Skin Rash

Rarely, a skin rash may develop in people who take ascorbic acid supplements. Ruskin,[19] and Anderson, et al.,[20] report that the buffered salt of sodium ascorbate, when substituted for ascorbic acid, eliminates skin rash in those people who are otherwise sensitive to megadose vitamin C. For this reason Cathcart recommends a mixture of ascorbates with ascorbic acid, while other doctors who administer IV-C prefer straight sodium ascorbate during pre- and post-IV-C therapy. All are in agreement, however, that sodium ascorbate is preferred for intravenous infusion rather than I.V. ascorbic acid.*

---

* Actually, all IV-C is prepared for use as sodium ascorbate, even when the label says ascorbic acid. Refer to Chapter 9 for explanation.

Interference With Results Of Clinical Laboratory Tests
　　　Various laboratory test results may be influenced by the concentrations of vitamin C in the material being tested. Because vitamin C is a chemical reducing agent, it may interfere with assays that require a redox reaction and depend on a change in color.[21] Some of these tests include blood sugar analysis using the orthotoluidine method, as well as stool tests for occult blood such as the quaiac test and the benzidine test. Again examining the Elliott study, it was noted that the addition of 3 grams of vitamin C per day for 12 weeks significantly changed a variety of blood parameters independently of the effect of vitamin C on the testing procedure itself. After 12 weeks the following blood values were noted:

INCREASED
- serum albumin
- serum ascorbic acid
- white blood cell ascorbic acid
- lactic dehydrogenase (LDH)

DECREASED
- alanine aminotransferase
- serum globulins
- serum sodium
- serum uric acid

　　　Dr. Elliott believes the increases and decreases in particular blood parameters were not due to any technical interference by vitamin C during the testing procedure. Instead, he feels the changes can be attributed to a healthful, positive effect on such parameters brought about by the influence of vitamin C loading on related body functions. The drop in blood uric acid, for example, can be accounted for by the rise in uric acid excreted through the urine. This relationship is consistent with the ultimate goals of treating gout and heart disease, since an elevated serum uric acid is associated with both conditions and must be lowered to reduce the risk.
　　　Although one can logically conclude that the risk for kidney stones is increased due to the resulting hyperuricosuria in patients taking megadose vitamin C, Bengt Fellström, M. D., Ph. D., a member of our medical and scientific advisory staff and an internationally recognized authority on kidney stones, is doubtful of a causal relationship. He says, "I can't recall ever seeing documentation on patients having formed uric acid stones by taking high doses of vitamin C." Thus, one can logically assume that the threat of forming uric acid stones, which is not a proven risk, can be maximally reduced by following the proposed lifestyle regimen to be discussed in Chapter 6.

Higher Levels of Blood Cholesterol
　　　Various studies indicate megadose vitamin C may cause no change, a drop, or a rise in blood serum cholesterol.[22,23] People who are at low risk to heart disease, who have a normal TSC before megadose vitamin C is administered, and who regularly supplement their diets with the RDA for vitamin C, experience the least change in TSC during megadose vitamin C therapy; some patients with an elevated TSC note a significant drop in TSC following megadose vitamin C therapy. The third option, that vitamin C may cause a rise in TSC, brings to light a basic point regarding interpretation of blood cholesterol levels. Almost every student of heart disease has been led to believe that any rise in blood cholesterol is a "bad" sign—an indication that the agent or food administered is doing bodily harm. This interpretation, however, may not be correct for every situation, as we will see in this scenario:
　　　Imagine for the moment that you have a serious blockage of your left coronary artery. Doctor X, who is both your friend and a noted researcher, has

just developed a magic bullet. The doctor promises you that the magic bullet will unblock your artery by removing the accumulation of cholesterol. Dr. X calls you into his office and explains the procedure. He will perform some baseline blood work and then administer to you the magic bullet. Uniquely, Dr. X will study changes in your blood cholesterol that may occur during the first few minutes, hours, and days following the treatment which, as he explains, will cause cholesterol to come out of the blockages throughout your arterial system. This being the circumstances, what do you suppose Dr. X is hoping to observe relative to your TSC? Of course, in due time he would expect TSC to lower, but as the cholesterol is first being removed from the blockage, Dr. X expects an initial <u>rise</u> in TSC.

Correctly, this phenomenon would be referred to as the "magic bullet effect," where regression of arterial blockages would cause TSC to at first rise, and then fall. Likewise, the magic bullet effect may explain, at least in part, the variable reports of the effect of vitamin C on TSC.

At this time, therefore, the relevance of a rise in TSC (in certain patients) following megadose vitamin C is questionable and should not be interpreted as a negative health effect.

Reduction in Vitamin B$_{12}$ Activity

Herbert and Jacobs[24] were first to suggest that megadose vitamin C may produce a vitamin B$_{12}$ deficiency by destroying the nutrient both in the G. I. tract and in the tissues. Hogenkamp[25] more recently determined that the sensitivity of vitamin B$_{12}$ to megadose vitamin C could be observed only in a few people suffering from one or more errors in vitamin B$_{12}$ metabolism. Even then it was determined that the sensitivity was limited to the least common of the cobalamins that comprise vitamin B$_{12}$ and that the major cobalamins in food and plasma are not affected. These findings suggested to Hogenkamp that it is unlikely that megadose vitamin C would have the capacity to cause a vitamin B$_{12}$ deficiency. To reduce this possibility even further, it has become common practice to instruct the patient to take vitamin C supplements between meals, and never with food.

Conditioned Scurvy

Irregular, on-again/off-again use of megadose vitamin C (any dosage that exceeds 250 mg/day) has been shown by dental researchers Siegel, et al.[26] to create a state known as conditioned scurvy. This is characterized by a conditioned increase in the rate of ascorbic acid catabolism and a corresponding increase in the urinary excretion of vitamin C. Following abrupt cessation of megadose vitamin C, the conditioned rate of vitamin C catabolism and excretion continues, thereby accounting for the onset of rebound scurvy. This was first noted in a patient with recurring periodontal disease. Researchers found that the patient's symptoms could be manipulated. The symptoms were corrected with vitamin C supplements, and returned again following abrupt withdrawal of the supplements.

While conditioned scurvy is a rare encounter—as with the previously described patient—it is likely that most people react similarly, although to a lesser degree. Using the experience of Siegel's group, symptoms of withdrawal can be anticipated one to one-and-a-half weeks after total cessation. Conversely, the withdrawal symptoms can be expected to clear one week after resumption of 1 gram of vitamin C per day. The works of Cochrane[27] in retrospect, and Siegel, suggests that special consideration should be given to expectant mothers when administering megadose vitamin C. The National Academy of Science agrees, and has warned that mothers taking oral vitamin C must provide their babies with supplements to prevent rebound scurvy in their infants.[28] Logically, the same reasoning would apply to infants of lactating mothers, assuming the mother was initially given megadose vitamin C post postpartum.

The message is clear. Any patient receiving IV-C must fully understand the importance of continuing with oral supplements for a significant period afterwards. They must also be made aware of the importance of a gradual reduction of dosage.

Complication of Existing Conditions Of Iron Overload

Vitamin C enhances the utilization of iron and, as demonstrated by Hallberg,[29] also enhances the absorption and bioavailability of iron. In addition, Fox,[30] in working with animals, reported that vitamin C and iron cooperatively block the absorption of cadmium. Yet this same beneficial mechanism at work in patients in whom iron overload is a feature of their condition (those with hemocromocytosis, polycythemia vera, and leukemia) may actually add to the problem. Therefore, as a general rule it is recommended that these people be discouraged from taking megadose oral vitamin C supplements. IV-C is the exception.

Dr. Robert H. Driesback, editor of the *Handbook of Poisoning*,[31] instructs that IV-C in the amount of 50 grams per 24 hours is an accepted chelating agent for iron overload, as the IV-C route aids in ridding the body of excess iron without enhancing further absorption. As the blood level of iron declines, approaching normal, IV-C loses its ability to chelate the mineral further, thereby serving as an ideal therapeutic for iron overload. Thus, while caution must be exercised to refrain from giving megadose oral vitamin C to patients with an iron overload, IV-C is an accepted method of treatment for the same. In addition, in those patients with a dual problem of iron overload and mercury poisoning, it may be necessary to repeat the IV-C several times. As you will recall from Step 3 in Chapter 2, it is necessary to keep the blood iron level at a minimum while treating chronic mercury toxicity. Otherwise, the iron may serve to mask a major symptom—fatigue—and make it difficult to rid the hemoglobin molecule of mercury.

Complications of Existing Condition Of Metastatic Cancer

Cameron and Pauling learned from their experiences with the orthomolecular treatment of cancer that megadose vitamin C, and particularly IV-C, should not be administered too rapidly to patients with widespread metastasis.[32] Extensive necrosis and hemorrhage can occur. While a satisfactory explanation is not yet determined, the researchers have found that megadose vitamin C can be administered to these people as long as the dosage is increased slowly over a couple of weeks. IV-C may be administered also, and its value certainly warrants such action, but only following the second week of megadose supplements.

Drug Interactions

Because vitamin C serves as a detoxifying agent in the liver, the doctor must be aware of the potential for drug interference by IV-C. First, it has the potential to impair anticoagulant therapy. Rosenthal,[33] studying healthy individuals, and Smith,[34] studying patients taking anticoagulant therapy, demonstrated that vitamin C serves to normalize the activity of Prothrombin and other clotting factors. Therefore if the patient is taking Coumadin, or Dicoumarol, the prescribing doctor should be notified before administering IV-C.

Interference with tubular reabsorption of amphetamines and the antidepressant drugs may also occur. Milne,[35] studying the effect of vitamin C on the efficacy of commonly used drugs, noted that vitamin C interfered with tubular reabsorption of many of the popular psychotropic agents, particularly amphetamines and the antidepressants. Milne's observations are especially important to this discussion, since mental disorders are among the commonly reported symptoms of chronic mercury toxicity. Patients who are candidates for IV-C, therefore, and who have been doctor-hopping in search of answers, may be taking psychotropic drugs. If so, it is again wise to notify the prescribing doctor of the treatment plan.

IV-C may also interfere with insulin treatment of Type I diabetes. Free and Free,[36] while demonstrating that megadose vitamin C may interfere with results of urine glucose determinations, suggested that ascorbic acid may also mediate the action of insulin. The researchers believed this was due to inactivation of glucose oxidase. While there have since been no serious reactions during insulin therapy that were vitamin C-related, prudence dictates that IV-C should not be administered to anyone with Type I diabetes, unless the potential benefit warrants the risk.

Scarlett, et al.,[37] noted that while megadose vitamin C may adversely affect insulin therapy of Type I diabetes, it does not affect glucose tolerance in normal people, nor does it significantly alter their fasting glucose level. In fact, as determined by Arendt and Pattee,[38] nondiabetic obese people taking megadose vitamin C respond with a lower insulin requirement, as evidenced by a decrease in the glucose tolerance curve. While these reports are somewhat conflicting, they indicate that megadose vitamin C may interfere with insulin therapy of Type I diabetes, but that IV-C may have either no effect or a beneficial effect in Type II, non-insulin dependent diabetes.

POTENTIALLY LIFE-THREATENING SITUATIONS

Glucose-6-Phosphate Dehydrogenase (G-6-PD) Deficiency

Campbell, et al.,[39] at the University of Mississippi Medical Center, reported on an adult black male who was admitted with acute kidney failure. He had been treated elsewhere with 80 grams of IV-C on two consecutive days for second-degree burns of the hand. Because the patient was anuric, hemodialysis was begun on admission with little change in status. Three weeks later the patient died. Laboratory data showed that the complete shutdown of the patient's kidneys was precipitated by intravascular hemolysis, followed by an episode of disseminated intravascular coagulation (DIC). Further analysis showed that the actual cause of hemolysis, followed by DIC, was a preexisting deficiency of erythrocyte G-6-PD.

G-6-PD is an enzyme that is normally contained within the plasma membrane of red blood cells (RBC's) where it serves to prevent hemolysis. G-6-PD is required because RBC's, unlike other body cells, are metabolically deprived and vulnerable to oxidative stresses. G-6-PD therefore prevents reducing agents, such as bacteria and certain drugs, from destroying the RBC's. Vitamin C is likewise a reducing agent, having the unfortunate potential for causing widespread hemolysis in people with serious G-6-PD deficiency. For similar reasons, according to Goldstein,[40] but without a history of fatalities, IV-C may promote hemolysis and exacerbate the inherited condition of sickle-cell anemia, as well as any disease that promotes red blood cell fragility.

The University of Mississippi Medical School experience indicates that it is important to identify those patients with RBC fragility, including sickle-cell anemia, thalassemia (the so-called Mediterranean anemia), and especially G-6-PD deficiency, prior to IV-C administration. G-6-PD deficiency (and thalassemia in general) is commonly associated with people of white, Mediterranean descent. Yet blacks are especially vulnerable, mostly because sickle-cell anemia is unique to the black race, and the prevalence of G-6-PD deficiency is more common among black males than among whites—about 1 in every 10. The severity of G-6-PD deficiency is also greatest in the black race. In fact, the condition among Caucasians has never been found to be as severe as it is among blacks, which probably accounts for the lack of reported fatalities among whites. Nevertheless, a few frightening episodes have occurred.

Dr. Warren M. Levin of New York City, who has had extensive experience with treating mercury-toxic patients, recounted a recent case history of G-6-PD deficiency. Over the years Dr. Levin has administered IV-C to thousands of people with no mishaps. On one occasion, shortly after administering IV-C, his patient (a Caucasian female) developed an acute, severe, hemolytic anemia crisis with jaundice. While the patient recovered, and did not require a transfusion, the experience was an eye-opener. "It simply isn't feasible to do a test for G-6-PD on everyone," says Dr. Levin, "yet there really isn't any other way of knowing for sure."

An ironic twist to the fear of G-6-PD deficiency was revealed by Snell, et al.,[41] who found that chronic methylmercury toxicity itself can (in some people) be a cause of depressed G-6-PD activity. Upon examining the patient's history and routine laboratory data, if G-6-PD deficiency is suspected (the greatest risk being for black males, followed by Jewish men and others of Mediterranean descent, or anyone with a diagnosis of chronic mercury toxicity), the doctor may elect to order a blood test (normal value: 7.1 to 9.7 IU). If G-6-PD is indeed deficient in the same patient who is suspected of being mercury-toxic, the doctor may want to take particular steps to increase G-6-PD activity before administering IV-C, or oral megadose vitamin C. (Such steps would include supplementing with vitamin E which, as was explained in Chapter 2, serves to protect cell membranes from the harm caused by mercury; and implementing those aspects of the **IV-C Mercury Tox Program** that do not require vitamin C.)

Progression of Kidney Insufficiency To Kidney Failure

While kidney disorders are common among those suffering from chronic mercury poisoning, available research indicates that megadose vitamin C, and particularly IV-C, is unsafe in the early stages of treating the mercury-toxic patient if there are signs of kidney insufficiency or failure. Thus, IV-C is contraindicated in patients with acute mercury poisoning, and it <u>should</u> be contraindicated, I believe, in patients with evidence of kidney insufficiency. This point is best explained by reviewing four separate case studies:

Case 1 - Nephropathic Cystinosis. The use of megadose vitamin C in the treatment of serious kidney disorders began during the 1970's, and was used especially for treating children with nephropathic cystinosis—a congenital defect involving excessive accumulation of cystine in glomerular cells. During the normal course of this condition, affected children experience progressive kidney insufficiency. Death ultimately occurs at about age 10 due to complete kidney failure.

It was found during autopsy that children who had died with nephropathic cystinosis had 50 to 100 times more free cystine in their bodies than is normal, and that vitamin C in cell culture research had been found effective in lowering cystine content by over 50 percent. It was anticipated, therefore, that megadose vitamin C might serve as an effective and safe form of therapy for these children. To test the hypothesis, Schneider, et al.,[42] performed a multi-year, controlled study. The test group received 200 mg vitamin C per kilogram of body weight, given orally every 6 hours for two years.

Following evaluation of data, the researchers were surprised to learn that megadose vitamin C therapy in the test group served only to hasten the children's death (probably through formation of cystine stones), as compared to the control group that received no supplemental vitamin C. Furthermore, among those in the test group who lived, there was a need at an earlier age for dialysis and renal transplant. These findings led the researchers to conclude that megadose vitamin C offers little benefit to those children with nephropathic cystinosis. The findings also gave reason to warn that megadose vitamin C should be administered with caution to anyone with kidney insufficiency.

Case 2 - Nephrotic Syndrome. The nephrotic syndrome, simply defined, is a syndrome of unknown origin in which the kidneys fail. It may either be congenital or acquired, highlighted by an error in glomerular filtration and/or an increase in pressure in the venous system of the kidney due, usually, to thrombosis of the renal vein. The condition is characterized by considerable urine protein, reduction of blood albumin, edema, and excessive blood fats. Yet proteinuria may be the only <u>distinguishing</u> characteristic, as the three remaining characteristics are believed to be only a consequence of proteinuria. While the congenital form is nearly always fatal in infancy, the acquired form rarely progresses to complete kidney failure—the prognosis depending upon the underlying cause.

Buchet, et al.,[43] studying workers exposed to mercury vapor, determined that people suffering from elemental mercury poisoning are likely to develop the nephrotic syndrome characterized by a reduced creatinine clearance. The nephrotic syndrome caused by mercury is a benign disease, however, which rapidly improves after removal from exposure. The congenital form was studied by Dr. Reznik, et al.,[44] who described a situation in which his group believed oral vitamin C played a role in accelerating the progression of kidney insufficiency to complete renal failure. A recount of this case study is important because it may also apply to particular mercury-toxic patients with the nephrotic syndrome or who have a reduced creatinine clearance.

According to Reznik, an infant with congenital nephrotic syndrome was given oral vitamin C by his parents. The dosage administered was 1.8 to 2 grams daily for six months. Ultimately, the child became ill with edema, vomiting, and fever, and was admitted to the hospital for long-term peritoneal dialysis. At last account, reported the doctors, the affected child was being readied for a transplant. This scenario raised a question: Was the association of megadose vitamin C and congenital nephrotic syndrome coincidental in this infant with the early onset of kidney failure; or did megadose vitamin C play an active role in accelerating the transition?

In an attempt to answer their own question, the Reznik group cited one large study in Finland,[45] in which nearly half of the infants with congenital nephrotic syndrome died within the first six months of life. Death due to kidney failure, however, did not occur in any of the children studied before they reached the age of two. In their own case in California, the child was near death and recommended for a transplant before age one. Of course, as the doctors readily admit, the clear association of megadose vitamin C and accelerated renal disease does not prove a causal relationship. Yet their observation raised further suspicion that megadose vitamin C may play an active role in accelerating the rate of progression from kidney insufficiency to kidney failure without regard to the initiating cause.

Case 3 - Active/Preexisting Renal Insufficiency. This single case study, reported by McAllister, et al.,[46] at a tertiary care center in Clearwater, Florida, demonstrated the reality that megadose vitamin C administered to a patient with active kidney dysfunction may lead to permanent renal failure.

A 70-year-old man with a dysfunctioning kidney was admitted to a chelation therapy center for treatment of occlusive arterial disease of the limbs. The patient was given 2.5 grams of IV-C the day before he was to receive IV-Editic acid (EDTA) therapy. Twelve hours later he experienced severe bilateral flank pain, passed only 3 ml of bloody urine, and then became anuric. The stricken patient was transferred to McAllister's team at the above health center. A biopsy and histochemical analysis demonstrated calcium oxalate crystals within the tubular lumina and tubular epithelial cells. The vitamin C infusion, they believed, was responsible for the development of the oxalate stones which caused rapid progression of kidney dysfunction—from insufficiency to permanent renal failure. It became increasingly clear that patients with poor kidney function are poor candidates for IV-C.

Case 4 - Silent/Preexisting Renal Insufficiency. Only a year following the previous study, Lawton, et al.,[47] reported a case study of a lady with nephrotic syndrome who died following a single 45 gram dose of IV-C. The 58-year-old woman's symptoms included a growth in the kidney that resulted from primary amyloidosis.* She also had poor cardiac output and a long history of nephrotic syndrome.†

Upon entering the County Medical Center the lady was properly diagnosed and given drug therapy for primary amyloidosis. Following her discharge from the facility she entered another hospital for a second opinion and alternative therapy. She was treated with an additional four or five drugs with no improvement. IV-C was then considered. Knowing that the lady had a history of nephrotic syndrome, a serum creatinine determination was performed. The reading was "normal", so her kidney function status was

* A poorly understood complex of glycoprotein that may accumulate in various body tissues and contribute to a wide variety of ailments involving nerve tissue, multiple myeloma, and arterial narrowing.

† There is a very significant point to be made by reexamining the characteristics of this syndrome. As stated before, the acquired form rarely progresses to complete kidney failure. In fact, there may be long periods in the patient's history when the symptoms are "silent". Even so, the poorly-defined, underlying cause remains in conflict with the patient's health throughout his lifetime. Once the diagnosis is made, therefore, the patient's kidney function status should never be considered sufficient, even during those periods when the serum creatinine reads normal. Although this attitude can rightly be challenged in less-than-exceptional circumstances, it is the only safe attitude when considering the use of IV-C.

considered sufficient and capable of handling IV-C. Soon after the IV-C, her serum creatinine level began to rise well above normal, and her kidney function status was downgraded to "insufficient." On the eighth day following IV-C administration the lady was transferred back to the County Medical Center for treatment of acute kidney failure. She was nearly anuric. Hemodialysis was started, but she died on the fifth hospital day.

During the autopsy that followed, the doctors found extensive intratubular deposits of oxalate stones, plus a corresponding increase in serum oxalate and serum ascorbic acid. The doctors credited the lady's death and the appearance of stones to IV-C.

There is an additional, important point to be made from this experience. It is quite clear that having a history of nephrotic syndrome is sufficient reason to decline the use of IV-C. (This is most ironic since the nephrotic syndrome may be a consequence of elemental mercury, or mercury vapor poisoning.[48]) It is not necessary for the condition to be active in order to predict disastrous results from IV-C, nor is it necessary for the serum creatinine to be elevated in these people. It is also quite clear, from the previous case histories, that any degree of kidney insufficiency is substantial reason to decline the use of IV-C. Of course, in any situation, the doctor must weigh the predictable risks against the potential for benefit. A Beta-2-Microglobulin (BMG) test may be helpful to this end.*

Ohi, et al.,[49] learned that an elevated BMG associates with Minamata disease, but is not a positive diagnostic indicator. Even though five times more mercury can be found at autopsy in the kidney than in the brain, brain tissue is more susceptible to mercury than kidney tissue, so some people with Minamata disease do not have renal tubular damage. Women are less inclined to develop kidney dysfunction than men.

To explain the significance of this further: BMG is a subunit of HL-A antigen of many cells. It is excessively excreted by men when their renal tubules are damaged by metals, such as cadmium and mercury. If IV-C must be administered to a critical patient with silent nephrotic syndrome, regardless of the underlying cause, it might be helpful to determine beforehand the level of urine BMG. In theory, if the urine BMG level is elevated the risk is highest; if normal, the risk should be greatly reduced.

Acidosis And Oxaluria

While reviewing the safety of megadose vitamin C, Lewis A. Barness, M. D., a pediatrician at the University of South Florida College of Medicine, and our reviewing specialist of vitamin C safety, went about his task of assessing the validity of the most repeated claims. His concern: "Probably the two most frightening claims about the toxicity of ascorbic acid are the development of acidosis, and production of oxaluria."

---

* When mercury poisoning is suspected, and when there is reason to believe that kidney function may be altered, research from Japan suggests that the probability of risk might be lessened by screening for Beta-2-Microglobulin in the urine.[50] There are two main forms of proteinuria. Glomerular damage allows glomerular proteinuria; tubular damage allows passage of renal tubular epithelial antigen and BMG (a light chain immunoglobulin). The researchers argue that the ratio of these proteins to albumin can help detect mildly affected renal tubules when the creatinine clearance is normal. They contend it is an excellent index of nephrotoxicity, especially as it relates to mercury, since mercury more often affects tubular, rather than glomerular, cells.

Acidosis. While frightening in concept, Dr. Barness informs that acidosis is—in practice—a negligible problem. First, ascorbic acid is a relatively ineffective urinary acidifying agent when given alone. To lower pH it must be administered in doses of 3 to 6 grams per day in combination with antibiotics or the urinary antibacterial mandelamine. At this dosage, according to Murphy, et al.,[51] when mandelamine and other antibiotics are not being administered there is a negligible effect on blood pH. Travis, et al.,[52] found that even 8 grams a day has little effect on blood pH. However, if the doctor is concerned over the risk of acidosis in a particular patient, sodium ascorbate rather than ascorbic acid should be administered orally. (As explained in Chapter 9, IV-C is only available as sodium ascorbate.)

Thus, while this area of concern could benefit from additional research, and one of the goals of this book is to stimulate such research, the available evidence does not support the fear of megadose vitamin C as a cause of acidosis. However, it would seem prudent to withhold administering IV-C following discontinuation of mandelamine and/or any general antibiotic. This advice is accentuated when treating people for acute mercurial poisoning, for which IV-C is not indicated, because acute mercurialism has been reported to cause acidosis independently of other factors, by blocking cellular metabolism of carbohydrates at the pyruvic acid level.[53]

Oxaluria. As opposed to simple adult oxaluria, Barness contends, oxalosis in children may be due to particular enzymatic defects. He suspects that adult oxaluria may also be connected with some enzymatic defects. In these people, he believes, there are reasonable grounds for fear that megadose vitamin C may promote stone development. Studying the relationship of urinary enzymes and the risk of stone development, Azoury, et al.[54,55] determined that a low UGOT and UGPT were associated with a tendency toward stone development. A lack of these enzymes, as indicated by readings in the range of 2 to 20 IU, interrupted conversion of the amino acids L-aspartic acid and alanine, to L-glutamic acid, which serves as a stone inhibitor. On the other hand, readings that range from 22 to 60 IU indicate very low risk of stone formation due to oxaluria.

Commenting on the practicality of this information, Wright contends that the practice of performing a UGOT/UGPT analysis prior to administering IV-C has contributed greatly to his excellent safety record (100 percent) when using IV-C. Those patients who exhibit a low reading are either denied access to IV-C or (among other nutritional and lifestyle considerations) are given an oral supplement of L-glutamic acid beforehand. Oxaluria is otherwise controllable and preventable through the many nutritional and lifestyle changes that will be discussed in Chapter 6. This is important to the issue of safety because—as the reader will learn in the following chapter—oxaluria is one of the greatest risks to the development of kidney stones, and must be overcome.

SUMMARY:
USE OF PATIENT QUESTIONNAIRE

In conclusion, the information presented in this chapter suggests certain positive steps that should be taken in conjunction with administering IV-C, screening first for any life-threatening risks. Through a patient questionnaire, a sample copy of which is provided in Chapter 8, the doctor should first determine if the patient has a history of the conditions that follow.

High-Risk Conditions: Exclude as Candidate for IV-C
In general, people who respond with "yes" answers to any of the following should be denied IV-C:

- G-6-PD deficiency (Men at greater risk than women. Black men and males of Mediterranean descent, especially Jewish men, are at greater risk than men of other nationalities, and blacks are at ten times the risk of white Mediterranean men)
  - RBC fragility
  - Thalassemia
  - Sickle cell anemia
- Kidney dysfunction (males at greatest risk)
- Nephrotic cystinosis (congenital)
- Nephrotic syndrome (congenital or acquired)
  - active
  - silent
- Renal insufficiency
- Kidney stones (Recurring and single stone formers)

If the doctor feels the patient's condition warrants the use of IV-C even in the presence of high-risk conditions, which may in themselves be due to chronic mercury toxicity, preparing the patient through the program offered in Chapter 6 will be extremely helpful, as it will increase the chances for a successful outcome. If the patient has a tendency toward any form of hemolytic anemia, for instance, it would be wise to begin a supplementation program of 400 to 600 IU vitamin E daily. This has been shown to restore RBC integrity and reduce the chance for drug-induced hemolysis. After a period of improvement the patient can perhaps be treated (alternatively) for chronic mercury toxicity. Jaffe, et al.,[56] for example, has found that a reduction in creatinine clearance (an indication of renal insufficiency) indicates the need for treating as though it is an acute case of poisoning.* Thus, those with the nephrotic syndrome, and who are mercury-toxic, might likewise benefit from completing the patient questionnaire (even though they are refused the vitamin C aspect of the **IV-C Mercury Tox Program**), by being treated first with BAL, Penicillamine, or some other agent appropriate for chelating mercury (See Appendixes G and H).

Another benefit of the information gained from the patient questionnaire: Before administering a chelating agent, such as BAL, to a high-risk patient in whom impaired renal function is suspected due to mercury-induced tubular lesions (detected through use of the creatinine clearance and the Beta-2-Microglobulin [BMG] test), the findings of Schulte-Wissermann and Straub[57] suggest that L-Thyroxine therapy may be helpful in restoring tubular function. Following these and other corrective steps the patient may still be denied access to IV-C, or may ultimately qualify as a candidate for IV-C.

Medium-Risk Conditions: Candidate Acceptable for IV-C with Appropriate Consultation and Monitoring
The patient questionnaire may likewise reveal medium-risk conditions, for which the doctor would want to take appropriate action to minimize the risk. A patient who answers "yes" to Type I, insulin-dependent diabetes, for

---

* A bibliography for the treatment of acute poisoning can be found in Appendix G.

instance, should be allowed to receive IV-C only after consulting the doctor who is treating the diabetic condition, and only after arranging to monitor his or her condition as indicated. The same cooperative spirit should be maintained in handling all the medium-risk conditions, which include the following conditions:

- Type I, insulin-dependent diabetes
- Iron overload
  - Hemochromocytosis
  - Polycythemia vera
  - Leukemia
- Presently taking any of the following medications:
  - Anticoagulant therapy, especially coumadin
  - Insulin, either injectable or oral agents for diabetic control
  - Antibiotics
  - The urinary antibacterial, mandelamine
  - Psychotropic drugs, especially antidepressants and amphetamines

In addition to the patient questionnaire, and the doctor's usual course of history-taking and physical examination, it is important when establishing risk that a minimum of laboratory work be performed. The minimum laboratory work-up should include the following:

- Routine urinalysis with 24-hour creatinine clearance
- UGOT/UGPT determination
- Serum uric acid
- Serum creatinine
- BUN
- CBC

Low-Risk Conditions

The low-risk patient should have answered "no" to all of the higher-risk conditions, and laboratory data should confirm the same. Yet even with abnormal laboratory values the patient remains a candidate for IV-C, so long as appropriate action can be—and is—taken to correct the problem.

If the patient is declared a candidate for IV-C, begin the program a few days (preferably a week) before IV-C, instructing him to take the prescribed amount and source of vitamin C daily. Whichever source and vitamin C regimen is decided upon, the chosen source should be taken between meals in 1 gram doses. This plan will aid in maintaining a steady blood level and will also avoid any conflict with vitamin B_{12} absorption.

IV-C candidates should be made aware that oral vitamin C must be taken at least a few days before IV-C is administered, and that to avoid the risk of rebound scurvy it is the patient's responsibility to continue taking the prescribed dosage of oral vitamin C for a specified period afterwards. They, or their guardian or disability sponsor, will sign to this effect at the conclusion of the patient questionnaire.

Before the patient begins taking megadose oral vitamin C, in preparation for IV-C, it may be advantageous for future evaluation to first obtain baseline laboratory data. Particularly include those blood, urine, and stool determinations with which megadose vitamin C has been shown to interfere. These would include:

- Stool occult blood
- TSC
- Blood A/G ratio
- Serum LDH
- Serum sodium
- Blood and urine glucose

Chapter 5 has discussed the causes of death that have been attributed to vitamin C, showing that stone development has been the cause of death in three of the four people who have died, to date. This, I believe, would not have happened had the doctors had this source book available to them at the time, and had they taken the necessary steps to either avoid or reduce risk. In other words, these disasters with vitamin C would have not have happened had the doctor had a plan for reducing such risk, or for establishing a basis for denying high-risk patients access to IV-C or megadose vitamin C.

If the patient with renal insufficiency is still to be regarded a candidate for IV-C, it is vital that the issue of kidney stones be addressed in order to assure a successful outcome. The next chapter will address the abnormalities that are predictive of stone disease, but which are subject to diet and lifestyle intervention. Based upon the caution delivered in this chapter, most patients would benefit from the lifestyle instruction developed in Chapter 6.

As its history of use indicates, the risk of vitamin C is exceedingly small. By taking seriously the lifestyle errors believed to foreshadow stone development, the doctor and the patient together will have maximally reduced whatever risk that vitamin C may present. In following this program the doctor and patient together will have planted the seeds for the best possible outcome to the **IV-C Mercury Tox Program** and the treatment of any other disease for which IV-C is indicated. They will have launched an ideal program for preventing heart disease, as well as laying the groundwork needed for a lifetime of optimal health.

LITERATURE CITED

[1] J.J. Burns, J.M. Rivers, and L.J. Machlin, eds., *Third Conference on Vitamin C*, Volume 498, 1987.

[2] R.F. Cathcart, "Vitamin C: The Nontoxic, Nonrate-Limited, Antioxidant Free Radical Scavenger," *Med Hypo*, 18: 61-77, 1985.

[3] J.V. Wright, *Dr. Wright's Book of Nutritional Therapy*, Rodale Press, Inc., Emmaus, PA, 1979.

[4] F.R. Klenner, "Observations on the Dose and Administration of Ascorbic Acid when Employed Beyond the Range of a Vitamin in Human Pathology," *J Applied Nutr*, 23: 61-88, 1971.

[5] E. Cameron and L. Pauling, "Supplemental Ascorbate in the Supportive Treatment of Cancer: Prolongation of Survival Times in Terminal Human Cancer," *Proc Natil Acad Sci USA*, 73: 3685-89, 1976.

[6] A. Hoffer and H. Osmond, "Scurvy and Schizophrenia," *Diseases of the Nervous System*, 24: 273-85, 1963.

[7] E. Cheraskin, W.M. Ringsdorf, Jr., and E. Sisley, *The Vitamin C Connection*, Harper & Row, Publishers, Inc., NY NY 10022, 1983.

[8] First Edition; The AMA Drug Evaluations, *JAMA*, 3: 391, September 1971.

[9] W.R. Korner and F. Weber, "Tolerance for High Doses of Ascorbic Acid," *Int J Vitam Nutr Res*, 42:528-544, 1972.

[10] L.A. Barness, "Safety Considerations With High Ascorbic Acid Dosage," *Ann NY Acad Sci*, 258:523-528, 1975.

[11] D.H. Hornig and U. Moser, "The Safety of High Vitamin C Intakes in Man," *Vitamin C (Ascorbic Acid)*, eds. J.N. Counsell and D.H. Hornig, New Jersey, Applied Science Publishers, p.225, 1981.

[12] M.A. Sestili, "Possible Adverse Health Effects of Vitamin C and Ascorbic Acid," *Seminars in Oncology*, X(3): 299-304, September 1983.

[13] L.H. Smith, *N Eng J Med*, 287: 412-413, 1972.

[14] H.C. Elliott, "Effects of Vitamin C Loading on Serum Constituents in Man," *Proc Soc Exp Biol Med*, 169: 1982.

[15] E.E. Selkurt and C.R. Houck, "The Effect of Sodium and Potassium Chloride

on the Renal Clearance of Ascorbic Acid," *Am J Physiol*, 141: 423-430, 1944.

16 T.W. Kurtz, H. A. Al-Bander, and R.C. Morris, Jr., "'Salt-Sensitive' Essential Hypertension in Men: Is the Sodium Ion Alone Important?" *N Eng J Med*, 317 (17): 1043-8, October 22, 1987.

17 T.W. Kurtz, and R.C. Morris, Jr., "Dietary Chloride as a Determinant of 'Sodium-Dependent' Hypertension," *Science,* 222: 1139-41, 1983.

18 S.A. Whitescarver, et al., "Salt-Sensitive Hypertension: Contribution of Chloride," *Science,* 223: 1430-2, 1984.

19 S.L. Ruskin, "High Dosage Vitamin C in Allergy," *Am J Digest Dis*, 12: 281-313, 1945.

20 T.W. Anderson, D.B.W. Reid, and G.H. Beaton, "Vitamin C and the Common Cold: A Double-Blind Trial," *Can Med Asso J*, 107: 503-508, 1972.

21 D.S. Young, L.C. Pestaner, and V. Gibberman, "Effects of Drugs on Clinical Laboratory Tests," *Clin Chem*, 21: lD-432D, 1975.

22 R.J. Morin, "Arterial Cholesterol and Vitamin C," *Lancet*, l: 594-595, 1972.

23 T.W. Anderson, D.B.W. Reid, and G.H. Beaton, "Vitamin C and Serum Cholesterol," *Lancet*, 2: 876-877, 1972.

24 V. Herbert and E. Jacobs, "Destruction of Vitamin B_{12} by Ascorbic Acid," *JAMA*, 230: 240, 1974.

25 H.P.C. Hogenkamp, "The Interaction Between Vitamin B_{12} and Vitamin C," *Am J Clin Nutr*, 33:1-3, January 1980.

26 C. Siegel, B. Barker, and M. Kunstadter, "Conditioned Oral Scurvy Due to Megavitamin C Withdrawal," *J Periodontal*, 53 (7): 453-455, July 1982.

27 W.A. Cochrane, "Overnutrition in Prenatal and Neonatal Life: Can it Cause a Problem?" *Can Med Assoc*, 93: 893, October 23, 1965.

28 *Recommended Daily Allowances*, 9th Ed., Washington, DC, National Academy of Sciences, p 75-77, 1980.

29 L. Hallberg, "Effect of Vitamin C on the Bioavailability of Iron from Food, in Vitamin C (Ascorbic Acid)," eds., J.N. Counsell and D.H. Hornig, *Applied Science Publishers*, New Jersey, p 49, 1981.

30 M.R.S. Fox, *Ann NY Acad Sci*, 258: 144, 1975.

31 R.H. Driesback, ed., *Handbook of Poisoning*, Larry Medical Publications,

1981.

[32] E. Cameron, and L. Pauling, "The Orthomolecular Treatment of Cancer: Reevaluation of Prolongation of Survival Times in Terminal Human Cancer," *Proc Natl Acad Sci USA*, 75: 4538-42, 1978.

[33] G. Rosenthal, "Interaction of Ascorbic Acid and Warfarin," *JAMA*, 215: 1671, 1971.

[34] E.C. Smith, et al., "Interaction of Ascorbic Acid and Warfarin," *JAMA*, 221: 116, 1972.

[35] M.D. Milne, "Influence of Acid-Base Balance on Efficacy and Toxicity of Drugs," *Proc R Soc Med*, 58: 961-963, 1965.

[36] H.M. Free and A.H. Free, "Influence of Ascorbic Acid on Urinary Glucose Tests," *Clin Chem*, 19:662, 1973.

[37] A. Scarlett, et al., "Acute Effect of Ascorbic Acid Infusion on Carbohydrate Tolerance," *Am J Clin Nutr*, 29: 1339-1342, December 1976.

[38] E.C. Arendt, and C.J. Pattee, "Studies in Obesity. III. Effect of Ascorbic Acid on the Insulin-Glucose Tolerance Curve," *J Clin Endocrinol Metab*, 16: 653, 1956.

[39] G.D. Campbell, Jr., M.H. Steinberg, and J.D;. Bower, "Ascorbic Acid-Induced Hemolysis in G-6-PD Deficiency," *Ann Int Med*, 82 (6): 810, June 1975.

[40] M.L. Goldstein, *JAMA*, 216: 332-333, 1971.

[41] K. Snell, S.L. Ashby, and S.J. Barton, "Disturbances of Perinatal Carbohydrate Metabolism in Rats Exposed to Methylmercury *in utero*," *Toxicol*, 8: 277-83, 1977.

[42] J.A. Schneider, et al., "Ineffectiveness of Ascorbic Acid Therapy In Nephropathic Cystinosis," *N Eng J Med*, 300 (14): 756-759, April 5, 1979.

[43] Buchet, et al., "Assessment of Renal Function of Workers Exposed in Inorganic Lead, Calcium or Mercury Vapor," *JOM*, 22: 741-750, 1980.

[44] V.M. Reznik, et al., "Letter to the Editor: Does High-Dose Ascorbic Acid Accelerate Renal Failure?" *N Eng J Med*, 302 (25): 1418-1419, June 19, 1980.

[45] O.P. Huttunen, "Congenital Nephrotic Syndrome of Finnish Type, *Arch Dis Child*, 51: 344-348, 1976.

[46] C.J. McAllister, et al., "To the Editor: Renal Failure Secondary to Massive Infusion of Vitamin C," *JAMA*, 252 (13): 1684, October 5, 1984.

[47] J.M. Lawton, et al., "Acute Oxalate Nephropathy after Massive Ascorbic Acid Administration," *Arch Intern Med*, 145: 950, May 1985.

[48] K. Iesato, et al., "Renal Tubular Dysfunction in Minamata Disease: Detection of Renal Tubular Antigen and Beta-2-Microglobulin in the Urine," *Ann Int Med*, 86: 731-7, 1977.

[49] Iesato, ibid.

[50] G. Ohi, et al., "Urinary Beta-2-Microglobulin does not Serve as Diagnostic Tool for Minamata Disease," *Arch Environ Health*, 37 (6): 336-341, November/December 1982.

[51] F.J. Murphy, S. Zelman, and W. Mau, "Ascorbic Acid as a Urinary Acidifying Agent. II," *J Urol*, 94: 300-303, 1965.

[52] L.B. Travis, et al, "Urinary Acidification with Ascorbic Acid," *J Pediat*, 67: 1176-1178, 1965.

[53] E.A. Natelson, et al., "Acute Mercury Vapor Poisoning in the Home," *Chest*, 59: 677-678, 1971.

[54] R. Azoury, et al., "Retardation of Calcium Oxalate Precipitation by Glutamic-Oxalacetic-Transaminase Activity," *Urol Res* , 10: 169-72, 1982.

[55] R. Azoury, et al., "May Enzyme Activity in Urine Play a Role in Kidney Stone Formation?" *Urol Res*, 10: 185-9, 1982.

[56] K.M. Jaffe, et al., "Survival after Acute Mercury Vapor Poisoning," *Am J Dis Child*, 137: 749-51, August 1981.

[57] H. Schulte-Wissermann and E. Straub, "Effect of L-Thyroxine on Renal Excretion of Water and Electrolytes in both Normal and Mercury-Intoxicated Rats," *Urol Res*, 8: 189-96, 1980.

CHAPTER 6

Kidney Stones

"Medicines are nothing in themselves, if not properly used, but the very hands of the gods, if employed with reason and prudence."

~Herophilus [fl. 300 B.C.]

Clearly, the first 50 years of use of megadose vitamin C demonstrates one of the best safety records of any nutrient or drug given in pharmacological amounts. Yet the history of use of megadose vitamin C, particularly IV-C, has always carried with it the fear of kidney stone development. Following the release of Dr. Linus Pauling's book, *Vitamin C, the Common Cold, and the Flu* (W.H. Freeman & Company, 1971), many editorials focused on this possibility. The May 1971 issue of *The Medical Letter*, for instance, warned that very large doses of vitamin C should be avoided in patients with a tendency toward gout and oxaluria, formation of urate stones, or cystinuria. Dr. Pauling maintained that vitamin C does not cause stones.

What we've since discovered is that both are correct. Stones do not develop if the doctor who prescribes vitamin C gives consideration first to factors that predispose the patient to stone development. A thorough review is made herein of the relationship of vitamin C to these factors, and to kidney stones in general.

Three of the four life-ending experiences linked with usage of megadose vitamin C, as related in Chapter 5, began with preexisting renal insufficiency. In each case the cause of death could be credited to complete renal failure, due to occlusive stone formation. While fatalities from stones have not been recorded among presumably healthy people regularly taking megadose vitamin C, and while healthy people pose no risk to developing stones,[1] the risk of stone development in mercury-toxic people is nevertheless real. Therefore, a preventive program has been designed for the IV-C candidate to minimize the risk for stones from megadose vitamin C. A thorough review of kidney stones is essential to such a program. Without this knowledge, IV-C cannot be safely and confidently administered.

The research conducted in recent years indicates there are many diet and lifestyle factors that may influence the development of stones independently of vitamin C. Lifestyle behavior problems must be overcome before vitamin C is administered, or megadose vitamin C may indeed increase the risk of stones in select individuals. Quite naturally, some of these factors are more or less important than others. In the pages that follow, an attempt has been made to prioritize relative risk while realizing that biological individuality and individual circumstances may warrant a change in the rating system. With these limitations in mind, it is believed that the preventive program that is summarized in the following discussion will significantly reduce the risks connected with IV-C administration.

While this program is not designed to solve the problem of kidney stones in general, the information presented will likely be helpful in doing so. There is an added bonus for those who are interested in lifestyle counseling. By continuing beyond IV-C with the pre-IV-C lifestyle, as outlined, the patient will reap additional health benefits. Most importantly, the steps taken to prevent kidney stones are significant for the prevention of heart disease as well. This will become more clear as the text develops.

THE HISTORY, INCIDENCE, AND RISK OF STONES IN THE GENERAL POPULATION

In an early review by Gershoff,[2] archaeological evidence was cited indicating that urinary stones are among the oldest afflictions of man, dating back at least several thousand years. Like many diseases, kidney stone development may have a genetic influence, but is primarily an acquired, adult-onset disease and the culmination of decades of poor lifestyle practices. Gershoff demonstrated that stones among children in developed countries account for no more than 1 of every 100 diagnosed cases. In contrast, the occurrence of stones in children from developing countries, where poorer lifestyle practices are in effect, may be equal to that of adults.

Gershoff's findings seem to be substantiated by the findings of Boyce.[3] In order to determine the incidence of stones within the population, which is important to the doctor planning to administer IV-C, Boyce reviewed data from autopsies performed in major hospitals in the U. S. and England. They indicated that kidney stones are the cause of less than one percent of all hospital deaths. Yet the incidence of stones found in people who died from other causes is greater than one percent. These stones developed mostly in men, as women seemed to have the protection of hormones.* In addition, Boyce learned that urinary stones are the cause of one percent of all hospital admissions—a figure both he and Gershoff believe does not reflect the extent to which the remaining population is afflicted, especially if one considers that 85 percent of the people who have stones are able to tolerate their problem without hospitalization. Based upon Boyce's hospital data and his own experience, as well as that of Gershoff's, as many as 5 to 10 percent of the adult (mostly male) population will develop stones at some point in their lives. The objective, therefore, is to learn how stones develop and to propose a method of prevention.

In 1936, Randall[4] was first to suggest that the appearance of stones was more accurately a symptom of another problem than a distinct disease entity. Gout, for instance, may encourage the development of kidney stones by promoting uricosuria, an event which commonly follows the rise in blood uric acid seen in gout patients. Heart disease may also follow gout and, if one observes the association closely, it is apparent that kidney stones, gout and heart disease have a mutual link: All three have multifactorial causes, and all three are influenced by underlying factors that relate to lifestyle. In fact, several lifestyle factors have been found during the 20th century to be common contributors to each, and especially linked to the rise in incidence of kidney stones.[5,6,7,8]

A major shared risk of these three is a diet high in animal protein (100 grams and more per day; the association is not nearly as pronounced when total daily protein intake is moderate, between 50 and 70 grams). This relationship is consistent throughout the Western World. During a period of comparison (1900 to 1975) when the incidence of heart disease and kidney stones mutually increased, the average daily consumption of meat rose steadily from 7 to 11 ounces per person.[9] At this time, there were subsequent rises in the incidences of elevated urine protein and calcium, and average levels of uric acid in both

---

* A suggested mechanism for this protection is presented later in the chapter.

blood and urine. It has since been noted that the appearance of each of these serves independently as risk factors in heart disease and kidney stone development. The rise in urine uric acid, secondary to serum uric acid, accounts greatly for the onset of kidney stones in the individual at risk.

These and other factors relating to both heart disease and kidney stone development, such as the urine and dietary calcium relationship, will be discussed throughout the remainder of this chapter. Clearly, by minimizing the risk for kidney stones through lifestyle intervention, while preparing the patient for IV-C (which requires examination of the causes of gout and heart disease as well) the groundwork is laid for implementation of an ongoing program of lifestyle counseling.

DETERMINING THE MAKEUP OF STONES AND THEIR PROCESS OF FORMATION: THE FIRST STEP TOWARD PREVENTION

Pak,[10] studying healthy individuals, found that urine is normally supersaturated with a variety of metabolic by-products such as minerals, amino acids, vitamins, bacteria, and cellular debris. This data, combined with his own earlier findings[11] and the work of Robertson,[12,13] confirmed that the urine of healthy people is normally supersaturated with agents that tend to form stones. The most common of these agents are:
- ammonium ions
- uric acid
- calcium
- oxalate
- phosphate
- cystine

This prompted Pak to question why stones don't form in everyone. A possible answer may be found through the work of Nancollas,[14] who reported that the urine of stone formers has a higher degree of aminotransferase than those who are free of stones, especially higher levels of calcium,[15] magnesium,[16] and oxalate.[17] Thus, one of the objectives of this review is to examine factors that contribute to the higher level of supersaturation.

While excessive supersaturation of urine is a feature of stone development, it is not necessarily the cause. Pak states that the presence or absence of inhibitory agents is also an important and deciding factor. Citrate and several of the trace minerals that enhance citrate action, are good examples. These prevent the formation of kidney stones by blocking spontaneous colloid precipitation. Their absence may otherwise lead to the formation, growth, and aggregation of crystals that become stones. (See Figure 6:1)

Relying on this concept, Fellström and colleagues[4] formulated an important rule for stone development:

"The propensity for crystal formation, growth, and aggregation depends on the balance between urinary supersaturation and inhibitory activity."

Fellström's rule provides the framework within which the preventive program herein is formulated. The problem will be approached by addressing three categories of physiological risk:

Risk Category 1 (Influencing Factors). We will examine factors that, according to Pak, contribute to stone development with respect to agents that inhibit stones or supersaturate the urine, but which may nevertheless influence supersaturation and the effectiveness of inhibitory agents.

Risk Category 2 (Supersaturation). We will search for factors required for reducing the urinary content and supersaturation of the major stone-forming agents.

Risk Category 3 (Inhibition). We will look at factors responsible for increasing or decreasing the urinary content of stone-inhibitory agents.

Robertson, et al.,[18] prioritized the major risks from among the three categories of physiological risks. In order of decreasing importance they are:

- Reduced urinary output
- Oxaluria
- A reduction of stone inhibitors
- Extreme urine acidity or alkalinity
- Calciuria

He further noted a difference in risk among men, women and children:

- Men are at high risk
- Women are at lower risk
- Children are at the lowest risk

Looking still further, Robertson noted differences in risk according to medical history:

- Recurrent stone formers are at the highest risk level
- Single stone formers are at high risk
- Those with no history of stones are at low risk

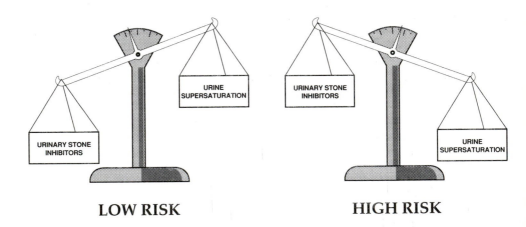

LOW RISK   **HIGH RISK**

Figure 6:1   Risk of stone development. As the urinary inhibitors of stones increase in concentration relative to urinary supersaturation (left), urinary supersaturation becomes less of a factor. Conversely, when the concentration of urinary stone inhibitors is inadequate (right), urinary supersaturation carries greater weight and becomes an important determinant of stone formation.

Knowing the risks of stone disease, and the priority of such risks, allows the doctor to more accurately conduct a risk assessment of the patient who aspires to be an IV-C candidate. Throughout the following review each of these risks will be discussed as they relate to the administration of IV-C. They will also be highlighted in the summary, along with suggestions for reducing these and other such risks prior to and immediately following IV-C administration. Near the chapter's conclusion will be found some important alternatives in the treatment of difficult patients.

RISK CATEGORY 1: FACTORS THAT CONTRIBUTE TO STONE DEVELOPMENT, WITH OR WITHOUT RESPECT TO INHIBITORY AGENTS AND URINE COMPOSITION

Beginning with a review of circumstances that are predictive of stones without regard to supersaturation or stone inhibition (Risk Category 1), and progressing to a review of factors that influence supersaturation (Risk Category 2) and stone inhibitory agents (Risk Category 3), but with some necessary overlap, the following will indicate the major predictors of stones, followed by a list summarizing the suggested solutions:

Predictors of Risk Category 1

- Urine pH (either extremely acid or extremely alkaline urine)
- Urinary tract infections
- Cystinuria
- Low urine output

Urine pH. When the composition of urine in stone formers was compared with the urine of people who were free of stones, Pak noted that an extremely acid or alkaline urine was an excellent predictor of stone development. He reasoned that both extreme acidity and extreme alkalinity reduce the extent of supersaturation that is needed to form stones, and also hinder the effect of the stone inhibitors. It is this notation that has prompted scientists such as Pauling[19] to place kidney stones into one of two classes—acid stones and alkaline stones. Stones from the alkaline class tend to form in extremely alkaline urine, whereas acid stones tend to form in extremely acid urine. For simplicity, the following may be helpful:

Alkaline Stones
- calcium phosphate
- magnesium ammonium phosphate
- calcium carbonate
- mixtures of the above

Acid Stones
- calcium oxalate
- uric acid
- cystine

Consistently with this concept, Pak noted that dehydration and urinary tract infections tend to form ammonium phosphate stones, through production of ammonium in an alkaline medium. Stones that form as a consequence of excess uric acid tend to do so in an extremely acid urine.

Pauling, therefore, suggested a remedial approach. A good way to raise the pH of an extremely acid urine, he believes, is to administer vitamin C in the form of sodium ascorbate. Citrate food sources such as oranges, lemons, limes, and grapefruit, also have a tendency to raise the urine pH. To acidify an extremely alkaline urine he prescribes 1 or more grams of ascorbic acid daily. If the patient with an alkaline urine is taking 3 grams of vitamin C daily, for instance, as he would prior to and following IV-C, it may be helpful to split the dosage forms; i.e., 1 gram sodium ascorbate plus 2 grams ascorbic acid. For acidifying extremely alkaline urine, straight ascorbic acid as recommended by Cathcart seems appropriate. High citrate foods may also be consumed along with ascorbic acid, to counter an extremely alkaline urine, as the citrate inhibitor is an even more important inhibitor of calcium phosphate stones (which form in neutral to alkaline urine) than acidic calcium oxalate. For more information see Risk Category 3.

While the before-mentioned remedy of altering extremely acid or alkaline urine through dietary means and through varying the form of vitamin C administered seems logical, Fellström warns that these attempts may have only a transient effect, as the findings reported in Chapter 5 would indicate. He explains that urine contains very potent buffers which make it difficult to affect urine pH by oral intake of salts of weak acids such as ascorbic acid, or citric acid. It is difficult, therefore, to affect urine pH by giving the acids *per se*. Often high amounts of citrate are needed in order to raise the urine pH. He has also found that, in patients with renal acidification dysfunction, it is very difficult to lower urine pH with ascorbic acid, hippuric acid or ammonium chloride. Very high doses are sometimes needed and the effect is again temporary. Therefore, while consideration of diet and the form of vitamin C to be administered represent a positive means of altering urine pH, the doctor can not rely solely on these means for control of extreme urine acidity or alkalinity.

Urinary Tract Infections. An overgrowth of bacteria in the urinary tract can readily cause stones through several mechanisms involving both urease-producing bacteria and nonurease-producing bacteria, although stones formed from the latter seem to be the most common. The least common stones (the infectious, struvite type comprised of magnesium ammonium phosphate and/or calcium carbonate) form in alkaline urine by the action of urease-producing bacteria on urea to form ammonium ions. Nonurease-producing bacteria may form stones irrespective of the urine pH by working as a nidus for precipitation of either calcium oxalate (in acid urine) or calcium phosphate (in alkaline urine). Furthermore, several strains of bacteria may promote stone formation by producing enzymes that break down the colloidal surface of epithelial cells within the urinary tract, which would otherwise work as a barrier against adhesion of calcium-containing microcrystals. In other words, bacteria tend to promote stones by providing the initial aggregate for attachment of stone forming agents, and by upsetting the colloidal balance.

Further complicating the issue, pre-formed calcium stones may actually be the cause of a patient's urinary tract infection, indicating that any candidate for IV-C who presents with a urinary tract infection should be examined for stones and cleared of such infection before the treatment is administered. Increasing urine output by drinking an adequate amount of water is also believed to be important in prevention of urinary tract infections.

Cystinuria. A medical history of cystinuria normally disqualifies the patient as a candidate for IV-C, although cystine stones, the consequence of a genetic defect in the tubular reabsorption of cystine, are rare, and account for no more than 3 percent of all stones. If the doctor and patient decide that the potential for benefit outweighs the risk, the patient's dietary intake of protein should be carefully controlled. While a high-protein diet does not contribute directly to significant cystinuria in a patient with normal renal function, cystinuria in combination with aciduria (which an excessive protein intake may contribute to) does represent a high risk situation that should be considered before IV-C administration.

Low Urine Output. Robertson determined that a low urine output was the most important risk factor in stone development. In contrast, an increase in the intake of fluid does a number of remarkably positive things, not the least of which is reduction of supersaturation. It lessens the extremes of urine pH, and reduces the chance for bacterial infection. Testing this concept, Pak reported a single case history of a patient who had a history of stones but would not take medication. He subsequently instructed the patient to drink plenty of water—at least 3 quarts each day. The aim was to bring about a persistent, daily urine output of two liters or more. The patient complied and formed no stones during the next ten years. Such a large amount of water benefits the patient by keeping urine composition at the lower stage of supersaturation, by reducing the likelihood of extreme urine acidity or alkalinity, and by greatly reducing the chance for urinary tract infection. Thus, it would seem prudent to instruct the patient to drink plenty of water a few days before, during, and a few days after IV-C administration.

Solution for Prevention of Stones due to Risk Category 1

- Instruct the patient to drink plenty of water. When addressing the high risk patient, Pak suggests up to 3 quarts per day. You may want to instruct the patient to drink water at night when the urine pH is normally at its low point.

- Clear up urinary tract infections before administering IV-C.

- Adjust for extremely acid urine by prescribing an alkalinizing agent. Pak suggests potassium citrate in patients with a high urine sodium (discussed under Risk Category 3). Otherwise, one can use ordinary baking soda, in increments of 1/8 teaspoon. One might also employ the use of sodium ascorbate as the oral vitamin C supplement, and/or a citrate-rich diet, although no more than a temporary effect should be expected.

- Adjust for extremely alkaline urine. While the doctor should expect no more than a transient effect from following Cathcart's recommendation (pure ascorbic acid as the oral vitamin C supplement), or Pauling's 2:1 formula (2 parts ascorbic acid to 1 part sodium ascorbate), and/or by following the recommendation for dietary citrates and protein, at least a positive step is being taken when combined with the recommended fluid intake.

- Deny IV-C access to patients who present with significant cystinuria.

RISK CATEGORY 2: THE MAJOR STONE-FORMING AGENTS AND FACTORS THAT CONTRIBUTE TO SUPERSATURATION

Often, because calcium oxalate stones are the more common stone type, it is believed that high levels of urine calcium and oxalate are equally the most significant features of active stone disease. Robertson pointed to an error in this perception. He found in his risk assessment study that an increase in oxalate was far more important. In support of Robertson's findings, Menon and Mahle[20] revealed that a high urine oxalate is 15 times more predictive of stone formation than the urinary content of calcium. In fact, their review demonstrates that a low urine calcium occurs just as often as an elevated urine calcium.

The lesser importance of urine calcium would lead one to believe (incorrectly) that dietary calcium and other dietary factors involved in calcium homeostasis have little to do with the process of stone development. In addition, being led to believe that the quantity of calcium in the diet does not affect oxalate excretion would likewise do nothing to correct a misconception that vitamin C is the major dietary contributor to urine oxalate, or that urine oxalate is generally a function of dietary oxalate. These commonly held misconceptions highlight the necessity of reexamining the relationship of vitamin C intake and stone development; of reviewing more thoroughly the mechanisms that jointly control calcium balance and affect oxalate absorption; and of learning how lifestyle may ultimately influence stone formation through the processes of inhibition and aggregation of urine calcium and oxalate. Several lifestyle predictors are apparent. There are three main topics with which we must concern ourselves in this category: oxaluria, calciuria, and uricosuria.

Oxaluria: the Greatest Risk to Developing Calcium Oxalate Stones

Predictors of Oxaluria
- Ingestion of megadose vitamin C without regard to the other predictors of oxaluria
- Vitamin B_6 deficiency (combined with deficiencies of folic acid and vitamin B_1)
- Excessive animal protein in diet
- Consumption of high oxalate foods
- Low calcium diet

Megadose Vitamin C: Hodgkinson,[21] in his text on oxalate stones, describes oxalic acid as a useless end product of metabolism. He indicates that urine oxalate may originate from a variety of dietary and metabolic pathways. Endogenous synthesis accounts for 45 to 85 percent, while dietary sources contribute 15 to 55 percent of urine oxalate. Vitamin C is one of the major dietary sources, accounting for as much as 40 percent of excreted oxalate. The normal metabolic pathway of vitamin C to oxalate occurs in the following manner:

L-ascorbic acid ⟶ L-dehydroascorbic acid

L-dehydroascorbic acid ⟶ 2,3 diketo L-gulonic acid

2,3 diketo L-gulonic acid ⟶ L-threonic acid + oxalic acid

The question that immediately comes to mind: Is the evidence of a metabolic pathway leading from vitamin C to oxalic acid also evidence of cause and effect? In other words, is megadose vitamin C the cause of oxaluria? An answer to this question can be found in a number of journal overviews and studies, and by reconsidering equilibrium position of the reducing redox potential for vitamin C: The healthful effects of vitamin C depend on a reducing redox potential equilibrium that tends toward the left of midline, i.e., ascorbic acid must be present in sufficient quantity to increase—above normal—the ratio of ascorbic acid to dehydroascorbic acid (plus other qualifying factors to be discussed). When dietary ascorbic acid is adequate, and when other conditions are suitable (such as the avoidance of an alkaline urine), the conversion of dehydroascorbic acid to oxalic acid is limited, and oxaluria is unlikely.

Other possible answers to this question can be drawn from the highly regarded critique by Sestili,[22] who concluded that the increase in oxaluria that sometimes follows megadose vitamin C is not in proportion to dosage administered, and that an underlying defect is evidently present in those who are oxalate responders. Patients with enteric hyperoxaluria are good examples. These people have a very high excretion of oxalate due to an enhanced oxalate absorption, and—drawing from Fellström's experience—may absorb 50 percent of ingested oxalate.

Barness[23] points to a wide array of studies that support an observation of the inconsistency of oxaluria and stone development following larger doses of vitamin C. Like Sestili, Barness could not build a case for cause and effect, although Fellström and other investigators report from their own experience that some patients do develop hyperoxaluria from the intake of more than a few grams of ascorbic acid daily. Fellström says, "In a calcium oxalate stone former (who is normally not considered a candidate for IV-C) the following rule should be strictly followed: Ascorbic acid (IV-C) should not be given unless it has been shown that the patient's oxalate excretion does not increase by the given (oral) amount of ascorbic acid. This can be done by monitoring urinary oxalate. Furthermore, if kidney stones do develop while treating the patient with vitamin C, the treatment must be stopped."

In healthy people not taking vitamin C supplements, Briggs[24] noted that the normal intake and biosynthesis of oxalate accounts for the excretion of approximately 50 mg oxalate per 24 hours. Yet, as was cited by Hodgkinson, no more than half of this output can be credited to the normal metabolism of vitamin C. Much of the variation can be explained by sexual differences.

Women, according to Hagler and Herman,[25] tend to excrete less urine oxalate than men. Estrogen accounts for the difference here. Its protective action in women lowers oxalate excretion by reducing the activity of the liver's oxalate-forming enzyme, glycolic acid oxidase (GAO). In men, GAO is significantly increased by the dominating influence of testosterone, which amplifies the excretion of urine oxalate.

In accordance with the findings of Briggs and Schmidt,[26] most people who consume megadose vitamin C do not show an increase in oxalate excretion. Swartz,[27] in observing the effects of megadose IV-C during total parenteral feeding, found that a limit is soon reached for total oxalate production. Beyond a particular point vitamin C is not metabolized, as expected, to oxalic acid and oxalate salt. A similar finding was reported by Swartz in a study of healthy persons. IV-C did not promote oxalate production in a dose-dependent fashion. The researchers conclude that, in healthy people, the conversion of ascorbic acid to oxalic acid is interrupted at some point.

These observations may help explain why healthy, vitamin C-producing mammals are relatively free of stones, in spite of the fact that they produce, in human standards, ultra-megadose vitamin C every day. A protective mechanism is at work for them which limits oxalic synthesis. Cathcart contends that the 'protective mechanism' can partially be explained by the animal's always having megadose vitamin C available, which at some point discourages any further conversion of dehydroascorbic acid to oxalic acid by promoting a shift in equilibrium favoring the reducing redox potential.   His many years of experience in administering megadose vitamin C without a single patient developing stones would seem to confirm that this same protective principal applied to people. Additionally, perhaps, the varying oxalate response among humans to megadose vitamin C reflects differences in lifestyle and the status of health prior to administration of the vitamin.

Hagler and Herman, for instance, in a study of healthy humans, found that 4 grams of vitamin C daily were required just to produce a slight oxaluria; whereas Roth and Breitenfield[28] found that 1 gram of vitamin C daily, as supplemented in the diet of clinic outpatients, led to a two- to three-fold increase in oxaluria and development of stones. In still another study,[29] Takenouchi and colleagues observed that, among people whose diet and usual lifestyle were otherwise undisturbed, 3 grams per day were required to effect a two-fold increase in oxaluria, and 9 grams per day for a three-fold increase.

Swartz, commenting on his own findings and those of other researchers, concludes that a dose-dependent excretion of oxalate can be seen only in sick people who are also consuming an unbalanced diet. His conclusion implies that illness and an unhealthy lifestyle predisposes the oxalate response to megadose vitamin C. Confirmation of this can be derived from Sestili's observation that in each case study the basal level of urine oxalate prior to the administration of megadose vitamin C was predictive of oxaluria afterwards. Simply stated, those patients who had normal amounts of urine oxalate before megadose vitamin C was administered, were least likely to develop oxaluria afterwards; whereas patients who had varying degrees of oxaluria before megadose vitamin C was administered demonstrated a correspondingly greater oxaluria afterwards. This has led to the speculation that kidney stones are more likely to occur in men, women, and children alike when urine oxalate is excessive prior to administering IV-C.

While many clinicians fear a cause and effect relationship between megadose vitamin C and stone development, solid proof for this is lacking. The risk, if there is indeed a risk, is perhaps more accurately tied to the underlying diet and lifestyle factors that create the initial oxaluria. Thus, the potential dangers of stone development following IV-C are more accurately related to factors other than vitamin C—factors that cause an excess of urine oxalate prior to administering IV-C. Even so, one must pay careful attention to Fellström's mandate that IV-C should not be administered to patients with a history of stones unless it has been shown, through monitoring urinary oxalate in response to oral vitamin C, that the patient's oxalate excretion does not increase by the given amount of ascorbic acid. Furthermore, if kidney stones do develop while treating the patient with vitamin C (whether that patient has been targeted as a stone former or not) the treatment must be stopped. While stone formers are normally denied access to megadose vitamin C, the secret to overcoming this danger in high risk patients is to determine effectual ways of minimizing oxaluria before, during, and immediately following IV-C.

Vitamin B$_6$ Deficiency: In the normal course of events, glycine from animal protein is converted to glyoxylic acid, which may then either revert back to glycine or form oxalic acid. According to the findings of Gershoff and Prien,[30] the availability of vitamin B$_6$ is a major determinant of the fate of glyoxylic acid. When vitamin B$_6$ is adequate, which is true in most cases, glyoxylic acid is preferentially reverted back to glycine, thereby preventing a high urine oxalate. When vitamin B_6 is deficient, which rarely occurs, glyoxylic acid is converted to oxalic acid and excreted in the urine as oxalate.

Balcke, et al.,[31] proposes that when the quantity of vitamin B_6 is sufficient, its active metabolite—pyridoxal-5-phosphate—serves to stimulate GOT enzyme activity that promotes conversion of glycine to glyoxylic acid and back to glycine. When vitamin B_6 is deficient, the GOT enzyme activity is insufficient to reverse the reaction back to glycine, thereby promoting the formation of oxalate. Testing this concept in patients with elevated urine oxalate, Balcke's group demonstrated that urine oxalate decreased by an average of 30 percent in response to 300 mg per day of oral vitamin B_6 supplements. A deficiency of vitamin B_6 caused a marked increase in oxaluria.

In a supportive manner, folic acid and vitamin B_1 are also involved. Gershoff, et al.,[32] and Buckle,[33] respectively, noted that folic acid and vitamin B_1 exert a positive and synergistic effect on the function of pyridoxine in preventing the conversion of glyoxylic acid to oxalic acid. Acting in harmony with pyridoxine, these two agents limit urine oxalate formation even more than vitamin B_6 acting alone.*

The primary dietary sources of folic acid are vegetables. The richest sources of Vitamin B_1 are almonds, cultured milk products, broccoli, and organ meats (although the latter will be discouraged in conjunction with administration of IV-C).

An Excess Of Animal Protein in the Diet: In considering the various origins of urine oxalate, Elder and Wyngaarden[34] found that a high animal-source protein diet is a greater determinant of oxalate synthesis than vitamin C. Fellström, et al.,[4] found that an exceptionally high animal-source, high-protein diet (142 grams daily) increased the risk of kidney stones in a variety of ways, not the least of which was its promotion of urine oxalate through glycine metabolism when vitamin B_6 was deficient. Yet the importance of animal protein for development of hyperoxaluria is not quite clear. Results of Fellström's studies of patients who consumed an extremely high protein intake, as well as other studies, showed no increase in oxalate excretion. Biochemical individuality seems to play an important role here. The general recommendation would therefore be to have a moderate intake of animal protein. Regardless, in those select studies where researchers have noted an association between protein intake and oxalate excretion, there are at least four possible reasons for their observations:

- Large amounts of glycine from a high protein diet discourage conversion of glyoxylic acid to glycine in the liver, thereby permitting uninterrupted biosynthesis of oxalic acid.

- Hydroxyproline, an animal collagen protein, also increases urinary oxalate. This again may be due to its exceptionally high content of glycine.

* These findings suggest that a B-complex supplement may be helpful as a prophylactic measure. Yet, putting this action into proper perspective, Fellström questions the value of a B-complex supplement for most patients. He has found Vitamin B_6 of value mostly in patients with primary hyperoxaluria—patients having an inborn error of metabolism, in whom vitamin B_6 may be an advantage—but he has found no solid evidence of the value of vitamin B_6 in patients not suffering from primary or secondary hyperoxaluria.

- Unless supportive foods are carefully chosen, the large quantity of methionine provided by a high animal-source, high-protein diet may indirectly contribute to an increase in urine oxalate by depleting the availability of vitamin B_6. The normal metabolism of methionine forms homocysteine, which must then be quickly detoxified by vitamin B_6. If not, the homocysteine is free to act as an angiotoxin, becoming a cause of arterial lesions. This greater demand for vitamin B_6 by a high animal-source protein diet could reduce its availability to a point that would favor oxalate synthesis rather than the normal conversion of glyoxylic acid back to glycine.

- Calcium homeostasis is decidedly upset when consuming a diet rich in animal source proteins, particularly red meats, promoting a rise in urine oxalate for a number of reasons (to be discussed).

Consumption of High Oxalate Foods and a Low Calcium Diet: Hagler and Herman, in 1973, provided the historic groundwork for our present level of understanding the effects of diet on urine oxalate excretion. They determined that the level of oxalate in the diet is important because it adds to the level of oxalate to be excreted. Their findings specify the foods which are the greatest contributors of dietary oxalate. As a general rule, the effects of limiting oxalate food sources are marginal, except in patients suffering from enteric hyperoxaluria where a hyperabsorption is present. Yet if the doctor is to put as many odds in his or her favor as possible, then it may be wise to restrict high and medium-to-high oxalate foods before and immediately following IV-C. (A list of these foods will be found later in this chapter.)

Kasidas and Rose,[35] comparing high oxalate foods, determined that spinach is the single greatest contributor of dietary oxalate. They found that a 5 ounce serving (200 g) of spinach yields 1 gram of oxalic acid. Menon and Mahle showed that in healthy people only about 15% (+/- 10%) of ingested oxalate enters the blood. This means that about 150 mg of the spinach oxalate would be absorbed per 5 ounce serving. Of the 850 mg of oxalate that remains, 50% (425 mg) is destroyed by intestinal bacteria, while 212 mg (25% +/- 10%) is excreted via the intestines. What is found in the urine depends on several factors, including the amount of oxalate absorbed, plus additional elements to be discussed. The amount of dietary oxalate absorbed and excreted, for instance, appears to be related to dietary calcium intake.

Because most kidney stones are comprised of calcium and oxalate, it is normal to assume that restriction of high-calcium, high-oxalate foods would maximally reduce the urine content of calcium and oxalate. Yet, Nordin and associates,[36] in 1972, showed this assumption to be unfounded. When habitual stone formers were placed on a low calcium diet (400 mg/day), with moderate oxalate restriction (60 mg/day), it served only to increase their oxaluria. Bataille, et al.,[37] made a similar observation of people who presented with oxaluria from an unexplained cause but who had no history of stones. A question that arose from these findings may be of greater than academic importance: Are some patients with enteric hyperoxaluria actually manifesting their hyperoxaluia simply from an error in choice of dietary combinations?

Following the revelation that a low-calcium, low-oxalate diet failed to reduce oxaluria, as previously assumed, it became necessary to reexamine the relationship. Menon and Mahle showed that calcium serves to control oxaluria by limiting oxalate absorption. It does this by binding with oxalic acid in the gastrointestinal tract, thereby promoting excretion of oxalic acid—as calcium oxalate—through the intestines. Similarly, calcium binds with excesses of phosphate, phytate, and sulfates. For this protective action to occur, the high-oxalate (sulfate, phosphate, or phytate) food source must contain a calcium and oxalic acid ratio that favors calcium, such as 2:1 or better, or the required calcium: oxalate ratio must be met in the same meal through combining foods.

Dr. Philip Washko, of the Department of Food Science and Human Nutrition at Michigan State University agrees.[38] The doctor, when interviewed by Sharon Faelten and the editors of *Prevention*, stated that consumption of greens high in oxalic acid probably does not pose a problem in a typical American diet, since few people would make a habit of consuming a diet that was high in oxalate and low in calcium. This most likely would occur only in Third World countries where first- and second-degree malnutrition is common. Yet, the evidence presented earlier would seem to suggest this <u>can</u> happen and, to speculate further, it probably <u>does</u> happen most often among people who tend to form stones.

Bataille and associates became curious, and wondered what the outcome would be of a diet low in calcium, while high in oxalate (above 90 mg/day). How, they wondered, would it effect urine oxalate? Their findings revealed that urine oxalate responded to a low-calcium, high-oxalate regimen with a 100% increase in oxaluria. (Though revealing, their finding wasn't a total surprise. This same observation has long been noted among malnourished children in areas of Thailand.[39]) Then, in a separate but related study, Barilla, et al.[40] performed the same experiment using a high-calcium diet of 1 gram per day. It was learned that a high-calcium, high-oxalate diet reduced oxaluria by 80%, but there was still one more combination to be tested.

Finch,[41] having previously performed studies similar to those of Bataille, elected to determine the calciuric and oxaluric effect of a diet combination of high-calcium (1 gram/day), low-oxalate (limited to 60 mg/day). His data of normally healthy people showed substantial evidence that the high-calcium, low-oxalate regimen, which reduced oxaluria by 100%, was the ideal dietary practice to follow before and immediately following IV-C.

The findings of Finch, Nordin, Barilla, and Bataille, demonstrated the importance of interviewing the IV-C candidate using a lifestyle questionnaire before treatment to determine nutritional status, as well as the importance of obtaining the patient's cooperation in strictly altering the diet a few days before administering IV-C.

Solution for Preventing, or Reducing, Oxaluria

- Supplement, if necessary, with up to 300 mg/day vitamin B_6, and/or a B-complex vitamin containing vitamin B_6, folic acid, and vitamin B_1. *Note: Vitamin B_6 has been used to prevent oxaluria mostly in patients with primary hyperoxaluria, i.e., patients having an inborn error of metabolism, in whom vitamin B_6 supplementation may be an advantage. In patients not suffering from primary or secondary hyperoxaluria there is no solid proof of the advantage of vitamin B_6 supplementation.*

- Supplement with 200 to 400 mg magnesium (Dr. Fellström recommends magnesium hydroxide; many other doctors prefer magnesium oxide).

While this doesn't necessarily aid in preventing or reducing oxaluria, a rationale will be offered later under Risk Category 3 for the role that magnesium plays in increasing the solubility of urine oxalate.

- Limit total protein intake to 50-75 g per day, keeping animal protein at about one-half this amount.

- Limit oxalate food sources. (A list of these foods can be found in the summation pages of this chapter under **Minimum Lifestyle Behavioral Changes for all Patients Regardless of Risk.**)
  Note: As mentioned before, the effects of limiting oxalate food sources are marginal, except in patients suffering from enteric hyperoxaluria where hyperabsorption is present.

- Include 1 gram calcium in the diet daily, particularly from cultured dairy products, since this is the source of calcium already recommended for countering the effects of mercury. As a guideline, 300 mg calcium is equal to one 8 oz serving of milk, 1-1/2 oz of cheddar cheese, 2 cups of cottage cheese, 1 cup of yogurt; 5 oz of salmon (with bones), or 1 cup of greens.

Calciuria: a Secondary Risk for Developing Calcium Oxalate Stones
      Robertson, in his risk analysis, determined that urine oxalate provides a much greater risk for stones than urine calcium. This may seem surprising since calcium is the principal constituent of most kidney stones, including calcium oxalate. In fact, calciuria by itself was determined to be one of the least significant risks. Yet, as Robertson states, "the odds of being a stone-former increase as urinary calcium increases, the curve rising sharply above an excretion of 10 mmol/day." Thus, calciuria remains important to the doctor who wishes to administer IV-C, most likely because the steps required to correct calciuria significantly influence supersaturation due to other urinary agents, as well as the stone inhibitory activity of urine. It is therefore wise to follow those steps known to decrease calciuria, and to identify the lifestyle factors known to influence excessive urine calcium.

Predictors of Calciuria
- An imbalance in calcium homeostasis
- An excess of active vitamin D and dietary vitamin D
- A diet excessively high in calcium (above 1500 mg/day)
- A diet deficient of calcium (500 mg/day or less), especially of cultured dairy products
- Low phosphorous intake
- High protein diet
- Excessive phosphate intake relative to dietary calcium
- Excess sodium (as sodium chloride)
- Caffeine abuse

      <u>An Imbalance in Calcium Homeostasis:</u> Drs. Lyles and Drezner,[42] in their excellent review of calcium control mechanisms, remind us that calcium is the most abundant cation in the human body. In order to prevent a net loss, the diet must contain a minimum of 3.2 mg calcium per kilogram of body weight, or about 200 mg daily. Yet even when one consumes as much as 400 mg a day many

body functions suffer, indicating either that dietary calcium is more efficiently used by the body than stored calcium, or that the excretion rate of calcium accounts for the greater dietary need. It is likely that both of these possibilities are valid. This greater need has prompted the National Research Council to set the RDA for calcium at somewhere between 600 and 800 mg per day, and a range between 800 mg and 1 gram is being considered.

Dietary Vitamin D: The kidneys' involvement as a site of calcium control has been studied extensively. While the kidneys filter about 10 grams of calcium daily, less than 200 mg daily appears in the urine of a healthy person. Over 98 percent is reabsorbed. Calciuria is recognized when urine calcium greatly exceeds 200 mg/day. Renal factors which control the amount of calcium excreted are urine pH and the level of active vitamin D* synthesized by the kidneys but mediated by the parathyroid hormone. The greater the quantity of active vitamin D, the greater the quantity of calcium that will appear in the urine. Orthophosphate, which decreases the output of active vitamin D, has been prescribed for some of those patients with hypercalciuria. An overproduction of active vitamin D may, however, be equally corrected through selected lifestyle changes.

Dietary vitamin D (vitamin D_2) is quite often associated with an exceptionally high intake of animal protein (100 grams or more per day, particularly from meat, milk, and eggs), which may then be a factor in stimulating the parathyroid hormone. This promotes calciuria in either of two ways: by enhancing the gastrointestinal absorption of calcium, thereby creating a greater demand for dietary calcium; or by stimulating the synthesis of active vitamin D.

Robert P. Heaney, M. D.,[43] a professor at John A. Creighton University, Omaha, Nebraska, suggests that hidden supplements of vitamin D, such as those found in fortified breakfast cereals, red meats, and milk, may be the greatest contributor to calciuria. Since 1947, when scientists first learned to synthesize vitamin D through irradiation of crystalline dehydrocholesterol, vitamin D has been added to as many foods as possible, including animal feed to ensure a faster rate of growth. While the amount of vitamin D added to meat today is substantially less, Holmes and Kummerow[44] only a few years ago demonstrated that Americans were consuming 14,000 lbs a year of vitamin D because of the practices, or 90 micrograms (3600 IU) per capita daily. This was nine times the RDA for vitamin D. While their findings led to the meat industry's decision to correct this error—to significantly reduce the amount of vitamin D added to animal feed—the total vitamin D added today to all foods, and food supplements, is still excessive. This practice may not only contribute to calciuria, but also may enhance uptake of unwanted lead (Chapter 2).

Heaney believes there is sufficient reason to suspect that most adults do not require supplemental vitamin D beyond age 22, when bone development is fairly complete. A combination of sunlight (15 minutes direct exposure daily) and dietary sources (mainly eggs, saltwater fish, and liver) provides adequate vitamin D for most adults. The exceptions are elderly people who spend much of their time indoors; people who live in climates where there is limited

* The inert, dietary source of vitamin D is vitamin D_2, as opposed to vitamin D_3 from sunlight. Vitamins D_2 and D_3 are together converted to 25 hydroxy (OH) vitamin D, which is the major circulating form of vitamin D. Under particular circumstances the parathyroid hormone signals the kidneys to convert 25 (OH) D to the active form of vitamin D, which is 1, 25 (OH) D.

sunshine; and people at risk to contracting tuberculosis (a recent finding of Dr. A.J. Crowle at the University of Colorado Health Sciences Center in Denver). For adults who regularly consume milk and fortified breakfast cereals, and who also consume nutritional supplements fortified with vitamin D, there is serious risk of heart disease from getting more vitamin D than is required for health (See Appendix D). Thus, for the purpose of limiting vitamin D intake while preparing for IV-C therapy, it is recommended that red meats and fortified breakfast cereals be consumed in moderation, that vitamin D supplements be avoided altogether, and that cultured milk products be substituted for whole milk.*

Dietary Inconsistencies of Calcium and/or Phosphorous: A dietary excess of calcium (1.5 grams or more, daily) has long been known to be a cause of calciuria. A dietary deficiency of calcium (0.5 gram or less, daily) may also be a cause of calciuria. A partial explanation can be found in the works of Chausmer, et al.[45] and Borle,[46] who demonstrated that a low-calcium diet has the greatest stimulating effect on the parathyroid hormone. Parathyroid hormone is released to conserve body stores of calcium, which stimulates the kidneys to convert vitamin D to active vitamin D, in turn encouraging a higher rate of absorption of dietary calcium. For some unknown reason, in the process of stimulating the kidneys there is also a decrease in the tubular reabsorption of calcium, promoting calciuria. The remedy requires an increase of dietary calcium to at least satisfy the RDA. The recommendation for calcium, established earlier for the purpose of administering IV-C, is 1 gram per day.

Heaney related calciuria to a deficiency of phosphate in the diet and/or an imbalance of calcium and phosphorous. He explained that the body requires calcium and phosphorous in a 1:1 ratio—approximately 800 mg per day each. A diet that exemplifies an imbalance in the calcium: phosphorous ratio is characterized mainly by a diet restricted of dairy foods, which tend to possess a balancing influence, and a diet restricted of fish, red meats, and eggs, which are all excellent sources of phosphorous. This profile, in particular, characterizes many vegetarians. Inclusion of cultured dairy products in the diets of these people, as a balanced source of calcium and phosphorous, is important to minimize their risk of oxaluria.

Either a dietary excess or deficiency of phosphate may alter the absorption and excretion of calcium.[47] Either may stimulate the parathyroid hormone independently of the amount of dietary calcium, resulting in calciuria.

---

* Data from the National Health Survey, (Series ll, Number 227, March 1983) shows a direct relationship between total serum cholesterol (TSC) and the serum level of calcium. This was an unexpected finding, and doctors who assessed the data suggested it was not related to dietary calcium, or to abnormal calcium homeostasis. Rather, they believed it reflected the calcium component of lipoproteins responsible for the rise in TSC. The finding, however, is consistent with the hypothesis that vitamin D excess is an important underlying cause of TSC, as well as arterial disease, in which calcium serves to complicate the lesion. In support of this concept, *The Merck Manual* (page 593, 14th edition) states that an elevated serum calcium (12 to 16 mg/100 ml) is a constant finding when toxic symptoms of vitamin D occur. Can not one logically assume, therefore, that a vitamin D level that is less than the recognized level where toxicity is acknowledged, may cause certain subtle changes in biochemistry, including a slight elevation in serum calcium? If so, then the direct relationship between an elevated TSC and the serum calcium level among the 20,000 participants in the National Health Survey may reflect a dietary excess of vitamin D, making this discussion all the more important.

A low-phosphorous diet, which usually occurs in malnutrition and/or when the individual is excluding dairy foods, fish, red meats, and eggs from his diet, has the gravest consequence. When the diet contains an excess of phosphate relative to dietary calcium, such as may occur among those people who are marginal consumers of dairy products, and who consume more than two high-phosphate soft drinks daily, a high urine phosphate may occur as well as calciuria. The solution would be to eliminate soft drinks from the patient's diet, and to encourage consumption of more cultured dairy products.

While dietary calcium is needed each day in greater amounts than previously believed essential,* the healthy body continually eliminates endogenous calcium, either through the urine or intestines (originating mostly from digestive secretions and sloughed off mucosal cells). In this manner the average healthy person excretes an average of 350 mg daily; 200 mg per 24 hours via the urine, and 150 mg through the intestines.

Dietary phytates from whole grains aid in preventing hypercalciuria by binding with intestinal, endogenous calcium and promoting its excretion. (Phytates also bind with exogenous calcium, thereby accounting in part for the high daily requirement for calcium to attain a positive calcium balance.) Dietary phosphorous is a limiting factor. When phosphorous and whole grains are adequate in the diet, the amount of endogenous-source calcium excreted through the intestines rises from 150 mg to about 200 mg at the expense of urine calcium. Thus, there exists an inverse relationship between dietary phosphorous and calcium, and urine calcium. A diet sufficiently rich in fiber, phosphorous, and calcium prevents calciuria; whereas, a diet that is deficient of phosphorous, or deficient of phosphorous relative to calcium and fiber, prompts a decrease in the amount of calcium lost through the intestines while promoting calciuria.

The need for maintaining the relative relationship between dietary calcium and phosphorous has become one of the arguments against calcium supplements as the practice relates to preparing the patient for IV-C. It is also a reason why cultured milk products are preferred as a source of calcium and phosphorous, and a reason why the recommended daily intake of total calcium, prior to IV-C, is limited to 1 gram total, including whatever may be contributed from hard water sources. A diet that provides just the right balance of phosphorous and calcium, and includes whole grains, promotes a greater excretion of intestinal calcium with a simultaneous reduction in urine calcium. Cultured dairy products, which are excellent sources of calcium and phosphorous (as well as magnesium) and contain lesser amounts of supplemental vitamin D than whole milk, are necessary to this end, to protect against kidney stones.

Dr. Heaney states that excesses of sodium chloride (table salt) and caffeine represent additional factors that tend to increase urine calcium, and may therefore contribute to calciuria. His disclosure provides further reason for moderating the intake of table salt (Kurtz, et al. showed that various other sodium salts actually cause a decrease in calciuria, whereas sodium chloride promotes calciuria). Heaney recommends reducing the patient's intake of tea, coffee, and soft drinks before and immediately following IV-C.

---

* The connection between calcium metabolism and the development of arteriosclerosis and hypertension has been studied extensively during the last few years. Calcium, it seems, has another influence than what was previously believed. A positive calcium balance by a high dietary intake tends to reduce the risk of high blood pressure, which may be related to a reduction in PTH secretion.

High Protein Diets and Protein Deficiency: Protein excess and protein deficiency alike contribute in different ways to an imbalance of calcium and phosphorous, thereby promoting calciuria. Calciuria caused by a low phosphorous intake is a feature of protein deficiency. At the other extreme, a diet high in animal- source protein (in excess of 100 grams of total protein daily) is usually consumed at the expense of phytate-containing whole grains, which are normally required to enhance the gastrointestinal excretion of endogenous calcium. As a consequence, the endogenous calcium that normally exits the body via the intestines, exits the body as calciuria. There are other factors that may account for the protein link with hypercalciuria: the sodium and phosphate content of a high-protein diet; the diuretic and glomerular filtration-stimulating effect of protein metabolites; and the acid ash content of protein diets, which may cause a bone resorption of calcium.   Additionally, as previously explained elsewhere, an excessive amount of animal-source protein usually brings with it an excess of vitamin D—a further cause of calciuria. Through one or any combination of these mechanisms calciuria may result from extremes of high and low protein intake.

Solution for Preventing, or Reducing Calciuria

- Restrict vitamin D intake, keeping it below 400 IU. This is accomplished most easily by following the protein recommendation, by avoiding whole milk, and by disallowing vitamin D supplements.

- Steer patient away from a high protein diet of 100 g or more daily. The ideal is 50-75 g per day, with at least 25, but not more than 35, of those grams coming from animal sources.

- Maintain phosphorous intake to keep pace with calcium intake. The minimum for both is 800 mg daily; ideally about 1 gram. Cultured dairy foods ideally supply phosphorous and calcium in a 1:1 ratio, and in adequate quantities with a minimum of vitamin D.

- Restrict caffeine (tea, coffee, cola).

- Restrict visible sodium chloride intake, such as table salt, salted french fries, and salted nuts. (It's the chloride in combination with sodium [not sodium *per se*] that is most responsible for the hypercalciuria that is commonplace among heavy users of table salt.)

Uricosuria and Hyperuricosuria Significantly Promote Uric Acid, Calcium Oxalate, or Cystine Stones
Predictors of Uricosuria
- Extreme urine acidity
- Hyperuricemia* (see note on following page)
- Gout* (see note on following page)
- Nondifferentiated arthritis
- Megadose vitamin C without consideration of other predictors
- High consumption of aspirin
- Lead poisoning* (see note on following page)
- Excessive consumption of purine-rich foods
- Alcoholism, or excessive alcohol consumption

- Obesity
- A diet lacking in vitamin B$_3$ (whole grains, seeds, peas, and beans)
- Excessive intake of animal protein/high acid ash diet

Urine Acidity: The appearance of uric acid in the urine is a serious concern for the doctor planning to administer IV-C, especially when the patient has a history of stone disease. Hyperuricosuria, along with high urine sodium, increases the risk of stones by affecting the inhibitors of calcium oxalate formation. It also lowers the pH, in turn enhancing development of uric acid-mediated stones. Either of these changes alone enhances the risk of stone development, but when hyperuricosuria and extreme acidity occur in the same patient, the risk is even greater. Coe and Parks,[48] studying stone formers, found that critical urine pH was 5.5; any additional acidity promoted stones, while any pH reading higher than this was preventive. The cause of extremely acid urine, according to Pak, can often be credited to a diet high in animal protein. These figures have been correlated worldwide.[49]

Hyperuricemia, Gout, and Arthritis: Under healthful conditions, uric acid is a harmless end product of purine metabolism. It is filtered by the kidneys and excreted in the urine, causing uricosuria. However, in instances of abnormal purine metabolism contributed from animal protein, hyperuricemia may ensue in varying degrees, highlighted by a diminished renal clearance. The blood level of uric acid must reach a very high level before the patient experiences painful gout or gouty arthritis. In most situations, however, there is only a slight or moderate rise in blood uric acid and the patient is without symptoms. This lack of pain can present an obstacle to the doctor who wishes to administer IV-C, since uricosuria may be present beforehand without suspicion. By the same token, a patient who complains of arthritic-like pain, but who has not been diagnosed as having arthritis, should not be given IV-C until tested for gout and hyperuricosuria.

Megadose Vitamin C: Reflecting on Elliott's study (Chapter 5) of the effect of megadose vitamin C (3 g/day) on serum constituents in healthy adults, a significant drop in the blood uric acid was noted for the study group as a whole following a 12-week period. The same observation was made for the group with normal baseline readings as for the group who showed elevated readings on the pretest analysis. The drop in serum level was accounted for by a rise in the average daily urinary excretion rate of uric acid in the total group.

Berger, et al.,[50] was first to report this relationship. He suggested that vitamin C competes with uric acid for renal tubular reabsorption. Through this mechanism, he believes, when megadose vitamin C is administered to a patient with an elevated level of blood uric acid, the kidneys tend to retain vitamin C and excrete uric acid. His conclusion was based upon his own observations, and the work of Gershon and Fox[51] who noted two years earlier that another weak acid, nicotinic acid (vitamin B$_3$), may likewise serve to modify renal clearance of uric acid, promoting a similar increase in uricosuria. (This finding is important, and will soon be covered.)

Stein and Fox,[52] studying the effect of vitamin C therapy on the uric acid of patients with symptomatic and asymptomatic hyperuricemia, revealed

---

* Gout and hyperuricemia are not necessarily associated with hyperuricosuria. Quite the contrary, either condition may develop with notable hypouricosuria. Lead poisoning is nearly always associated with hypouricosuria. It's inclusion here is important only when the patient is undergoing therapy for hyperuricemia, which develops in lead poisoning due to a disturbance in the tubular secretion of uric acid.

that vitamin C is corrective of a problem associated with hyperuricemia. It lowers the blood level of uric acid by restoring renal clearance, but the increase in uricosuria that ensues may cause the patient to be at increased risk to kidney stones (although urate stones have not been reported in the literature as a consequence of taking vitamin C). Looking more closely, Stein's group noted that the degree of uricosuria was dose-related. They observed no effect up to two grams of vitamin C per day, then uricosuria increased 200 percent on four grams within the same time period. While it is important to somehow rid the body of uric acid while reducing the blood content, the potential risk of kidney stones that follows is nevertheless disturbing, even though stones have never been reported via this scenario. Fortunately, there are ways of adjusting the patient's lifestyle before IV-C that will significantly reduce that potential.

Use of Aspirin: Elliott[53] was first to observe that aspirin prevented the uricosuric response to megadose vitamin C. Spector,[54] and Loh, et al.[55] agreed that small-dose acetylsalicylic acid apparently modulated the competitive action for tubular reabsorption of uric acid and vitamin C. Aspirin is currently being prescribed for this purpose. However, Myers[56] explains, when too large a dose is administered, aspirin may in some manner amplify the stone-promoting effect of uricosuria, indicating that aspirin may also present an undetermined risk. Thus, while the use of aspirin may be acceptable to the experienced practitioner, the potential risk when used in conjunction with IV-C suggests there is need for a continued investigation of the roles that nutrition and lifestyle play in the onset and prevention of gout, hyperuricosuria, and kidney stones. The objective here is to help overcome hidden pitfalls and put as many odds in the doctor's favor as possible before administering IV-C.

An excellent review of the effect lifestyle has on the development of gout and hyperuricosuria has been written by J. T. Scott.[57] He explains that obesity, excessive alcohol intake, and a diet high in purine-rich foods* all contribute strongly to gout. All of these lifestyle factors affect normal liver function, and thereby alter the course of purine metabolism. The risk from alcohol becomes greatest when consumed as homemade whiskey, since homemade whiskey is quite often a source of lead poisoning, and gout is a classic symptom of lead poisoning. Yet, hyperuricemia, gout, and lead poisoning are not necessarily associated with hyperuricosuria. Hyperuricemia and gout may develop due to deficient renal excretion of uric acid, in which case hypouricosuria is evident rather than the expected hyperuricosuria.

It is noteworthy that high concentrations of alcohol (enough to cause intoxication) produce an elevation of lactic acid in the blood. In turn, lactic acid inhibits the excretion of uric acid, just as aspirin, vitamin C, and vitamin B₃ do.† Unlike vitamins B₃ and C, however, the effect of alcohol-generated

---

* Foods rich in purine include organ meats, particularly sweetbreads, and fish roe. Foods which contribute moderately to purine nitrogen include all red meat and meat extracts, poultry, fish, eggs, and legumes. When consumed heavily, beer may also serve as a high purine food.

† Lactic acid from healthful foods, such as cultured milk products and sauerkraut, does have a beneficial effect, however slight. From healthy sources it serves to modulate the rate at which uric acid appears in the urine. This does not occur when derived from alcohol. Blood lactic acid, from foods and anaerobic energy production, is converted in the kidney to citrate and excreted in the urine, where it raises the pH above 5.5 and becomes one of the major inhibitors of stone development (discussed later in this chapter under its own heading).

lactic acid is not good. Alcohol unnecessarily and unnaturally raises the blood level of uric acid in people who might otherwise show a normal reading, setting the stage for hyperuricosuria and unusual risk during IV-C. On the other hand, one might expect to reap benefits from placing hyperuricemic individuals on lactic acid-producing foods prior to IV-C.

Scott believes that abstinence from alcohol and fasting can be an effective means of reducing the risk of hyperuricosuria prior to IV-C. There is evidence that the benefit to be derived from these measures is most pronounced when the patient is both obese and a heavy drinker.

Obesity: Further evidence of the association of lifestyle with gout, uricosuria, and asymptomatic hyperuricemia, was indirectly assessed from data from NHANES I. From the 20,000 people examined, it was determined that the uric acid concentration of blood was related directly and independently to obesity, measured in terms of body mass index (BMI) and alcohol consumption. When foods high in purine (limited to glandular meats, meat extracts, poultry, fish, and legumes in this study) were assessed for the group as a whole, there was no consistent association between purine intake and serum urate levels. The association became evident only when combined with other variables, such as BMI and alcohol consumption.

While high-purine foods contributed 0.5 to 1 gram urate per day in these people, it seems evident that the average healthy person has a means of coping with dietary purine. Only people who simultaneously engaged in other lifestyle practices that adversely affected health were inclined to develop hyperuricemia and hyperuricosuria.

A further review of the NHANES I data showed that for progressively higher levels of serum urate, the SGOT enzyme concentrations were significantly higher. Because both alcohol ingestion and SGOT served independently to affect serum urate levels, it was proposed that subtle hepatic inflammation resulting from poor lifestyle practices indicates a healthy liver is required for normal purine metabolism.

Vitamin B$_3$: The idea of liver involvement in hyperuricemia suggests that we again look at the work of Gershon and Fox. In their study of nicotinic acid, they had demonstrated that vitamin B$_3$ inhibited renal clearance of uric acid. Their evidence suggested also that vitamin B$_3$ prevents a further increase in blood uric acid, supporting the concept that a healthy liver is required for normal purine metabolism, and that dietary changes or supplemental vitamin B$_3$ may be important to this. (Some foods high in vitamin B$_3$: whole grains, seeds, peas and beans, liver, brewer's yeast.) While the RDA for B$_3$ is 13 to 19 mg, the higher dosage employed by Gershon and Fox (50 mg) suggests the practical approach to supplementation is prescription of a good B-complex. The symptoms of facial flushing that are a common side effect, due to its vasodilating action, usually do not occur before the dosage reaches 100 mg daily. Additionally, a dosage higher than 50 mg is contraindicated in patients with gout and hyperuricemia. By prescribing a daily B-complex vitamin containing 50 mg vitamin B$_3$ the doctor will be able to satisfy all additional requirements for the B vitamins. The body seems to handle a complete source of the B vitamins better than a selection of individual B vitamins, all of which (as a complex) are known to contribute to improved liver function.

Proteinuria and Excessive Protein Intake: This chapter has highlighted several mechanisms by which an excessive intake of animal source protein may serve to promote kidney stones, taking the stand that the patient's diet should be corrected accordingly before administering IV-C. Inconsistencies

may lead to calciuria (a high-acid ash diet such as results from excessive protein intake promotes calciuria because of the necessity for buffering the organic
acids), oxaluria, and (rarely) proteinuria.

As explained in Chapter 5, there are two main forms of proteinuria:
glomerular and tubular. Glomerular proteinuria does not occur from occasional
excesses of dietary protein, as is often assumed. Quite the contrary, proteinuria
is usually an indication of a glomerular disease, which is more likely to lead to
development of renal insufficiency than tubular proteinuria. The only time a
high-protein diet might be a cause of glomerular proteinuria is in a patient
with reduced renal mass. Glomerulosclerosis may develop in these patients
following years of excessive protein intake, but in such cases switching to a low-
protein diet does nothing to correct the patient's proteinuria. Tubular proteinuria, on the other hand, is especially a feature of nephrotoxicity, in which case
the urine creatinine is usually elevated. If the urine creatinine is normal, then
the proteinuria may be reflective of altered kidney function, however subtle,
due to mercury poisoning. To distinguish this, Japanese researchers have suggested determining the ratio of urine Beta-2 Microglobulin (BMG) to urine albumin. A higher ratio than normal would suggest some degree of renal damage
from chronic mercury toxicity in an otherwise healthy person, and the patient
should be excluded as a candidate for IV-C.

Solution for Prevention of Uricosuria

- IV-C and megadose oral vitamin C should not be administered without considering the patient's lifestyle, and medical circumstances
  that may relate to uricosuria.

- For extreme hyperuricosuria doctors commonly prescribe sodium
  bicarbonate, sodium ascorbate, and citrate to maintain the pH above
  6. Both prescription and dietary sources of citrate will be discussed.

- Purine-rich foods should be excluded from the patient's diet.

- The patient should consume foods high in vitamin B3. Nicotinic acid
  improves purine metabolism and modulates renal clearance of uric
  acid.

- With exception of patients who present with gout and hyperuricemia
  (conditions for the findings of Gershon and Fox suggest that mega-
  niacin therapy, 130 to 190 mg daily, or more, is contraindicated), the
  patient's diet should be supplemented daily with up to, but not exceeding 50 mg vitamin B3.

- The patient should drink plenty of water: an increase in urine volume
  will lower supersaturation, raise urine pH, and aid in excretion rate
  of sodium and uric acid.

- Avoid aspirin to counter hyperuricosuria. Utilize changes in nutrition
  and lifestyle instead, which has the same advantage of effectiveness
  as aspirin without risking the potential for development of stones due
  to an incorrect dosage.

- The patient should consume sauerkraut and cultured milk products. The lactic acid derived from these foods, however slight, aids vitamin B3 in modulating renal clearance of uric acid, if only minimally, while also contributing to urine citrate. This helps to keep the pH above 5.5 and thereby serves as a stone inhibitor.

- Abstention from alcohol is recommended, especially a few days before and following IV-C. In some people, alcohol may contribute to hepatic inflammation and altered purine metabolism, becoming a major potential cause of hyperuricemia. Be wary if the patient is suspected of being an alcoholic. Warn the family of the danger and seek everyone's cooperation. Hospitalization or confinement may be required. If the patient habitually consumes homemade whiskey, thereby causing lead poisoning, hyperuricemia may develop in the absence of uricosuria (due to a disturbance in the tubular excretion of uric acid).

- If obese: if time allows, and if the patient is hyperuricemic, enter the patient in a weight loss program. If the time factor is crucial, gain the patient's cooperation in participating in other lifestyle changes that are reasonable and attainable beforehand.

- Follow previous guidelines for control of urine oxalate and calcium, and for factors discussed previously under Category 1.

- In patients who are experiencing uricosuria from a high generation of uric acid due to purine break-down, and who do not respond to the above steps, Dr. Fellström recommends treating with the hypoxanthine oxidase inhibitor, allopurinol.

RISK CATEGORY 3: URINARY AGENTS THAT SERVE AS STONE INHIBITORS, THE LACK OF WHICH CONTRIBUTE TO STONE DEVELOPMENT

Predictors of a Deficiency of Urinary Stone Inhibition
- Diet lacking in citrate and potassium-rich foods.
- Extremely acid urine
- Dietary deficiency of magnesium
- Diet lacking in cultured milk products* (see note on following page)
- Diet lacking in iron or chromium
- Dietary excess of animal protein
- Physical inactivity
- Protein deficiency* (see note on following page)
- Vitamin C deficiency* (see note on following page)
- Dietary deficiency of phosphorous
- A cloudy, particulate urine
- Amino acid imbalance (dietary deficiency of glutamic acid and/or alanine)
- Diet lacking in vitamin B6.* (see note on following page)

Again, Fellström's rule for stone development states: The propensity for crystal formation, growth, and aggregation depends on the balance between urinary supersaturation and inhibitory activity. To satisfy this requirement for prevention of stones, Pak had established three criteria: 1) urine pH must be neither unusually acid nor alkaline; 2) the urine supersaturation of stone-forming agents must be kept low; and 3) the urinary excretion of stone inhibitors must be sufficient to inhibit crystallization and aggregation of stone-forming salts.

In accord with Robertson's assessment of risk, as presented immediately before the discussion of Risk Category 1, the significance of a deficiency of stone inhibitors is a risk described as being only slightly less than the risk due to an increase in urine oxalate, and more significant than urine pH. Stone inhibitors are small molecular weight substances, such as citrate and pyrophosphate, and macromolecular weight substances, such as glycosaminoglycans. In addition to the action of stone inhibitors, there are nutrients that support this action, such as iron, magnesium, chromium, and vitamin B_6.

Citrate: Citrate in the urine is perhaps the best understood stone inhibitor. Its beneficial function can be credited to two primary actions: Pak noted its ability to lower the saturation of urine through formation of soluble complexes of calcium/citrate/oxalate, or calcium/citrate/phosphate; and Meyer and Thomas[58] report that citrate serves as a chemical buffer to keep the urine pH from extreme acidity. In fact, the researchers contend that the excretion of citrate and the level of plasma citrate are good indicators of the acid-base status of the individual. The opposite may also be true. Extreme acidity (pH 5.0, or less) would suggest that the patient's urine is deficient of citrate, and without adequate urine citrate the acid-base balance is upset, giving rise to stone development.

Lemons, limes, and oranges are the primary sources of dietary citrate. These may be supplemented through the diet, by use of products such as 100 percent pure lemon juice concentrate. The frozen brands that contain only water, lemon juice concentrate, and lemon oil are recommended because they are as close to natural as can be found, and are prepared without preservatives. Instruct patients to read labels when grocery shopping.

Lemons and lemon concentrate, in addition to being an excellent source of citrate, are one of the better sources of potassium. Potassium, as explained by Chulkaratana,[59] has a highly positive influence on the action of citrate in rendering calcium oxalate soluble. His explanation largely accounts for the popular use among doctors of potassium citrate, as a source of alkali for preventing stones and correcting extreme acidity of urine. Pak reports there is something unique about potassium preparation versus sodium preparation. He has noted that sodium promotes calcium stones. Even sodium bicarbonate does this in some people, while potassium citrate has a preventive action. Thus, it would seem advisable to instruct the patient to add a squeeze of lemon to drinking water, or a tablespoon of lemon concentrate per quart of water, a week or two before and after the IV-C.

Miller, et al.,[60] determined that an excess of citrate can cause extreme alkalinity and thereby promote the development of calcium phosphate stones. His group further determined that the addition of supplemental magnesium prevented this from happening. Thus, with respect to IV-C, it is believed important to supplement the patient's diet beforehand with at least 100 mg

---

* These predictors, while hypothetically of value, can not be supported by solid evidence as being reliable predictors of deficiency of urinary stone inhibition. They are nevertheless included here because each is included in other aspects of the **IV-C Mercury Tox Program**, which makes these steps of value even if the effect in this category is minimal.

magnesium daily.   The patient should also be instructed to include high
magnesium food sources, such as whole grains, in the diet. An additional rationale for magnesium is given later under the heading <u>Magnesium and Vitamin
B</u>6.

Dietary sources of citrate other than citrus fruits are derived from
high-lactate foods, such as cultured milk products (cottage cheese, yogurt, and
buttermilk) and fermented foods, such as sauerkraut. The lactic acid derived
from these foods, however slight, is converted in the kidneys to citrate and excreted in the urine. Foods that support the action of citrate are those high in
iron and chromium.

Meyer and Thomas found that a 1:1 ratio of a high molecular weight
complex of iron and citric acid was even more effective on stone inhibition than
citrate acting alone. In fact, the ratio of iron to citric acid in urine determined
the extent of the effectiveness of the calcium/citrate/oxalate complex. The
lower ratio (1:1) effectively inhibited stone development even when the pH
was as low as 5.0; whereas an unbalanced ratio was less effective and reinforced
the importance of maintaining urine pH at about 6, or just below neutral.
Chromium also enhanced the action of citric acid, helping to maintain the
acid-base balance of urine. Traces of chromium proved to be an effective inhibitor even when citric acid was absent, or markedly reduced. In this case it
worked best at pH 7.4. Thus, supplementation of iron in addition to citrate may
be important to patients whose urine is extremely acid, as is supplementation of
chromium and citrate in those people who have an extremely alkaline urine.

On the other hand, a diet that is exceptionally high in animal protein
(over 100 grams per day) may have a depressant effect on urine citrate. Research by Tschope, et al.,[61] suggests that such a diet serves to depress urine citrate production and effectiveness. In contrast, he reports that a low-protein
diet of approximately half this amount (he used 57 grams daily) improves the
output of urine citrate and restores its inhibitory role. Tschope credits the reduction of effectiveness of citrate to a rise in the serum levels of uric acid,
glycine, and methionine. An increase in these three, as a consequence of excessive protein intake, is known to reduce the effectiveness of citrate, with or
without a change in the quantity of urine citrate. Tschope believes the protein
excess causes an upset of the acid-base balance, perhaps because an overabun-
dance of animal protein favors aerobic rather than anaerobic metabolism,
thereby decreasing lactic acid output. In contrast, a low protein diet favors
anaerobic over aerobic metabolism, causing a rise in the serum level of lactic
acid. The kidneys, in turn, convert lactic acid to plasma and urine citrate,
which aids in stabilizing the acid-base balance. A further examination of the
process of anaerobic glycolysis suggests that a portion of urine citrate can also be
credited to regular and sustained muscular exertion.

According to Hermansen and Vaage,[62] although 75 percent of the lactate produced during maximal exercise is resynthesized to muscle glycogen, 10
percent or better is deposited in the blood stream. This amount of lactic acid,
however small, is available for conversion by the kidneys to citrate and excreted in the urine, supporting the belief that the habit of regular physical exertion, coupled with adequate fluid replacement, is a factor in maintaining the
acid-base balance, and thereby of benefit in the overall program for preventing
stones.

<u>Pyrophosphate:</u> Pyrophosphate, similarly to citrate, is a small
molecular weight substance that serves as a stone inhibitor. Unlike citrate,
however, very little is known about its origin, although pyrophosphate in the

urine has recently been credited to dietary practices. Suphakarn, et al.,[63] studied the effect of pumpkin seeds on the tendency toward stone development among malnourished, high-risk children of Thailand. He noted that pumpkin seeds provided a rich and inexpensive source of phosphorous and potassium (necessary to these people, who are much too poor to afford meat and eggs as their primary sources of protein and phosphorous). Following 4 days of dietary supplementation of 60 mg phosphorous per kg body weight per day (the equivalent of 13 ounces roasted seeds daily for a 150 lb adult), the researchers noted several significant and healthful changes. They noted an increase in urine potassium and glycosaminoglycans, and a threefold increase in urinary pyrophosphate (measured using an enzymatic method that they believed to be most accurate). This was very important, as previous studies using other methods of detection had not demonstrated a change of this magnitude for pyrophosphate. The increase in glycosaminoglycans and potassium was a pleasant surprise also, indicating that pumpkin seeds, as a single dietary source, had the potential to improve directly and indirectly the urine's capacity to inhibit stones.

In addition to the observed response to pumpkin seeds, the researchers noted also a significant reduction in urine calcium, as was previously reported by other researchers. Their observation helps to explain the association of a high urine pyrophosphate and the lesser tendency toward stone development. The corresponding reduction of urine calcium could reflect the influence that the high phosphorous content of pumpkin seeds has on active vitamin D, which is known to be suppressed by an adequate intake of phosphorous. A positive change first became obvious in the urine's appearance, which was grossly cloudy before the pumpkin seeds were administered, and clear afterwards. The combination of effects was not only dramatic, but encouraging for those doctors who desire to administer IV-C safely.

While doctors practicing in the U.S. and other high-tech countries are less likely to see patients who are as severely deficient of phosphorous, potassium, and protein, as the children seen by doctors in Thailand, it is still not unusual to encounter patients who, due to their illnesses, present with some degree of malnutrition. The evidence indicates these people may benefit from pumpkin seed supplementation just as the children of Thailand. However, the dosage should be somewhat smaller than what was administered to the Thai children—not to exceed the nutritional requirement for phosphorous, especially since pumpkin seeds are such a poor source of calcium. In the average doctor/patient encounter, assuming the patient is following the previous recommendation of 50-57 grams of protein and three servings of cultured dairy foods daily, it is not likely that pumpkin seeds would be necessary, except in rare instances. When the situation warrants, however, it's reassuring to know that pumpkin seeds are relatively inexpensive and readily available in most health food stores. The equivalent of 1 to 2 ounces daily of roasted pumpkin seeds should be more than adequate for the average 150 lb adult.

Glycosaminoglycans: Glycosaminoglycans are long-chain, high molecular weight polymers. Due to their physicochemical property of extreme viscosity and adhesiveness, they help provide a stable environment for tissues. According to Cameron,[64] hyaluronic acid is the principal glycosaminoglycan, along with varieties of chondroitin (mucopolysaccharides found in connective tissues, especially cartilage, and in the cornea). In the former, which serves to contain cell proliferation, the cellular release of the enzyme hyaluronidase is essential to initiate and sustain cell division. Cameron believes the control of this mechanism—important to the onset of cancer, scurvy, and collagen diseases as well—is a function of vitamin C. Vitamin C protects by limiting the activity of hyaluronidase. When adequately provided in the diet, vitamin C aids to control cell proliferation and, by protecting cellular glycosaminoglycans from uncontrolled destruction, serves to maintain the integrity of cell structure. While this proposed mechanism is speculative and unproven, it implies that a deficiency of vitamin C would contribute to a deficiency of urine glycosaminoglycans; whereas, when dietary vitamin C is sufficient urinary glycosaminoglycans are more apt to be plentiful. Through this indirect action megadose vitamin C may have a role in maintaining the stone inhibitory activity of urine.

Magnesium and Vitamin B$_6$ were studied by Gershoff and Prien.[65] Their classic report states that magnesium salts have been used effectively, since the early part of the century, to prevent urinary stones. This is surprising to those who fear the effect of urine calcium, since magnesium is known to promote calciuria.[66] Only in recent years, they report, has the protective mechanism been understood. A group of German investigators, in 1964, showed that hard water, high in magnesium, increased the colloid stability of urine irrespective of calciuria.[67] Hammarsten,[68] in 1956, reported that dietary magnesium decreased urine oxalate, and that along with vitamin B$_6$, it offered protection when citrate was deficient.[69] (Miller, as you recall, reported also that magnesium prevented calcium phosphate stones in an extremely alkaline medium, when dietary citrate was excessive.)

As has been previously discussed, a low urine citrate may be the simple consequence of a diet exceptionally rich in animal protein. In their own study of 60 patients, in which Gershoff and Prien put these concepts to practice, it was determined that daily oral supplements of 100 mg magnesium oxide and 10 mg pyridoxine (vitamin B$_6$) successfully held calcium oxalate in solution and prevented further stone development. Fellström's research team has found through extensive clinical experience that magnesium oxide is poorly absorbed; whereas, magnesium hydroxide is absorbed much more easily and is excreted in the urine while it exerts its effect. As a prophylactic measure, Fellström has found that a dosage of 200 to 400 mg magnesium hydroxide is required. Furthermore, as noted by Gershoff and Andrus, a synergistic effect on stone inhibition occurs in people who regularly include magnesium, vitamin B$_6$, and a source of citrate in their diets.

An Imbalance of Amino Acids with Vitamin B$_6$ Deficiency: A novel explanation has recently been proposed to show how either a low protein diet, a diet of imbalanced amino acids, and/or a deficiency of vitamin B$_6$ contribute toward reducing the stone-inhibiting capability of urine. It began with McGeown,[70] who was first to test the stone inhibitory capabilities of each amino acid. By adding glutamic acid to the food of rats inclined to form stones, he demonstrated a marked reduction in the incidence of stone formation. McGeown then demonstrated a similar finding among patients with idiopathic stone disease, who have lower than normal amounts of urine amino acids.[71] Glutamic acid, he concluded, was a significant inhibitor of stones. Chow,[72] several years later, reported the same observation with alanine. A group of four Israeli scientists was then able to complete the explanation.

Azoury, et al.,[73] determined that the source of urinary L-glutamic acid was not from diet alone. It was also the consequence of enzymatic action on alanine and L-aspartic acid. The group determined that the enzyme UGOT (plus cofactors) was required to convert L-aspartic acid to L-glutamic acid, while

UGPT, a related enzyme (plus cofactors), converted urinary alanine to L-glutamic acid. Through these sources, in addition to diet, they hypothesized that glutamic acid in normal urine served as an important stone inhibitor.[74] To test their hypothesis, they studied the UGOT and UGPT levels of normal people and compared the results with those of patients who were inclined to form stones. The control subjects, they found, expressed a range of 22 IU to 60 IU for both. The urine of patients who tended to form stones contained only 2 to 20 IU of UGOT and UGPT. They concluded that a deficiency of the enzymes interrupted conversion of the amino acids L-aspartic acid and alanine to L-glutamic acid, and thereby contributed to the tendency toward stone development, while normal readings placed the patient at very low risk of developing stones.

Commenting on the applicability of this information, Wright has stated that he believes his practice of performing a UGOT/UGPT analysis* prior to administering IV-C has contributed greatly to his excellent safety record when using IV-C. Those patients who exhibit a low reading are either denied access to IV-C or (among other nutritional and lifestyle considerations) are given an oral supplement of L-glutamic acid beforehand.

While Wright's approach does indeed solve the problem of deficiency of the urinary stone inhibitor—glutamic acid—it still leaves open the question of why some people do or don't have adequate UGOT and UGPT. A partial explanation is found by reexamining the work of Balcke, et al.

Balcke's group proposed that when the quantity of vitamin B_6 is sufficient, its active metabolite—pyridoxal-5-phosphate—serves to stimulate GOT enzyme activity, promoting conversion of glycine to glyoxylic acid and back to glycine. I believe it also contributes to the total UGOT enzyme activity required for maintaining an adequate, protective urine level of glutamic acid. When dietary vitamin B_6 is deficient, the GOT enzyme activity is deficient also, and is incapable of not only reversing the reaction from glyoxylic acid back to glycine, thereby promoting the formation of oxalate, but may also be a significant cause of the decreased level of UGOT noted in high-risk patients. In a supportive manner, a deficiency of folic acid and vitamin B_1 may also be responsible for the decrease in UGOT (just as in the formation of urine oxalate) and/or the decrease in UGPT noted in these same high-risk patients. It thus seems likely that a supplement of vitamin B_6, administered either orally prior to IV-C, or parenterally with IV-C; and concurrently with glutamic acid, would serve to increase the UGOT level and significantly reduce the patient's risk for stones. With respect to IV-C, reliance upon synergisim is the best approach to prevention.

Solution for Restoring Urinary Stone Inhibitors

- The diet must be adequate in citrate-rich foods like lemons, limes, oranges, and grapefruits. Lactate-rich foods are slight, indirect sources of citrate. They include sauerkraut and cultured milk products, such as cottage cheese, yogurt, buttermilk, and soft cheeses. Regular physical exertion may also provide an indirect source of citrates, through the lactic acid produced by anaerobic metabolism.

*If a laboratory that performs this test is not available in your area, you can contact the Meridian Valley Laboratories of Seattle, Washington. See Appendix E for address.

- A squeeze of lemon should be added to drinking water, or a tablespoon of lemon concentrate added to each quart of water. Lemon is the citrus fruit of choice because it also contains an ample quantity of potassium.

- If the urine is extremely and persistently acid, potassium citrate may be used as an alkalizing agent. This, however, should be a last resort, as it can make some people feel nauseated.

- Prescribe a dietary supplement of 100 mg magnesium. Magnesium will guard against the risk of extreme alkalinity due to an excess of citrate, and it will serve also as a potent stone inhibitor independently of citrate.

- For patients with an exceptionally low urine pH, supplement the diet with 20 mg ferrous iron daily, along with the suggestions mentioned previously. Take into account the warning in Chapter 2 that supplemental iron may mask an important symptom of mercurial poisoning, making it difficult afterwards to accurately assign credit for the patient's improvement. If the patient is a stone former, or at high risk for other reasons, Fellström recommends treating beforehand with orthophosphate.

- For patients with an exceptionally high urine pH, supplement the diet with 30 mcg chromium daily. You might also borrow a few suggestions from Risk Category 1, such as resorting to the ascorbic acid form of oral vitamin C, or a mixture of ascorbic acid and sodium ascorbate, although the benefit is only transient.

- Moderate total dietary protein (50 to 70 grams daily).

- If the patient is malnourished, and deficient of protein and phosphorous, supplement with 1 to 2 ounces per day of dry roasted pumpkin seeds, in addition to the other recommendations for protein, calcium, and phosphorous from Risk Categories 1, 2, and 3.

- If the total UGOT/UGPT level is below 22 IU, supplement orally with 1 gram glutamic acid daily.

- Supplement the diet with 10 to 50 mg vitamin B_6 per day, for low- and medium-risk individuals, and up to 300 mg per day if the recipient is a high-risk candidate. Parenteral vitamin B_6 may, as an alternative approach, be added to the IV-C infusion.

- Continue to adjust the patient's lifestyle until the urine is no longer cloudy.

The evidence presented in Chapters 5 and 6 indicates that the frightening aspects of megadose vitamin C are related not to vitamin C, but to a lack of doctor awareness of recognized and heretofore unrecognized contraindications for IV-C. Whatever the risk, it can be greatly minimized in nearly all patient situations through corrective lifestyle practices. To paraphrase the words of one researcher, when the truly important aspects of lifestyle are put

into practice they together exert a synergistic, protective effect. It is this concept upon which the patient questionnaire has been designed. The intent is to
provide an instrument for giving relative significance to medical history, and
for identifying lifestyle practices that predictably increase the risks. This
questionnaire is provided in Part III, Chapter 8.

A Summary of Risks and Solutions for Preventing Stones

By responding to the patient's medical history, and by making the
proper lifestyle adjustment before administering IV-C, one will have maximally minimized the risk for kidney stones. A safe and effective treatment
outcome will largely depend on your evaluation of the answers provided by the
patient questionnaire that relate to stone development. In general, a "yes" answer, or laboratory data that signals any of the following, would indicate increased risk. Any combination of danger signals would increase the risk still
further, requiring the doctor to either reject the patient as a candidate for IV-C,
or demand that the patient follow instructions closely before and following IV-
C.

High Risk Conditions

- Obesity (20% or more above ideal weight for age and height). This
  will be considered medium risk if other predictors of gout that follow
  are not apparent.
- Alcohol consumption (averaging two or more ounces per day of any
  type alcohol).
- Hyperuricemia (with or without symptoms of gout or gouty arthritis).
- Hyperuricosuria (demonstrated by observing uric acid crystals on
  urine microscopic examination).
- Calcium oxalate crystals (observed during urine microscopy).
- Urinary tract infection.
- Dehydration, highlighted by high urine saturation and extreme
  acidity (urine cloudy; pH 5.0 or less).
- Severe malnutrition, highlighted by a protein deficiency.

Medium Risk Conditions

- Extremely alkaline urine
- Proteinuria: While proteinuria is not accepted normally as a risk
  factor or risk indicator for stone formation, its presence may be an in-
  dicator of renal insufficiency (whether due to chronic mercury toxicity
  or otherwise) which must be looked into further before IV-C can be
  safely administered
- Unbalanced diet:
  - A daily intake of low-calcium, high-oxalate foods
  - A diet exceptionally high in animal protein, with total daily
    protein intake above 100 g
  - A diet exceptionally low in total protein and/or deficient of
    glutamic acid
  - A diet void of cultured milk products and high in whole milk
  - A diet low in citric acid and fermented foods (other than cul-
    tured milk)
  - A diet deficient of grains and foods high in the B vitamins
  - An excess of dietary sodium, especially as table salt (4,000 mg
    daily, or more)

- Consumption of one ounce (two drinks) of (any type) alcohol daily
- Heavy consumption (2 or more cups per day) of high caffeine beverages, such as coffee, tea, and cola
- A total UGOT/UGPT level of 22 IU or less
- Specifically, heavy dependence on cola beverages high in phosphate (2 or more colas per day)
- Physical inactivity
- Dependence upon foods high in refined sugar, void of chromium
- Habitual (daily) use of aspirin
- Excessive calcium supplementation, raising total daily calcium intake above 1000 mg

Minimum Lifestyle Behavioral Changes for all Patients, Regardless of Risk

For those patients with no history of renal insufficiency, gout, hyperuricemia, or uricosuria, who presently are free of a urinary tract infection, and who are presently not taking an antibiotic or an antibacterial for a urinary tract infection, the following list summarizes a minimum of lifestyle practices that should be followed at least 36 hours (unless otherwise specified) prior to and following IV-C:

- Have the patient drink 6-8 glasses of water daily. 2-3 glasses of this should be taken during the IV-C procedure, which generally takes from 2-1/2 to 3 hours. The patient won't have to be told more than once, as IV-C will make him quite thirsty.

- Restrict all alcohol.

- Add a squeeze of lemon to each glass of water, or take 1 tablespoon concentrated lemon juice the day before IV-C. Take an additional teaspoon of lemon juice during the IV-C, followed the next day by another tablespoon. Thereafter, for the next 30 days, the patient should become conscious of the need to include a squeeze of lemon daily, added either to salad or water.

- Restrict high oxalate foods, although only limited effects can be expected from such restriction (with exception of patients with enteric hyperoxaluria who may absorb 50% of the ingested oxalate), and limit medium-to-high oxalate foods:

High Oxalate Foods

- spinach
- beet greens
- rhubarb
- Swiss chard
- leaf tea
- instant coffee

Medium-to High Oxalate Foods

- chocolate
- cocoa
- strawberries
- red currents
- celery
- kale
- parsley
- haricot
- asparagus
- noncitrus fruit juices
- white wine
- nuts (especially peanuts)
- sorrel
- turnip greens
- mustard greens
- collard greens
- broccoli

(Unacceptable, high oxalate food sources have up to eight times more oxalic acid than calcium. Once the mercury issue has been resolved, or following an IV-C given for other reasons, the patient should be instructed to include a serving of cultured dairy foods for every serving of the above.

Acceptable, medium-to-high oxalate food sources, but ones which should be limited prior to IV-C, would include turnip, mustard, and collard greens; kale; and broccoli. These are oxalate-rich foods in which the calcium/oxalate ratio ranges from 2:1 to 42:1. Again, to limit oxalate absorption it is important to consume adequate calcium, preferably via cultured dairy foods.)

• Restrict all caffeine. Cola, tea, and coffee drinkers should find it acceptable to switch to caffeine-free herbal teas and natural, non-sweetened citrus juices.

• Restrict whole milk. Do, however, include 1 g dietary calcium daily, particularly from cultured dairy foods. As a guideline, 300 mg calcium equals 1-1/2 ounces of mozzarella cheese, 1 cup of yogurt, 2 cups of cottage cheese or 1 cup of broccoli. Have the patient cease taking calcium supplements.

• Supplement the patient's diet with a B-complex nutrient at least two days (and preferably a week) before and following IV-C. Continue thereafter as the situation dictates.

• Supplement the patient's diet with 100 mg magnesium daily, at least two days (and preferably a week) before and following IV-C.

• Moderate total protein intake at about 50-60 grams per day, two days before and two days following IV-C, while maintaining animal protein intake at about one-half this amount.

The minimum pre-IV-C testing should include the Patient's Medical History/Risk Analysis Questionnaire, and the Patient's Lifestyle Questionnaire. The patient will have also completed the Informed Consent. (Sample forms of all these can be found in Part III, Chapter 8.) The results of the patient questionnaires will serve as a directive for further testing. The minimum laboratory workup should include:

• Serum uric acid
• Routine urinalysis:
  - urine pH
  - urine microscopic
  - urine protein
• Total UGOT/UGPT determination
• 24-hour urine creatinine clearance
• Serum calcium and magnesium
• Urinary calcium, magnesium, sodium
• Urinary potassium, uric acid, oxalate, and citrate

The laboratory findings* may reveal facts about the patient's health that

---

* The protocol now being used for testing varies slightly from doctor to doctor. To illustrate these differences, a sample protocol was provided by the team of Robert Rowen, M.D., and Pat Hayes, R.N. (see Appendix E). They suggest screening for kidney function by determining the level of serum creatinine and blood urea nitrogen (BUN). IV-C is not given when the creatinine is above 1.6, or when BUN is over 30.

would require a reassessment of risk, and a more aggressive attitude toward lifestyle changes, perhaps in combination with drug therapy. For instance, the urine analysis of an otherwise normal patient may reveal an abnormal amount of bacteria in the absence of an active or a diagnosed urinary tract infection. This would then be correlated with the urine pH. If extremely alkaline, the doctor would follow the instructions at the conclusion of the discussion of Risk Category 1.

Suggested Lifestyle Behavioral Changes for Medium Risk Patients

The objective here is to improve the patient's lifestyle in a specific manner that would reduce the risk category from medium to low. Ideally, one would want to follow these instructions for 2 weeks before and following IV-C, rather than only a couple of days:

- Follow first the steps listed previously for the minimum lifestyle behavioral changes. Extend the period for following each and every recommendation from 2 days to 2 weeks before and following IV-C. This and other recommendations can be amended as need dictates.

- Adjust the dosage of the B vitamin supplement to fit the situation.

- If the patient is alcohol-dependent, or borders on alcohol dependence, the family's help will be needed to enforce the requirement of alcohol-restriction.

- Absolutely do not allow calcium supplements, or any dietary supplement that contains vitamin D. The restriction of calcium supplements would include calcium ascorbate. Calcium ascorbate as a source of vitamin C provides an excess of calcium (124 mg calcium/gram vitamin C, or 2,480 mg/20 grams), which adversely affects the treatment program.

- Restrict high purine foods: organ meats, including kidney, liver, and sweetbreads; and fish roe.

- While restriction of sodium isn't absolutely necessary, it would be helpful to limit dietary sodium (as table salt) to 2,000 mg daily.

- Supplement the diet with 750 mg glutamic acid daily.

- Have the patient limit consumption of sugary foods, especially those sweetened with refined sugar. These tend to raise the requirement for two trace minerals: chromium and magnesium. A chromium supplement should be used if the urine is extremely alkaline; iron if the urine is extremely acid. Monitor same weekly, two days before, and once on the day that IV-C is administered.

- Unless the patient is physically handicapped, it would be wise for him to engage in a daily walking program, or a comparable physical exertion program.

The laboratory testing should be tailored to fit the patient's specific risk. The patient should be clear of urinary tract infections before administering IV-C.

Suggested Protocol and Lifestyle Behavioral Changes for High Risk Patients
Normally, a patient who shows medium and high risk conditions, as discussed in Chapter 5, and who demonstrates a high risk lifestyle, is denied access to IV-C. The decision to administer IV-C, however, is the doctor's and patient's. To assist the doctor in assessing the risk analysis, obesity and excessive alcohol consumption represent a high risk situation only when either or both are combined with hyperuricemia, hyperuricosuria, extreme urine acidity or alkalinity, calciuria, or oxaluria, or any combination therewith. A simultaneous urinary tract infection adds to reasons for concern. Of course, the risk for stone development from lifestyle must be multiplied by the high or medium risk conditions discussed in Chapter 5. If the doctor and the patient together choose the IV-C treatment regimen (the doctor knowing full well that he's dealing with a high risk condition and a high risk lifestyle), it is vital to the expectation of a successful outcome that the full extent of modification of lifestyle be instituted before administering the intravenous infusion. Even then, in all likelihood, there remains a substantial risk. It's a matter of weighing the risk vs. the potential for benefit.

- Utilize the total programs previously outlined for **all patients** and for **medium risk patients**.

- Increase water intake to 3 quarts per day.

- If time permits at all, enter the patient in a weight control program that considers overall health needs, rather than a crash program of sudden weight loss.

- One possible option to negate dietary influence is to have the overweight person begin a fruit juice and water fast 36 hours before administering IV-C, continuing for 24-36 hours afterwards, while taking his prescribed dietary supplements and lemon juice concentrate.

- If time permits, enter a confirmed alcoholic patient in an alcohol rehabilitation program. Otherwise, it may be necessary to institutionalize the patient to monitor their behavior before and immediately following IV-C.

- Beyond the previously suggested supplement of B vitamins, include a daily vitamin/mineral supplement program that provides up to 50 mg vitamins B_6, B_1, and B_3 (the findings of Gershon and Fox suggests that a dosage greater than 50 mg is contraindicated in patients with gout and hyperuricemia), 0.4 mg folic acid, 30 mcg chromium, and 100 mg magnesium. A ferrous iron (20 mg) supplement should be considered, but only when the urine pH is extremely acid, as supplemental iron may mask the symptom of fatigue that associates with mercury poisoning. In those patients who present with poor absorption, the doctor may want to consider parenteral vitamin and mineral supplementation concurrently with the IV-C.

- If the pH of an extremely acid urine cannot be raised to pH 6.0 or above using the previously mentioned lifestyle practices, consider the use of potassium citrate. Consult with a urologist who has had experience with its use.

- Perform the minimum laboratory workup, plus whatever is decided upon with the consulting urologist. Appropriate tests may include the enzyme, G-6-PD, RBC fragility, serum and urine osmolality, total UGOT/UGPT level, serum creatinine, BUN or a kidney function profile, to include an IVP (intravenous pyelogram).

- Supplement with 1 gram daily of glutamic acid to start, and recheck UGOT/UGPT. Increase the dosage accordingly if indicated, or if necessary.

- In a calcium oxalate stone former (who is normally not considered a candidate for IV-C) the following rule should be strictly followed: Ascorbic acid (IV-C) should not be given unless it has been shown that the patient's oxalate excretion does not increase by the given (oral) amount of ascorbic acid. Furthermore, (it goes without saying) if kidney stones do develop while treating the patient with vitamin C the treatment must be stopped.

- Establish clearly, for yourself and for your office staff, an incident management protocol (Chapter 7).

Many doctors report that on difficult and high-risk patients it is nearly impossible to impose lifestyle behavioral changes as a mode of treatment. For these people it may be necessary to resort to medical therapeutics. If such is the case it is recommended that you consider the following therapeutics in accordance with the patient's problem, and in accordance with the recommendation of a consulting urologist:

- Thiazides
- Orthophosphate
- Magnesium hydroxide
- Allopurinol
- An oral glycosaminoglycan analogue
- An oxalate binder

In the chapters to follow I propose a method of motivating patients to overcome the objection of poor patient compliance to lifestyle treatments. Putting the concept of informed consent to practice—actively involving the patient and his family in the treatment program—will, I believe, greatly reduce the need for medical therapeutics.

Clearly the many years of use of megadose vitamin C demonstrates one of the best safety records of any nutrient or drug given in pharmacological amounts. The doctor who regularly administers megadose vitamin C, therefore, seldom needs the information provided in Chapters 5 and 6. In fact, it would be a rare patient indeed who actually needed all of the precautions suggested in these two chapters. Yet death and disability have occurred, which can be credited equally to indiscriminate use and the broad lack of awareness of the dangers imposed by such treatment. Lacking this information, there is reason to believe that death and disability will eventually strike again. The program outlined here, while extensive, was designed to prevent this from happening, by helping the doctor to identify the patients at risk, and by helping to design a preventive lifestyle before administering IV-C. It is believed, by so doing, that IV-C will provide the doctor with a safe and effective adjunct therapeutic in a variety of disease conditions, including the management of the patient who is mercury-sensitive and the patient who suffers from chronic mercury toxicity. In addition, the program suggested here, if applied generally to the lifestyle of all patients (regardless of what treatment they are receiving, or for what condition) is believed to be an enhancement to the treatment regimen—all the while offering the doctor a basis for preventing any and every disease that commonly afflicts man.

LITERATURE CITED

[1] J.M. Rivers, "Safety of High-level Vitamin C Ingestion," *Ann NY Acad Sci*, 498: 451, 1987.

[2] S.N. Gershoff, "The Formation of Urinary Stones," *Metabolism*, 13 (10): 875-887, October 1964.

[3] H.W. Boyce, et al., "Incidence of Urinary Calculi among Patients in General Hospitals—1948 to 1952," *JAMA*, 161: 1437, 1956.

[4] A. Randall, "An Hypothesis for the Origin of Renal Calculi," *N Eng J Med*, 214: 234, 1936.

[5] B. Fellström, et al., "Dietary Animal Protein and Urinary Supersaturation in Renal Stone Disease," *Proc EDTA*, 20: 411-416, 1983.

[6] "Data from the National Health Survey, Series ll, No. 227," *DHHS Publication No. (PHS)*, 83-1677; U.S. Dept. of Health and Human Services, National Center For Health Statistics, March 1983.

[7] W.G. Robertson, et al., Finlayson, ed., "Urinary Calculus," in *Brockis*, PSG Publishing Company, p. 3-12, 1981.

[8] B. Ferrie, et al., "A Prospective Study of the Development of Hypertension and Renal Stone Disease in Subjects with Increased Blood Urate," *Urol Res*, ll: 211-213, 1983.

[9] D.A. Anderson, author, A. Hodgkinson and B.E.C.Nordin, eds., "Historical and Geographical Differences in the Pattern of Incidence of Urinary Stones Considered in Relation to Possible Aetiological Factors," in *Renal Stone Research Symposium*, London, J.A. Churchill, Ltd., 1968.

[10] C.Y.C Pak, "Formation of Renal Stones may be Prevented by Restoring Normal Urinary Composition," *Proc EDTA*, 20: 371-385, 1983.

[11] C.Y.C. Pak, *J Clin Invest*, 48: 1914, 1968.

[12] W.G. Robertson, et al., *Clin Sci*, 34: 579, 1968.

[13] W.G. Robertson, et al., *N Eng J Med*, 294: 249, 1976.

[14] G.H. Nancollas, "The Mechanism of Formation of Renal Stone Crystals," *Proc EDTA*, 20: 386-397, 1983.

[15] R.W. Marshall, et al., *Clin Sci*, 43: 433, 1972.

[16] R. Hartung, et al., "Proc IV International Symposium," *Urol Res*, Plenum Press, NY p.28, 1981.

[17] R. Hautmann, et al., *J Urol*, 123: 317, 1980.

[18] W.G. Robertson, et al., "Risk Factors in Calcium Stone Disease of the Urinary Tract," *Brit J Urol*, 50: 449-454, 1978.

[19] L. Pauling, *Vitamin C the Common Cold and the Flu*, W.H. Freeman and Company, San Francisco and Reading, England, p.111, 1971.

[20] M. Menon and C.J. Mahle, "Oxalate Metabolism and Renal Calculi," *J Urol*, 127: 148-151, January 1982.

[21] A. Hodgkinson, *Oxalic Acid in Biology and Medicine*, Academic Press, London, 1977.

[22] M.A. Sestili, "Possible Adverse Health Effects of Vitamin C and Ascorbic Acid," *Seminars in Oncology*, X (3): 299-304, September 1983.

[23] L.A. Barness, Safety Considerations with High Ascorbic Acid Dosage," *Ann NY Acad Sci*, 258: 523-528, 1975.

[24] M. Briggs, "Vitamin C-Induced Hyperoxaluria," *Lancet*, l:154, 1976.

[25] L. Hagler and R.H. Herman, "Oxalate Metabolism II," *AJCN*, 26: 882-889, August 1973.

[26] K.H. Schmidt, et al., "Urinary Oxalate Excretion after Large Intakes of Ascorbic Acid in Man," *AJCN*, 34: 305-311, 1981.

[27] R.D. Swartz, et al., "Hyperoxaluria and Renal Insufficiency due to Ascorbic Acid Administration during Total Parenteral Nutrition," *Ann Intern Med*, 100: 530-531, 1984.

[28] D.A. Roth and R.V. Breitenfield, "To the Editor: Vitamin C and Oxalate Stones," *JAMA*, 237 (8): 768, February 21, 1977.

[29] K.K. Takenouchi, et al., "On the Metabolites of Ascorbic Acid, Especially Oxalic Acid, Eliminated in Urine, Following the Administration of Large Amounts of Ascorbic Acid," *J Vitaminol*, 12: 49-58, 1966.

[30] S.N. Gershoff and E.L. Prien, "Effect of Daily MgO and Vitamin B6 Administration to Patients with Recurring Calcium Oxalate Kidney Stones," *AJCN*, 20 (5): 393-399, May 1967.

[31] P. Balcke, et al., "Pyridoxine Therapy in Patients with Renal Calcium Oxalate Calculi," *Proc EDTA*, 20: 417-420, 1983.

[32] S.N. Gershoff, et al., "Effect of Pyridoxine Administration on the Urinary Excretion of Oxalic Acid and Related Compounds," *AJCN*, 7: 76, 1956.

[33] R.M. Buckle, "The Glyoxylic Acid Content of Human Blood and its Relationship to Thiamine Deficiency," *Clin Science*, 25: 207, 1963.

[34] T.D. Elder and J.B. Wyngaarden, *J Clin Invest*, 39: 1337, 1960.

[35] G.P. Kasidas and G.A. Rose, *J Hum Nutr*, 34: 255, 1980.

[36] B.E.C. Nordin, et al., "In Urinary Calculi," *International Symposium Renal Stone Research*, Madrid, Karger Publishing, Basel, p 170-176, 1972.

[37] P. Bataille, et al., "Critical Role of Oxalate Restriction in Association with Calcium Restriction to Decrease the Probability of Being a Stone Former: Insufficient Effect in Idiopathic Hypercalciuria," *Proc EDTA*, 20: 401-406, 1983.

[38] S. Faelten, *The Complete Book of Minerals for Health*, Rodale Press, Inc., Emmaus, PA., p 31, 1981.

[39] A. Valyasevi, et al., "Dietary Habits, Nutritional Intake, and Infant Feeding Practices Among Residents of a Hypo- and Hyperendemic Area," *AJCN*, 20: 1340-51, 1967.

[40] D.E. Barilla, et al., "Renal Oxalate Excretion Following Oral Oxalate Loads in Patients with Ileal Disease and with Renal and Absorptive Hypercalciurias," *Annals J Med*, 64: 579, 1978.

[41] A.M. Finch, et al., *Clin Science*, 60: 411, 1981.

[42] W.L. Lyles and M.K. Drezner, "An Overview of Calcium Homeostasis in Humans," *Urologic Clin N America*, 8 (2): 209-226, June 1981.

[43] R.P. Heaney, "Calcium Bioavailability," in *Contemporary Nutrition*, General Mills Nutrition Department ll (8): 1986.

[44] R.P. Holmes and F.A. Kummerow, *J Amer Col Nutr*, 2: 173-199, 1983.

[45] A.B. Chausmer, et al., *Endocrinol*, 90: 633-672, 1972.

[46] A.B. Borle and T. Uchikawa, *Endocrinol*, 102: 1725-1732, 1978.

[47] S. Dhanamitta, et al., "Effect of Orthophosphate and Fat Free Powdered Milk Supplementation on the Occurrence of Crystalluria," *AJCN*, 20: 1387-91, 1967.

[48] F.L. Coe and J.H. Parks, "Hyperuricosuria and Calcium Nephrolithiasis," *Urologic Clinics of North America*, 8 (2): 227-244, June 1981.

[49] W.G. Robertson, et al., "Dietary Changes and the Incidence of Urinary Calculi in the United Kingdom Between 1958 and 1976," *J Chron Dis*, 32: 469, 1979.

[50] L. Berger, C.D. Gerson, and T. Yu, "The Effect of Ascorbic Acid on Uric Acid Excretion with a Commentary on the Renal Handling of Ascorbic Acid," *Am J Med*, 62: 71-76, 1977.

[51] S.L. Gershon, and I.H. Fox, "Pharmacologic Effects of Nicotinic Acid on Human Purine Metabolism," *J Lab Clin Med*, 84:179-186, 1974.

[52] H.B. Stein, et al., "Ascorbic Acid-Induced Uricosuria. A Consequence of Megavitamin Therapy," *Annals Int Med*, 84: 385-388, 1976.

[53] H.C. Elliott and H.V. Murdaugh, "Effects of Acetylsalicylic Acid on Excretion of Endogenous Metabolites," *Proc Soc Exp Biol Med*, 109: 333-335, 1962.

[54] R. Spector and A.V. Lorenzo, "Ascorbic Acid Homeostasis in the Central Nervous System," *Am J Physiol*, 225: 757-763, 1973.

[55] H.S. Loh, et al., "The Effects of Aspirin on the Metabolic Availability of Ascorbic Acid in Humans," *Clin Pharmacol*, 13: 480-486, 1973.

[56] F.H. Myers, *Review of Medical Pharmacology*, Medical Publishers, Los Altos, California, 1972.

[57] J.T. Scott, "On Food, Drink and Gout: New Insights. Executive Health Report," *Executive Health Publications, Inc.*, PO Box 589; Rancho Santa Fe, CA 92067, XXI (8): May 1985.

[58] J.L. Meyer and W.C. Thomas, Jr., "Trace Metal-Citric Acid Complexes as Inhibitors of Calcification and Crystal Growth," *J Urol*, 128: 1376-1378, December 1982.

[59] S. Chulkaratana, et al., "Studies of Bladder Stone Disease in Thailand. Factors Affecting the Solubility of Calcium Oxalate," *Invest Urol*, 9: 246-50, 1971.

[60] G.H. Miller, et al., "Calcium Oxalate Solubility in Urine: Experimental Urolithiasis XIV," *J Urol*, 79: 607, 1958.

[61] W. Tschope, et al., "Different Effects of Oral Glycine and Methionine on Urinary Lithogenic Substances," *Proc EDTA*, 20: 407-409, 1983.

[62] L. Hermansen and O. Vaage, "The Quantitative Significance of the "Himwich-Cori Cycle" for Removal of Lactate During Recovery After Maximal Exercise in Man," in *Lactate: Physiologic, Methodologic and Pathologic Approach*, P.R. Moret, et al., eds., Springer-Verlag, New York, 1980.

[63] V.S. Suphakarn, et al., "The Effect of Pumpkin Seeds on Oxalcrystalluria and Urinary Compositions of Children in Hyperendemic area," *AJCN* 45: 115-121, 1987

[64] E. Cameron, "Biological Function of Ascorbic Acid and The Pathogenesis of Scurvy: A Working Hypothesis," *Med Hypotheses*, 2 (4): 154-63, July-August 1976.

[65] S.N. Gershoff and E.L. Prien, op. cit., pp. 393-399.

[66] F.F. Faragalla and S.N. Gershoff, "Interrelations among Magnesium, Vitamin B$_6$, Sulfur and Phosphorous in the Formation of Urinary Stones in the Rat," *J Nutr*, 81: 60, 1963.

[67] H.L. Du Mont, et al., "Uberlegungen und Untersuchungen zur Frage der Harnsteinprophylaxe: Magnesium," *Z Urol*, 58: 1, 1964.

[68] G. Hammarsten, *Etiologic Factors in Renal Lithiasis*, A.J. Butt, ed., Thomas, Springfield, IL, 1956.

[69] S.N. Gershoff, and S.B. Andrus, "Dietary Magnesium, Calcium and Vitamin B$_6$ and Experimental Nephropathies in Rats," *J Nutr*, 73: 308, 1961.

[70] M.G. McGeown, "The Urinary Amino Acids in Relation to Calculus Disease," *Urol*, 78: 318, 1957.

[71] M.G. McGeown, "The Urinary Excretion of Amino Acids in Calculus Patients," *Clin Sci*, 18: 185, 1959.

[72] Fu-Ho-C Chow, et al., "Control of Oxalate Urolithiasis by DL-Alanine," *Invest Urol*, 13: 113, 1975.

[73] R. Azoury, et al., "May Enzyme Activity in Urine Play a Role in Kidney Stone Formation?," *Urol Res*, 10: 185-9, 1982.

[74] R. Azoury, et al., "Retardation of Calcium Oxalate Precipitation by Glutamic-oxalacetic-transaminase Activity," *Urol Res*, 10: 169-72, 1982.

PART III

The IV-C Mercury Tox Program

CHAPTER 7

Professional Safeguards

The consultant's first obligation is to the patient..."
~Burton J. Hendrick [1870-1949]

The prospect of a lawsuit from any form of therapy is a reality that all doctors who practice within the U. S. health care system are aware of. Doctors all too often react to this threat by overdoctoring, or by practicing defensive medicine—both of which have contributed substantially to the escalation of health care costs. In spite of apparent negativism there are lessons to be learned from the courtroom experience which can provide safeguards for the doctor who wishes to administer IV-C safely and effectively. In a manner consistent with any good marketing concept, one observes and compiles first the court's data identifying the needs and desires of patient clientele, the law, and the medical profession; and then designs his or her services accordingly. If the analysis is valid, and the findings properly applied in the manner attempted here for doctors, it is logical to assume that these actions will greatly improve the standard of patient care and quality assurance. This, in essence, is what professional liability is all about—being professionally, morally, and legally responsible and accountable for understanding and implementing those practices that protect the patient.

"By law," says Alexander Straser,[1] "the courts hold doctors accountable for managing their professional practice." Professional liability, therefore, translates to little more than practicing a standard level of accountability as it relates to professional skill, the quality of patient care, and society's expectations. Negligence occurs only when the doctor departs from these standards, increasing professional risk proportionately.

While a doctor can never be assured that his patient won't initiate a lawsuit, malpractice happens only when the patient is injured as a consequence of negligence. Thus, if we may apply Straser's message to the use of IV-C, the decision to recommend IV-C—or any other adjunct therapy—to a patient carries with it a degree of professional risk related to professional skill and the corresponding levels of liability and accountability that are required.

As with any other form of therapy, professional liability in administering IV-C requires that the doctor learn the standard of care required for its safe and effective use. (It is wise to be absolutely sure of this standard of care, as it may vary in the U. S. according to state statutes and medical or dental specialty). Lacking such awareness increases professional risk. If the doctor concludes, as we have, that the current standard of care for administering IV-C fails to take into account the unfortunate incidents reported in recent years, then a revision is in order. You will agree that such a revision is necessary to ensure the patient's safety. After all, if improvement of patient care is the first priority, the medical-legal concern becomes secondary.

FULFILLING EXPECTATIONS OF LIABILITY IMPROVES PATIENT CARE WHILE PROTECTING THE DOCTOR

Elvoy Raines,[2] in reviewing professional liability, provided insight that can benefit any doctor who desires to administer IV-C. He says that the accountability required of doctors in fulfilling their professional liability (their obligations to society, to their profession, and to the law of the land), lends credibility to themselves as well as to their profession. Professional liability serves as a yardstick in fulfilling the doctor's obligation under the law— following recognized steps that constitute an accepted standard of care. It does not require, as is often misconstrued, that the doctor not make the patient's condition worse by his actions.

To better explain this, I sought the advice of Walter J. Murphy, Jr., a partner in the law firm of Welch, Murphy & Welch of Wheaton, Maryland and Washington, D. C., who specializes in medical legal affairs. Says Mr. Murphy, "Although the doctor may be acting in good faith and following accepted standards of practice, there obviously are many situations where adverse effects will be created and the patient will be made worse by the treatment itself. The issue is not whether the doctor has made the patient's condition worse, but whether he adhered to the accepted standards of practice in determining to undertake the treatment and the concomitant risks."

In compliance with these guidelines the doctor must take certain necessary steps and make the following decisions before administering IV-C:

- Determine whether IV-C is actually indicated for the condition he or she is planning to treat.

- Justify this action in accordance with the licensing authority of the health specialty. A professional license may or may not allow the doctor to administer IV-C, or treat chronic mercury toxicity.

- Determine whether the doctor is dealing with a high, medium, or low risk patient, as described in Chapters 5 and 6. A higher percentage of bad outcomes quite naturally results from taking on more difficult medical cases. (Normally, as stated, IV-C would not be administered to a high risk patient, and seldom to a patient demonstrating medium risk, unless the doctor and patient have jointly concluded that the potential for benefit far outweighs the known risk.)

- Require the patient to complete and sign an Informed Consent form.

- Establish an incident management protocol for the office and/or the health institution where IV-C will be administered.

With regard to the legality of the use of IV-C in general, and specifically for the treatment of chronic mercury toxicity, I spoke with Gerald Brunzie, Ph. D., Director, Documentation Control at Steris Laboratories, Inc.* Dr. Brunzie informed me that IV-C falls into the "B" category of drugs under FDA compliance policy guide 7132c.02. Category B indicates that a drug is generally safe when used as directed, and can legally be used as an adjunct

* Steris Laboratories is a major producer of IV-C. See Appendix E.

therapeutic in a broad range of disease conditions. Thus, a drug such as IV-C that falls into Category B does not require the user to submit a new drug application with the FDA before it can be administered, "provided the product meets certain conditions described in the compliance policy guide."

To further clarify the legal issue for the use of IV-C in treating the mercury-toxic patient, the FDA's Center for Drugs and Drug Regulations was contacted. Their spokesman said that megadose vitamin C and intravenous vitamin C fall under the "assumed to be safe" classification. This classification is of drugs that were generally in use prior to the FDA regulations of 1962. Because of their long standing records of safety and effectiveness, they are not required to undergo the same rigorous testing for a new indication, except as is deemed necessary. The package insert for these drugs will customarily list a number of recommended uses, but no one specific indication. Regardless of whether they are to be used for a new or old indication, the decision to administer is pretty much left to the doctors' professional judgement.

While the physician who is licensed to practice medicine can treat his patients for chronic mercury toxicity based solely on symptoms that relate to their medical histories, much more is required of the dentist. The dentist must relate the same to the patient's oral health; he must demonstrate a connection between the patient's expressed health problem and dental health through some manner of testing; and he must relate the two to his own dental specialty. In satisfying these requirements there is generally a more extensive protocol to be followed by the dentist than is required of the physician. One might therefore conclude that the use of IV-C in the treatment of chronic mercury toxicity seems to be approved as an adjunct therapy when used by a qualified doctor within his area of specialty in accordance with the package insert. These inserts generally read as follows:

Vitamin C is recommended for the prevention and treatment of scurvy, and for the symptoms of mild deficiency. These may include faulty bone and tooth development, gingivitis, bleeding gums, and loosened teeth, as well as hemovascular disorders, burns, delayed fracture and wound healing. Premature and immature infants require relatively large amounts of the vitamin. *Likewise, febrile states, chronic illness, and infection increase the need for vitamin C* (author's italics).

Chronic mercury toxicity certainly falls under the category of chronic illnesses. In addition, the propensity of mercury to cause a wide range of bodily dysfunctions could place it among any of the generally accepted conditions for which vitamin C is indicated.

UPGRADING THE STANDARD OF CARE FOR IV-C

While the findings reported in this book justify its use in the treatment of chronic mercury toxicity, IV-C is not indicated in acute mercurial poisoning. In fact, because affected patients often become anuric and suffer renal damage following acute mercurial poisoning, I believe that acute mercurialism should be listed as a contraindication. Under the present standard of care the package insert lists <u>no</u> contraindications to the administration of vitamin C. This suggested change is believed to be important enough that manufacturers are urged to take steps immediately to change the package insert.

The official list of warnings should also be amended. Until now, the package insert has generally warned the doctor of the following: "Diabetics, patients prone to recurrent renal calculi, those undergoing stool occult blood tests, and those on sodium-restricted diets or anticoagulant therapy should not take excessive doses of vitamin C over an extended period of time." The latest research indicates that the warning should be extended to encompass those conditions and circumstances discussed in Chapter 5. Through this action I believe that the possibilities of improper administration and adverse reactions can be greatly reduced.

THE IMPORTANCE OF INFORMED CONSENT

The implied doctor/patient contract requires that the doctor follow a professionally-accepted protocol. By doing so, the doctor demonstrates good faith in striving to not make the patient's condition worse through his actions, although an adverse outcome is allowable and sometimes unavoidable. The contract does not, however, demand that the patient show improvement following therapy. Yet, as was emphasized recently in a forum conducted for obstetricians at the National Institute of Health,[3] failure of the doctor to improve the patient's condition is the basis of many lawsuits—precipitated not by professional negligence, but by failure to communicate to the patient realistic expectations of the outcome. The participants at the forum concluded that very often a failed outcome could have been a successful outcome had the doctor solicited the patient's cooperation and transferred to them some of the responsibility for their treatment and the decision for treatment. The attendees concluded that two steps are necessary to more closely equalize the doctor's and patient's responsibilities:

1. Educate the patient as to risks, realistic expectations, and his own responsibilities.

2. Obtain a signed consent for the patient's care program, witnessed and understood by the patient, and the patient's family or disability sponsor.

These steps transcribe perfectly to the use of IV-C, as it is vitally important to a successful outcome that the patient carry through with the doctor's directives before, during, and immediately following the treatment program. To adapt this approach to each specialty, the doctor will need to develop a customized version of "informed consent" for administering IV-C in general and, specifically, for its use in treating chronic mercury toxicity. To this end, a thorough review of informed consent is necessary.

Informed consent, as explained by Lenke and Nemes,[4] is the doctor's responsibility for telling a patient about risks associated with a proposed treatment (not all risks, as will be elaborated on later, but only those which are material to the decision). Failure to do so constitutes negligence—a break from the accepted standard of care. Informed consent is used also as a means for stimulating the patient to ask further questions, while giving like opportunity to the patient's family or disability sponsor. In this manner the process of informed consent fosters two-way communication. It provides assurance that the patient understands what will occur and why, and the various alternatives and risks to consider. Of perhaps even greater importance, informed consent gets the patient actively involved in his own treatment. It explains early-on what's expected, and makes it perfectly clear that his cooperative participation is a key element in the treatment's outcome. If complications result, it is less likely that an antagonistic relationship will develop for not being informed of such likelihood. A great deal of data supports this assumption.

Douglas Der Yuen,[5] commenting from the viewpoint of a hospital's risk management committee, reported that patients who are involved in the decision making—through informed consent—are far more likely to perceive adverse reactions and negative outcomes as a "no-fault" situation. A similar conclusion was reached by James Herman,[6] who added that it is reasonable for the doctor and patient to share the decision-making responsibility. The doctor brings expertise and experience to the relationship, while a patient must live (or die) with the treatment outcome. In support of the concept's practicality, said Herman, "there is evidence that shared responsibility between the patient and the doctor creates better communication and promotes compliance and satisfaction with care."[7]

The elements of informed consent, which herein are applied to IV-C, have been outlined clearly by Walter Murphy.[8] He states that the courts have ruled in favor of the patient, and that the patient has a right to informed consent, and a right to sufficient information to make an intelligent decision on whether to accept or reject a treatment program. On the surface the ruling sounds simple enough, but one of the difficulties is in determining an acceptable definition for "sufficient information."

There are two standard tests: the <u>material risk test</u> and the <u>professional standard test</u>. To comply with the former, which looks at the judgement through the eyes of the patient, the doctor must have disclosed both the diagnosis and the prognosis, and he must have warned the patient about the material risks inherent in administering IV-C, as well as alternative therapies. "More simply," says Murphy, "the courts are saying that the doctor must reveal all risks which, to the average patient, would be material in determining whether to accept the treatment or not. To comply with the latter, which looks at the judgement through the eyes of the profession, the doctor who recommends IV-C must have revealed those risks and alternatives generally revealed by his fellow practitioners."

Murphy explains, "All risks need not be disclosed. Under the professional standard test the rule is not whether the doctor has explained all of the risks but whether he has explained the risks which a like practitioner would explain to a patient under the circumstances. There is a greater necessity to disclose information as the consequences of the risk become more threatening. Conversely, there is a consequent decrease in necessity to emphasize disclosure of risks that carry a smaller burden of harm. Both, of course, have to be weighed against the necessity for the treatment. Thus, a purely elective treatment using IV-C would probably require greater detail in disclosure than when IV-C therapy is necessitated by a diseased condition attributed to mercury or some other condition where IV-C is indicated. This is so because inherent in all of the concepts of informed consent is the idea of whether the patient would accept the risks in that therapeutic setting."

In compliance with these principles, the IV-C Informed Consent must establish the following:

- Indication of all of the pertinent risks of IV-C
- Alternative treatments, if any
- The patient has been given the opportunity to ask questions about the procedure and risks
- The patient is literate and understands the terminology

Murphy, citing a court case which demonstrated that patients tend to block out pertinent facts about risk during the doctor's oral disclosure of risk,[9] suggests that at least one member of the family should also be involved in the process of informed consent. Afterwards, by serving as a witness, that person should attest to having understood the patient's responsibility and expected level of involvement. It is important, says Murphy, that the doctor himself make the disclosure of the proposed therapy, the risks, and the alternatives— taking care not to delegate this duty. The time taken personally for complete disclosure will help the patient and his family retain the information, and will do much to reinforce the entire doctor/patient relationship. The risk disclosure may be omitted, but only rarely, when the doctor feels that being informed of such risks might make the patient worse.

In addition, the elements of informed consent should also include the following:

- Patient's diagnosis
- A statement of risk to be expected if the recommended treatment is rejected, or if an alternative treatment is chosen
- A statement attesting to the fact that the patient has had sufficient opportunity to discuss further questions with the doctor
- The form should be written in lay language, the doctor should explain it in lay language, and the patient must understand the terminology
- There must be some indication that the patient is of sound mind—sufficient to reasonably make the decision for treatment
- The completed form must contain the signatures of both patient and witness

But How Do Patients React to Informed Consent? It Requires So Much of Their Time and Energy...

A recent survey (1984-1985) by Louis Harris and Associates[10] revealed that while patients generally do not desire total control over medical decisions, 80 percent of 1,500 Americans queried believe the patient and doctor should agree on whether surgery is appropriate, and well over half felt they and their doctor should agree on any course of therapy. Bear in mind that these were not necessarily people who were unhappy with their doctors. Over 80 percent of those with a personal doctor gave that doctor a positive rating. So, in general, the average patient is quite happy with the doctor/patient relationship. He just wants a little more say regarding the treatment plan, adding support to the court's revelation that the use of informed consent not only protects the doctor but is consistent with the desires and wishes of the average patient.

The 1984-1985 survey also showed that over 80 percent of all Americans consider it important for a doctor to advise on ways of preventing illness or improving health, but that barely 50 percent gave their doctors a positive rating for this. The survey indicated that doctors fail to teach patients the art of healthy living. These are statistics that the majority of patients would like to change. These facts, therefore, give credence to the belief that most every patient will welcome the opportunity to participate in informed consent, regardless of the time and energy required, and the additional task of having to provide his medical history and complete a lengthy lifestyle questionnaire. The patient's willing participation also provides a high level of confidence that he will later embrace a suggestion for a continuing program of lifestyle counseling. Thus, the steps that are necessary to strengthen professional safeguards relative to administering IV-C, are the same steps that are being requested by today's informed patient.

A FINAL NOTE: SUCCESSFUL TREATMENT BEGINS WITH INCIDENT MANAGEMENT

Most reactions to IV-C are relatively minor, transient, and related to the rate of infusion; generally the only precaution given in the package insert. The minor, transient symptoms may include the feelings of being cold, dizzy, faint, light-headed, headachy, and/or thirsty. The practitioner should warn the patient of these signs and symptoms beforehand, and the patient should be instructed to report any such reaction immediately. Yet, as was stated in Chapters 5 and 6, a small number of patients may experience life-threatening reactions as well. While the medical history and patient questionnaire are designed to identify these high risk people beforehand, and remove them as candidates for IV-C, there always remains such risk.

The risk/benefit analysis for a critical patient may at times encourage the doctor, the patient, and the family to go ahead with the IV-C program, regardless of risk. So the doctor may, from time to time, elect to administer IV-C to high risk and medium risk candidates who would otherwise be excluded. Should a reaction occur, it is important to have a previously established protocol for incident management. In fact, according to Raines, incident management is perhaps the most critical element of professional liability. The action taken by a doctor in the first moments and days after an incident is an important determinant in maintaining patient confidence (and perhaps avoiding a claim). To this end it is important to inform the patient and family of such incident as soon as possible, and to go about the process of correcting the incident without delay—taking care not to be make matters worse.

As a general rule the doctor who administers IV-C should have resuscitation equipment readily available and workable; he should be skilled in its use and trained in CPR. The patient's chart information, including vital signs, should be close at hand. A working relationship should be established with a urologist and/or a urology clinic—preferably with dialysis capabilities. It might be wise to consult with them beforehand, asking for their assistance in setting up a protocol in case of emergency. The objective is to have a timely, positive response planned in advance. In this manner, if a reaction should occur the doctor will more likely be in a position to rescue the patient and to take effective steps to correct the defect, rather than "react" to the situation and possibly endanger the patient even more.

Following is a sample, all purpose copy of Informed Consent. It is presented in this chapter to give an idea of the basic elements of any Informed Consent, regardless of the form of therapy. A version tailored to fit the needs of the doctor who wishes to administer **The IV-C Mercury Tox Program** will be found in Chapter 8.

IV-C Mercury Tox Program®
INFORMED CONSENT (OR) REQUEST FOR TREATMENT

I hereby request of Dr._____
that he provide to me the following treatment:_____

_____

1. I understand the nature of the condition, or diagnosis, which calls for the treatment to be as follows:_____

_____

2. I understand the treatment is planned as follows:
    A. _____
    B. _____

3. I understand that the condition can be treated by alternative methods, which are:
    A. _____
    B. _____

4. I understand that the treatment recommended is recommended for me because it has the following advantages over the alternative methods of treatment:
    A. _____
    B. _____

5. I understand that this recommended treatment, like all treatments, has some risks. The risks of importance involved in my treatment have been explained to me. They are:
    A. _____
    B. _____

OR

(5. Alternate) I understand that the recommended treatment, like all treatments, has some risks. I, however, prefer not to be acquainted with the specific risks and accept the judgement of Dr. _____ as to the acceptability of any such risks.

6. I have been given the time and opportunity to discuss this proposed treatment and alternatives and risks with Dr. _____.

_____   _____
Signature of Patient or Guardian   Dated

_____   _____
Signature of Witness or Disability Sponsor   Dated

_____
Relationship of Witness to Patient

LITERATURE CITED

[1] A.L.Straser, "Lawsuits Must Be Curbed or Medical Profession Will Suffer," Editorial, *Occup Health & Saf*, 54 (10): 70, October 1985.

[2] E. Raines, "Professional Liability in Perspective," *Ob & Gyn*, 63 (6): 839-45, June 1984.

[3] E. Casselberry, "Forum on Malpractice Issues in Childbirth," *Public Health Reports*, 100 (6): 629-633, November-December 1985.

[4] R.R. Lenke and J.M. Nemes, "Wrongful Birth, Wrongful Life: The Doctor Between a Rock and a Hard Place," *Ob & Gyn*, 66 (5): 719-722, November 1985.

[5] D. Der Yuen, "A Large Community Hospital's Experience with an Obstetrics-Gynecology Risk Management Committee: Quality Assurance," *Am J Obstet Gynecol*, 154 (6): 1206-1210, June 1986.

[6] J.M. Herman, "The Use of Patients' Preferences in Family Practice," *J Fam Prac*, 20 (2): 153-156, 1985.

[7] S.A. Eraker, et al., "Understanding and Improving Patient Compliance," *Ann Intern Med*, 100: 258-268, 1984.

[8] W.J. Murphy, "Development of the Concept of Informed Consent," *Dent Clin of N Am*, 26 (2): 287-305, April 1981.

[9] Meyer vs. U.S., 638 F. 2dj. 155 (CCA 10 1980)

[10] S. Findlay, "Doctors and Our Health: We Want More of a Say—and More Advice," *USA Today*, 3D, Thursday, January 31, 1985.

CHAPTER 8

Preparing the Patient
for Treatment

"A careful physician...,before he attempts to administer a remedy to his patient, must investigate not only the malady of the man he wishes to cure, but also his habits when in health, and his physical constitution."

~Cicero [106-43 B.C.]

Throughout this book the emphasis on the use of IV-C encompasses three major areas of concern—the rationale (Part I), safety (Part II), and patient preparation (Part III). Part I first demonstrated that the use of megadose vitamin C and intravenous vitamin C as adjunct therapeutics in many disease conditions have had a long and remarkable history of safety and effectiveness. Part I also made clear that IV-C is enjoying a revival of use among doctors of every specialty, and for a variety of indications. It has become especially useful in the successful management of patients who have varying degrees of chronic mercury toxicity, ranging from slight sensitivity to subacute poisoning. These constitute the exciting aspects of IV-C use, a side which cannot be overemphasized.

IV-C has also had its dark side. In spite of a long standing record of safety and effectiveness, a handful of deaths and life-threatening reactions have been reported in recent years, owing perhaps to its growing popularity and widespread use. The careful accounting of these reactions, as examined in Part II, has made it possible to form a pattern of predictability that is most likely to occur in the presence of certain preexisting disease conditions. The aim of Chapters 5 and 6 was to aid the doctor in recognizing danger signals, and to reduce risk through modification of the patient's lifestyle.

Part III, beginning with Chapter 7, proposes an upgrade for the standard of care for administering IV-C, based upon the predicted dangers. Once accepted, as I fully expect it to be, the proposed change will benefit the patient and doctor alike. It will require the patient to become actively involved in his own therapy program, thereby greatly improving the odds for a successful treatment outcome. The risk of adverse reactions that now exists will be all but eliminated.

The concept of shared responsibility is not new; nor is informed consent. What's been done here, however, is merge the two and emphasize their importance. The combination allows patients to have a greater voice in their treatment programs, while providing the doctor with a basis for an introduction of lifestyle counseling as an added professional service. Chapter 8 is designed to encourage the doctor in making this transition, and to guide him through the process of completing the proper forms and preparing the patient for the **IV-C Mercury Tox Program**. Bear in mind, however, that while the chapter's emphasis is upon the process of treating chronic mercury toxicity, the forms that are provided can easily be adapted to IV-C treatment in general.

To reemphasize a point: The concept of shared responsibility holds the key to a successful treatment outcome using the **IV-C Mercury Tox Program**. A patient's full cooperation is required, and he must thoroughly understand this.

If made aware of the importance of this role from the beginning, the patient will be more accepting of the need for accuracy in recalling medical history and in completing the questionnaires concerning everyday diet and lifestyle patterns. The data will help the doctor in making the diagnosis of chronic mercury toxicity, it will help evaluate patient risk, and it will provide the confidence required when assessing risk vs. benefit with the patient. If the patient accepts the recommended treatment plan, and agrees to Informed Consent, and if both patient and doctor understand the level of risk that must be addressed before administering IV-C, then a protective lifestyle corresponding to this risk can be implemented successfully.

PROTOCOL FOR TREATMENT

The order of treatment first assumes that the patient does not have acute mercurialism, for which IV-C is not indicated. It also assumes that a diagnosis has already been made of chronic mercury toxicity, which includes hypersensitivity to mercury. In so doing the doctor must have linked the patient's symptoms with some previous, significant exposure to mercury, or the likelihood of repeated, low-level exposure to mercury. Dentists will have no problem in assessing the latter as it relates to the patient's dental history; physicians, on the other hand, will want to revise their medical history protocol to include the patient's dental history. To interpret the findings, it is recommended that the physician establish a working relationship with a local dentist, and that dentists make themselves available as consultants.

As indicated in Chapter 7: While the physician's license to practice medicine allows him to treat patients for chronic mercury toxicity based solely on symptoms that relate to the patient's medical history, a more involved protocol may be required of the dentist. The dentist generally must relate symptoms to his patient's oral health; demonstrating a connection between the patient's dental health and expressed health problem through some manner of testing; the two must then be related to dentistry and the dentist's own dental specialty. In satisfying these requirements prior to treating the mercury-toxic patient, there is generally a more extensive protocol to be followed by the dentist than is required of the physician. The first six protocol steps are outlined in this chapter. Steps 7 (how to administer IV-C) and 8 (follow-up and evaluation) are the primary topics of the next and last chapters.

Step 1. Patient Medical History/Risk Analysis

Dentists and physicians will already have their own forms for completing a medical history. The form provided herein for the patient's medical history and risk analysis will be helpful in either case. While it can be used in its entirety (as an addendum to the existing medical history form), the doctor will likely choose to blend this with his own forms. The data gained from this as well as the patient's lifestyle questionnaire, will give clues regarding mercury as a possible cause of the patient's symptoms. Suspicion should be heightened if the patient is engaged in a high risk profession.*

* See Appendix C for a list of high risk professions. Because the effects of mercury are accumulative, patients engaged in such professions are most likely to suffer health consequences from low-level exposure from other sources, such as mercurial fungicides, fish, and dental amalgam fillings. These are also the people most likely to demonstrate a sensitivity to mercury.

There should be even more concern if the patient gardens, regularly eats fish, and/or also has two or more silver fillings—and magnified still further if these fillings are old and fractured. When evidence from the patient's lifestyle is supported by symptoms that correspond with mercury poisoning, and whatever testing used, the data will be helpful in making the diagnosis. The patient's answers to the remaining questions will be helpful later when the doctor is ready to perform the risk analysis (Step 4).

(To be completed by the patient)

IV-C Mercury Tox Program®
PATIENT'S MEDICAL HISTORY/RISK ANALYSIS

<u>Please note:</u> Not all of these questions pertain to the medical problem at hand, and you are not required to answer any question you don't wish to. However, by completing the questionnaire thoroughly, you will enable the doctor to consider all aspects of your health, and not only treat your present condition, but also help prevent future potential problems. To assist the doctor in accurately and appropriately adjusting your diet and lifestyle prior to IV-C, it is important that you answer the following questions as completely as possible, and to the best of your knowledge.

Date_____

Patient's Name_____
Address _____ Home phone_____
_____Work   phone _____
City _____State_____ Zip_____
Marital status_____# Dependents _____ Ages _____
Race_____Sex_____ Age_____ Ht _____Wt_____

Education (Check all that apply)   grade school_____ high school_____
college_____ technical training_____ graduate school_____ doctorate_____

Occupation _____Employment Status _____

IN YOUR PRESENT JOB:
Are you exposed to any substances that could endanger your health, such as lead, cadmium, mercury, chemicals, dusts, fumes, or gases? Yes ___No___
If yes, please explain_____
_____

Have you been exposed to any of these in previous jobs? Yes ___ No___
Which?_____
Are you exposed to any work conditions that might endanger your health (for example: loud noise, extreme heat or cold, physical or mental stress, radiation)? Yes____No_____
Is there any risk of accident or injury at work? Yes____ No_____
Please explain _____
_____
_____

DENTAL WORK:
Do you now have silver fillings in your teeth? Yes___No___
If so, how long have they been there?_____
If no, have you previously had silver fillings that are no longer in place?
Yes___No ___ If so, how long ago were they removed?_____
Do you now have, or have you ever had, a metallic taste in your mouth?
Yes____ No ____

Please   explain _____
_____
_____
_____

ALLERGIES:
Please list any drugs that you are allergic to_____
_____

Please list any foods that you are allergic to_____
_____

Have you ever developed a skin rash from taking vitamin C? Yes____ No____
If yes, what form of vitamin C were you taking (if known)?_____
Have you ever experienced gastrointestinal disturbance after taking vitamin
C? Yes____ No____
If yes, what form of vitamin C were you taking (if known)? _____
Have you ever reacted to vitamin C supplements in a manner other than just in-
dicated? Yes ____ No_____
If yes, what bodily changes were noted?_____
_____
_____
_____

IMPORTANT: While large doses of oral vitamin C and intravenous vitamin C
are generally considered safe—as well as effective—therapeutics, for which
adverse reactions are extremely rare, there remains an element of risk that
must be considered. Isolated cases of death and serious health disabilities
have occurred when administered to people with certain preexisting disease
conditions. It is therefore of vital importance that you inform the doctor if you
now have, or have ever had, any of the following:

HIGH RISK CONDITIONS

KIDNEY PROBLEMS
   Serious kidney disease   Yes____ No____
   Acute kidney failure   Yes____ No____
   Insufficient kidney function   Yes____ No____
   Kidney stones   Yes____ No____
      If so, a single episode?   Yes____ No____
      Or recurring episodes?   Yes____ No____
   Nephrotic syndrome   Yes____ No____
   Nephrotic cystinosis   Yes____ No____
   Primary amyloidosis   Yes____ No____

BLOOD ANEMIAS
   Anemia other than simple iron deficiency anemia   Yes____ No____
   Sickle cell anemia   Yes____ No____
   Thalassemia   Yes____ No____
   Hemolytic anemia   Yes____ No____
   Red blood cell fragility   Yes____ No____
   G-6-PD (enzyme) deficiency   Yes____ No____

MEDIUM RISK CONDITIONS

The following conditions are considered of medium risk, in which case special considerations must be made before administering IV-C. Please indicate if you now have, or have ever had, any of these conditions, or if these health situations apply to you.

Diabetes	Yes____	No____
If so, are you now taking insulin?	Yes____	No____
Heart disease	Yes____	No____
If so, are you now on anticoagulant therapy?	Yes____	No____
Gout	Yes____	No____
If so, are you now taking medication for same?	Yes____	No____
Arthritis	Yes____	No____
If so, are you now taking aspirin?	Yes____	No____
Iron overload disease	Yes____	No____
If so, did the diagnosis include any of the following conditions?		
Leukemia	Yes____	No____
Polycythemia vera	Yes____	No____
Hemochromocytosis	Yes____	No____

PREGNANCY, the taking of ANTIBIOTICS, and acute KIDNEY INFECTIONS are in a category all their own. They are each considered to fall somewhere between high and medium risk.

Are you now pregnant? Yes____ No____ Not certain____
If you're not certain, please explain_____
_____
Are you now taking an antibiotic for any reason at all? Yes____No____
Are you being treated for kidney or urinary tract infection? Yes____No____
If not, do you have any reason to suspect that you now have a kidney or urinary tract infection (for example, a burning sensation when you urinate)?
Yes____ No____
Have you ever undergone kidney dialysis? Yes____ No____
If yes, for what reason(s)?_____
_____

MISCELLANEOUS:

Are you now under the care of a physician for any condition (including cancer) other than just mentioned? Yes____ No____
If so, please explain, including all special instructions pertaining to diet and lifestyle, such as low salt, low cholesterol, and low fat, or other precautions _____
_____
If presently under the care of a psychiatrist are you now taking either amphetamines or an antidepressant drug? Yes____No____
What medications are you now taking other than what has already been discussed? _____
_____

Step 2. Patient Lifestyle Questionnaire
    The answers a patient gives concerning lifestyle can offer valuable information for completing the risk analysis, and for designing a plan to reduce such risk. An example was shown in the March 1987 *Journal of the National Cancer Institute*, which contained the findings of several studies that related to urinary frequency with diseases of the bladder, particularly cancer. It was reported that men who are in the habit of urinating an average of six or more times per day have fewer urinary tract diseases than men who urinate less, and their urine is less concentrated than the latter. Data, therefore, may help determine if a patient's water intake needs to be increased; if he is suspected of having renal insufficiency; or if he needs counseling about the necessity of urinating more often in order to decrease the risk of developing stones (among other diseases).

    In about 7 of every 10 patients, doctors will find the profile of the mercury-toxic patient to follow a predictive pattern (the remaining patients will demonstrate at least half or more of these same traits). Because chronic mercury toxicity tends to alter the normal sensory, motor, and emotional responses, making the patient irritable and always anxious, and because it promotes food and chemical sensitivities, the patient's appetite tends to be sharply reduced (bordering on anorexia). The mercury-toxic patient is therefore likely to be thin and have an altered sleep pattern; he is likely to be impulsive, to smoke and to overindulge in alcohol and caffeine drinks; and is at risk for a variety of infections and contact dermatitis. Habitually, he skips breakfast; doesn't eat enough protein, and seldom eats large meals. When he does eat there is a tendency to consume junk food, or to rely more on one food group than another, causing nutritional deficiencies.

    Left to themselves these patients eat for convenience rather than for nutritional considerations; they characteristically consume a diet low in fiber, vegetables, fruits, and whole grains, while high in refined sugar and white bread. Seldom do they exercise; irritability mixed with shyness makes them emotionally unstable and withdrawn, and they are reluctant to spend time out of doors.

    The need is obvious, therefore, to provide them with lifestyle counseling and to solicit their families' support—not just to prevent the development of kidney stones from IV-C, but to provide them with the correct lifestyle regimen for ridding their bodies of mercury and other heavy metals. In this regard, patients who smoke, or who fish and/or live near industries that pollute the waterways, are at risk of being poisoned by cadmium and possibly lead, either of which is likely to become a cofactor in the patient's declining health status. The doctor must be prepared, therefore, to look for clues. A well-vacuumed house, for instance, is less likely to be a source of cadmium toxicity even if the person lives near a polluting factory; lead intoxication is less likely to occur in people who regularly consume dairy products. These lifestyle factors must be considered in conjunction with making the diagnosis and before starting the treatment program. To detect these traits, and to guide in suggesting the proper behavioral changes, we've designed the questionnaire that follows.

(To be completed by the patient)

IV-C Mercury Tox Program®
PATIENT'S LIFESTYLE QUESTIONNAIRE

Please note: Not all of these questions pertain to the medical problem at hand, and you are not required to answer any question you don't wish to. However, by completing the questionnaire thoroughly, you will enable the doctor to consider all aspects of your health, and not only treat your present condition, but also help prevent future potential problems. To assist the doctor in accurately and appropriately adjusting your diet and lifestyle prior to IV-C, it is important that you answer the following questions as completely as possible, and to the best of your knowledge.

SLEEP
Do you normally get a restful night's sleep? Yes____ No____
If not, to what do you credit the problem?_____
_____
How many hours do you normally sleep at night?_____ naps?_____

AIR QUALITY
Do you live within 10 miles of an industrial company that emits pollution into the air? Yes____ No____ Don't Know____
Is your home dusted and vacuumed regularly? Yes____ No____
If yes, how often? weekly ____biweekly ____ monthly ___other_____

EXERCISE
Do you exercise regularly? Yes____ No____
If so, what type(s) of exercise?_____
_____
How often for each type?_____
_____
_____

CIGARETTES
Do you smoke cigarettes? Yes ____No ____
If yes, how many packs per day?_____
Do you smoke or chew any other form of tobacco? Yes____No____
What kind? _____

ALCOHOL
How would you estimate the amount of alcohol you normally consume?
2 or more drinks per day_____ 1 drink per day ____ 3 drinks, or less, per week_____
Is this mostly wine____beer____spirits____or a combination___?
When was your last drink?_____
Have you ever had a drinking problem? Yes____No____

FOODS AND NUTRITION
How many cups of the following would you say you consume daily? hot black tea____ herbal tea____iced tea____coffee____iced coffee____instant coffee____ colas____

How often do you eat breakfast?
Every day ___ Nearly every day___ Sometimes ___ Rarely or never ___
What did your last breakfast consist of?_____
_____
_____

Which is generally your largest meal of the day?_____
What did your last large meal consist of?_____
_____
_____

Which of the following foods do you regularly eat and how often:

FOODS	HOW OFTEN	HOW MUCH
High Protein foods		
Beef	_____	_____
Pork	_____	_____
Poultry	_____	_____
Fish	_____	_____
Cheese	_____	_____
Eggs	_____	_____
Nuts	_____	_____
Whole grains	_____	_____
High calcium foods		
Sardines	_____	_____
Salmon	_____	_____
Milk	_____	_____
Buttermilk	_____	_____
Yogurt	_____	_____
Cottage cheese	_____	_____
Cheeses (soft)	_____	_____
Cheeses (hard)	_____	_____
Broccoli	_____	_____
High oxalate foods		
Spinach	_____	_____
Beet greens	_____	_____
Rhubarb	_____	_____
Swiss chard	_____	_____
High purine foods		
Liver	_____	_____
Kidney	_____	_____
Sweetbreads	_____	_____
Fish roe	_____	_____
High citrate foods		
Lemons (whole)	_____	_____
Lemon juice	_____	_____
Oranges (whole)	_____	_____
Orange juice	_____	_____
Grapefruit (whole)	_____	_____
Grapefruit juice	_____	_____

Which of the following five food groups do you prefer to eat the most of?
Meats, Eggs, and Beans_____ Fruits_____ Vegetables_____ Breads, Grains, and Cereals_____Dairy Products_____
Which of the following food groups would you be most likely to skip?
Meats, Eggs, and Beans_____ Fruits_____ Vegetables_____ Breads, Grains, and Cereals_____ Dairy Products_____
Do you normally include all the food groups in your diet daily? Yes___ No___
Do you take food supplements regularly?   Yes____ No____
Are you now taking vitamin B complex daily?   Yes____ No____
Are you now taking calcium supplements?   Yes____ No____
If yes, how much daily (in mgs)?_____
If yes, what is the brand name and source of calcium?_____
_____
Do you consciously restrict your sodium intake? Yes____No____
If yes, what is your approach? Avoid salt shaker____Avoid obviously salted foods____ Read labels for hidden salt____ Use a salt substitute, high in potassium____

WATER
How many glasses of water do you drink each day? _____
Is your source of drinking water soft____, hard____, or medium____?
Are you usually____, rarely____, or never____thirsty during your normal day?
During the day, do you urinate 3 or fewer times per day____ 6 or fewer times per day____ more than 6 times per day____?
At night, do you urinate frequently____, sometimes____, never____?

MISCELLANEOUS
How much time do you spend daily out of doors?
Less than 15 minutes____ 15 to 30 minutes____ 30 minutes or more____
Please explain the nature of your time spent outdoors (i.e., exercising, gardening, playing with the children, working, etc.) _____
_____
_____

Please check all that apply to you:
____I am consciously aware of the amount of fiber in my diet.
____I never pay much attention to fiber.
____I drink milk regularly.
____I don't like milk.
____I use a lot of milk on cereals and in cooking.
____All bread is enriched. It doesn't matter if it's white or wheat.
____I always try to select whole grain breads and pastries when I can.
____I have a sweet tooth.
____I never eat sugar when I can have honey.
____I'm a meat and potatoes person.
____I always try to eat something from the five food groups each meal.
____I always try to eat from the five food groups each day.
____I'm not consciously aware of eating from the five food groups normally.
____I'm always on a diet.
____I never diet.

Step 3: Clinical Laboratory Testing

As discussed in Chapter 3, laboratory testing based on methodology that is now available may or may not prove helpful in making a diagnosis of chronic mercury toxicity. If acute mercury poisoning is suspected, however, Drs. Goldfrank and Bresnitz,[1] who specialize in toxicological emergencies, make it clear that blood, urine, and hair analysis are required. Chapter 4 emphasized that IV-C is not indicated in such patients, for which the treatment regimens that now exist have proven to be quite successful. (IV-C, which is not indicated in acute mercurialism, is indicated only in chronic mercury toxicity, due either to repeated, low-level exposure, or to a single, significant exposure from which the patient was rescued. IV-C is indicated following rescue as soon as the doctor terminates the emergency drug program—that difficult point following acute mercurialism for which there has not previously been an accepted form of treatment.) A doctor would therefore not immediately accept a patient into the **IV-C Mercury Tox Program** whose symptoms and blood and urine mercury level were consistent with mercurial poisoning; but would accept him only after the patient had undergone the standard treatment for acute mercurialism.

Before administration of IV-C, the following, as outlined in Chapter 6, is the suggested minimum laboratory work-up for patients who do not report medium risk and high risk conditions:

- Serum uric acid
- Complete blood count (CBC)
- Routine urinalysis:
    - urine pH
    - urine microscopic
    - urine protein
- Total UGOT/UGPT level
- 24-hour urine for creatinine clearance
- Black males should have a blood test for G-6-PD deficiency

Ideally, the facilities to perform these tests would be available in the doctor's office or institution. If not, there is likely a commercial lab in the area, such as Metpath or National Medical Laboratories. The doctor would write the patient a prescription and instruct him to call the laboratory before arrival, since the lab may want to issue its own special instructions beforehand.

While most test results are self-explanatory, it is easy to forget the interpretation of a creatinine clearance. Creatinine clearance, a renal function test, is expressed in ml/minute. It is the volume of plasma that is completely cleared of creatinine in 24 hours, or the volume of plasma that must pass through the nephrons within 24 hours to provide 15-25 mg/kg creatinine. The rapid elimination of creatinine (104-125 ml/min) is a good sign, expressed as a high clearance; whereas, a reduction in creatinine clearance (0 to 100 ml/min) indicates some degree of renal insufficiency.

While chronic mercury toxicity may be the underlying cause, renal insufficiency is enough reason to reject the patient as a candidate for IV-C, but this doesn't mean the patient can't be treated for his mercury problem. The findings of Jaffe, et al.[2], for instance, as discussed earlier in Chapter 5, suggests that if the patient with reduced creatinine clearance is diagnosed as having chronic mercury toxicity, the doctor should consider treating as an acute case of poisoning. Before administering a chelating agent, such as BAL, the findings of Schulte-Wissermann and Straub[3] suggest that L-Thyroxine therapy may be helpful when impaired renal function is due to mercury-induced tubular lesions. Yet before administering L-Thyroxine, if uremia is present, Friedman, et al.[4] suggests administering 20 to 50 g daily of activated charcoal, which serves to reduce uremia and the hyperlipidemia that is normally associated with uremia.*

Normal reporting of all tests indicate the need for no more than a minimum of lifestyle adjustments. Any abnormal laboratory findings, however, other than creatinine clearance, would indicate a need to reassess risk, but do not necessarily mean that the patient is denied access to the IV-C program. On the contrary, many of the abnormal findings may serve as helpful indicators of poor eating habits correctable through diet and lifestyle changes. Urine pH, about which much was written in Chapter 6, is a good example. An alternating regimen of testing, followed by lifestyle correction, would continue until the risk is acceptable. On this basis the acceptance of any patient as a candidate for IV-C would depend upon final assessment of risk vs. benefit and the patient's continued commitment to making the lifestyle adjustments that are necessary.

Step 4: Risk Analysis

Upon completion of the questionnaires and laboratory work, the attending doctor is ready to study the data to perform a risk analysis, after which findings will be shared with the patient and risk vs. benefit determined together. If there is a lifestyle counselor on the staff, or if someone has been selected from the staff to assume those duties, he or she will need to be present during the patient interview, as they will need to know as much about the patient as possible.

High Risk. Although rare, high risk patients will be clearly identified by medical history. These people are normally rejected as candidates for IV-C unless their "yes" answers can be justified, corrected, and/or compensated for through medical and lifestyle adjustments. For instance, red blood cell (RBC) fragility may or may not be a clue to G-6-PD deficiency, sometimes indicating no more than simple vitamin E deficiency, in which case vitamin E-rich foods and supplements are corrective. Thus, through the risk analysis one is often able to facilitate improvement of a patient's health even without IV-C. If through implementing a change in lifestyle behavior the doctor can remove him from the high risk category then he has made another important inroad to better health. In essence, this is the manner through which an ongoing program of lifestyle counseling may continually benefit both the doctor and patient.

A patient who is discovered to have anemia, and who complains of weakness and fatigue, exemplifies how the **IV-C Mercury Tox Program** can accomplish this. These symptoms might be due to G-6-PD deficiency, but this is not likely, since symptomatic G-6-PD deficiency rarely occurs. It is more likely to be accounted for by cadmium and chronic mercury toxicity, in part or in full, or by iron deficiency, which itself may be due to chronic exposure to mercury or cadmium.

As with mercury, the risk due to cadmium is often correctable if the kidneys have not been functionally damaged, in which case the first objective would be to identify and remove the cadmium source. Check the questionnaires to see how the patient answered any of the following: "Do you smoke

---

* A large dosage such as this can be acquired directly from American Cyanamid Company, Pearl River, N.Y

cigarettes?" "Are you exposed to any substance that could endanger your health, such as...cadmium?" (Such would be the case, for example, if the patient worked for a firm that manufactured nickel/cadmium batteries.) "Do you live within 10 miles of an industrial company that emits pollution into the air?" "Is your home dusted and vacuumed regularly?"

Next, follow the program outlined in Chapter 2 for ridding the body of cadmium. This may be especially important if the patient also demonstrates other risks, such as hyperuricosuria, because cadmium may contribute to stone development in people who are already at risk.

If the patient has serious kidney disease, and if the doctor and patient still decide upon the **IV-C Mercury Tox Program**, being fully aware of risk, then it is absolutely necessary that the patient follow the diet and lifestyle measures outlined for high risk patients in Chapter 6. If all this seems complicated and time-consuming, remember that treating *all* underlying problems is <u>essential</u> for a successful outcome.

Medium Risk. The patient who answers "yes" to medium risk questions presents a special challenge. If he has been diagnosed as mercury-sensitive, or mercury-toxic, the doctor will want to do whatever possible to make him acceptable as a candidate for IV-C. Such being the case, he would want to cooperate with any other doctor who may be treating this patient for unrelated conditions. As many diet and lifestyle errors that might otherwise complicate the risk should be corrected as possible. Diet and lifestyle corrections, in many such cases, will compensate for risks that would otherwise be unacceptable. This is why it is so <u>very</u> important to impress upon the patient the significance of his own participation. The patient must be willing to fully cooperate.

What if chronic lead toxicity is also suspected? In this case the doctor would address the lead problem first, through diet (withholding EDTA therapy, if indicated, until after the patient has undergone the **IV-C Mercury Tox Program** [as explained in a footnote in Appendix H]), then cadmium, and then mercury. Chronic lead toxicity, like cadmium, exhibits many of the same symptoms as chronic mercury toxicity. If lead, cadmium, and chronic mercury toxicity coexist, the patient's lifestyle questionnaire will reveal low calcium intake and many of the other lifestyle errors discussed in Chapter 2. The patient who is fatigued, for instance, and who demonstrates symptoms of gout, and who is thereby at risk to forming stones, may actually be suffering from lead and cadmium exposure in addition to mercury. To treat, first follow the steps in Chapter 2 for ridding the body of lead and cadmium; then rid the body of mercury.

When assessing risk, particular dietary and lifestyle errors have the potential of increasing risk. Any combination of errors raises the risk one step higher. Through this formula a low risk becomes a medium risk; medium risk becomes a high risk; and a high risk becomes even higher. The most common of these risks would include:

- obesity
- excessive alcohol consumption
- insufficient water intake
- high oxalate food consumption
- abstention from citrate-rich foods
- substantial calcium intake (over 1 gram daily)
- low calcium diet (500 mg or less daily)
- calcium supplementation

- excessive milk consumption (two or more glasses daily)
- diet lacking in cultured milk products

For other diet and lifestyle considerations refer again to Chapter 6.

When assessing risk, remember that obesity and excessive alcohol consumption do not represent high risk conditions independently, but only when either or both are combined with hyperuricemia, hyperuricosuria, calciuria, or oxaluria, or any combination therewith. Of course, the patient with a history of single or recurrent stone disease, who expressed either or both of these lifestyle conditions along with any abnormal laboratory findings, would be classified at extremely high risk; and at an even greater risk (if that's possible) should his medical history include renal dysfunction, or insufficiency. The number of possible combinations are endless.

To further assess the risk for stones and other possible reactions imposed by the patient's diet and lifestyle, which will be considered along with laboratory findings, it may be helpful to refer again to Robertson's assessment of risk factors. In order of decreasing importance these were determined to be:

RISK FACTORS	RISK RATING
• Reduced urinary output	Highest
• Oxaluria	High
• A reduction of stone inhibitors	Medium
• Extreme urine acidity or alkalinity	Medium
• Calciuria	Low to Medium
• Men	High
• Women	Low
• Children	Lowest
• Recurrent stone formers	Highest
• Single stone formers	High
• Those with no history of stones	Low

Step 5: Patient Interview

Once the risk analysis is completed, the doctor is ready to meet with the patient and his family or disability sponsor. A decision must be reached regarding risk vs. benefit, in order to decide on a recommended course of therapy. All of the requirements of Informed Consent, as outlined in Chapter 7, must be satisfied. Thus, while it is important that the person designated as lifestyle counselor be present during the interview, professional liability requires that the doctor alone present the facts and options. In so doing the patient must be provided with full information, so that he can make an intelligent decision with respect to informed consent.

To satisfy the requirements of Informed Consent, four helpful documents follow. The **first**, a handout, informs the patient of commonly reported reactions that may occur during the IV-C infusion. Do go over these points with the patient, and then ask him to take it home to study further.

The **second** is a blank copy of the Informed Consent as applicable to the **IV-C Mercury Tox Program**. The patient should fill in all of the blanks, recounting in his own words what was learned in the interview.   Reassurance should be given that it is okay to ask questions. By answering these questions and having the patient record those answers in his own words, the learning process is facilitated. In fact, from the standpoint of patient education, by using this means of instruction the adult learner is best able to retain the important facts.

A **third** document is included: an Informed Consent with sample answers, designed to show the patient exactly what he must know. It is important to cover these points during the interview. This completed form gives an idea of the depth of knowledge a patient should have about his condition and treatment. It is acceptable to copy and use this form as an official Informed Consent: to be studied, completed, and signed by the patient. Its educational value is slightly less, though comparable to the method described in the preceding paragraph, so long as the patient expresses his understanding through the questions he asks. In this context it is equally correct to use either form. However, since no single form can possibly satisfy the needs of every doctor, one can also, based on the forms provided, design his or her own version of Informed Consent to satisfy each particular health specialty.

The **fourth** document, a Shared Responsibility form, is similar to the first form. It is to be signed and presented to the therapist on the day IV-C is administered. The patient should retain a copy as well. It will reinforce the responsibility that must be assumed in the treatment process, and it will help the therapist, doctor, and the lifestyle counselor determine to what extent the patient understands that role.

(To be read aloud and given to the patient)

IV-C Mercury Tox Program®
PATIENT INFORMATION

The following are commonly reported reactions that may occur during the I.V. Vitamin C infusion: Promptly report these or any other reactions you may have to the therapist.

- Sleepiness, lightheadedness, and/or a headache, may occur during and approximately 30 minutes after IV-C has been administered. If this happens please notify the therapist, who will want to observe you and adjust the rate of intravenous infusion. *Because of the possibility of this reaction it is recommended that you have someone with you to accompany you home afterwards.*

- Unusually persistent thirst is common during IV-C. The therapist will provide you with plain or lemon water.

- A slight chill is not uncommon during the IV-C infusion. As before, the therapist will want to know if this occurs. You will be provided with a blanket and the rate of infusion will subsequently be adjusted.

- An increased urge to urinate during the IV-C. This is good. It indicates the IV-C is working. Again, notify the therapist whenever necessary.

- A burning sensation in the arm in which the IV-C infusion is being administered, which is often accompanied by generalized pain. The therapist will adjust the rate of infusion, massage your arm, or take other appropriate actions, such as temporarily stopping the infusion.

The following possible reaction may occur if you abruptly stop taking vitamin C supplements before or after your treatment:

It has been reported that patients who abruptly quit taking oral vitamin C, or who refrain from taking the prescribed supplement of oral vitamin C following IV-C, may develop scurvy. Scurvy is a disease normally caused by a deficiency of vitamin C. For reasons not entirely understood, this condition may develop following your IV-C if you do not follow your supplementation program as directed. You must understand the importance of taking your prescribed supplements. Preceding the IV-C infusion and on the same day that IV-C is administered, you are to take oral vitamin C in the amount of 3 grams per day, or some other amount which you and the doctor have agreed upon previously, which is____ gram(s) per day. Afterwards you will continue taking your oral vitamin C for 30 days—gradually tapering the dosage to whatever is agreed upon between you and the doctor.

(To be completed by the patient)

IV-C Mercury Tox Program®
INFORMED CONSENT (OR) REQUEST FOR TREATMENT

I hereby request of Dr. _____ that he provide to me the following treatment: _____
_____

1. I understand the nature of the condition which calls for the **IV-C Mercury Tox Program** to be as follows: _____
_____

2. I understand the treatment is planned as follows:
    A. _____
    B. _____

3. I understand that the condition can be treated by alternative methods, which are:
    A. _____
    B. _____

4. I understand that the treatment recommended is recommended for me because it has the following advantages over the alternative methods of treatment:
    A. _____
    B. _____

5. I understand that this recommended treatment, like all treatments, has some risks. The risks of importance involved in my treatment have been explained to me. They are:
    A. _____
    B. _____
OR
(5. Alternate) I understand that the recommended treatment, like all treatments, has some risks. I, however, prefer not to be acquainted with the specific risks and accept the judgement of Dr. _____as to the acceptability of any such risks. Even so, I do_____(Please check) agree to follow my doctor's advice closely for a specified time period before and following IV-C, especially as it relates to necessary changes in my diet and lifestyle, since this is important to the outcome of the treatment.

6. I have been given the time and opportunity to discuss this proposed treatment and alternatives and risks with Dr. _____

_____   _____
Signature of Patient or Guardian   Dated

_____   _____
Signature of Witness or Disability Sponsor   Dated

_____
Relationship of Witness to Patient

(To be completed by the patient)
(Points to be covered by the doctor are written in italics)

IV-C Mercury Tox Program®
INFORMED CONSENT

I hereby request of Dr. _____
that he provide to me the following treatment: *A strict dietary program with an adjunct infusion of intravenous vitamin C, commonly referred to as "The IV-C Mercury Tox Program"*

1. I understand the nature of the condition which calls for the **IV-C Mercury Tox Program** to be *mercury sensitivity, or chronic mercury toxicity, sometimes referred to as chronic, low-level mercurialism, micromercurialism, or subacute mercurialism.*

2. I understand that the condition will be treated by the following means:

A. *The doctor will instruct me to follow a particular lifestyle starting a few days or weeks before the IV-C is to be administered and continuing a few days afterward. It will be based upon the doctor's Risk Analysis of my medical history and the answers that I provide in the lifestyle questionnaire.*

B. *The doctor will administer a very large amount of vitamin C through my veins, which will take about 2 and 1/2 to 4 hours; I should come to his office dressed warmly, and should arrange for someone to drive me home afterwards.*

3. I understand that the condition can be treated in the following alternative methods:

A. *The Doctor could bypass the use of IV-C, choosing instead megadose oral vitamin C in conjunction with the other major segments of the **IV-C Mercury Tox Program**.*

B. *The doctor could choose to treat only my symptoms, paying less attention to the underlying cause of such symptoms.*

C. *The doctor could choose to treat me using IM EDTA, oral DMPS, or DMSA.*

4. I understand that the treatment recommended is recommended because for me it has the following advantages over the alternative methods of treatment:

A. *The doctor cannot attain with oral vitamin C the blood and tissue level of ascorbic acid that is possible with IV-C, and a very high level is needed, however brief the time period, in order to most effectively reduce the toxicity of mercury in my body.*

B. *Treating only my symptoms does not necessarily address the cause of my condition; whereas,the proposed treatment plan has the potential for doing so.*

C. *Because of my mercury-toxic condition, IM EDTA may be toxic to my kidneys; DMPS is not yet available in the USA; and neither DMSA, IM EDTA, nor DMPS have the advantage of treating my health condition while reducing my body's burden of mercury. Otherwise, there is no other treatment proven safe and effective for my condition.*

5. I understand that the treatment projected, like all treatment, has some risks. The risks of importance involved in my treatment have been explained to me and are:

A. *If I should be pregnant I understand there is insufficient data to state with confidence that IV-C is safe and non-toxic to my unborn child.*

B. *If I am anemic or if my red blood cells are fragile, and should the cause not be known, I could have a condition that could bring about my death or cause serious disability. To this end my doctor has presented to me the analysis of my relative risk, which is low   ,medium   , or high   (check only one).*

C. *If my kidneys aren't functioning properly, or if I have a urinary tract infection, or if I have other predictors of kidney stone development, I am aware I could develop kidney stones and die, or experience serious disability. Based upon the laboratory data and the answers that I provided in my medical history and the lifestyle questionnaire, my doctor has presented to me an analysis of my relative risk, which is low   ,medium   , or high   (check only one).*

D. *I understand that there is risk of kidney stones developing even in apparently healthy people, Knowing this, I have completed the lifestyle questionnaire as accurately as I can, so that the doctor may assess my relative risk according to what is currently known about diet and kidney stones. In accordance with the risk analysis previously expressed, I agree to share the responsibility for the treatment outcome by expressing my preference of treatment, and by following the lifestyle recommended by my doctor for a prescribed period of time before and following IV-C.*

E. *During the period when I am receiving IV-C the commonly reported reactions (although not considered life-threatening) include thirst, a slight chill, headache, lightheadedness, and a frequent urge to urinate. Rarely, I might experience soreness, or a burning sensation in the arm where the IV-C is being administered; or backache, which can be a sign of a serious, adverse reaction. I am expected to report these or any other reactions promptly to the doctor or therapist,*

F. *Following the IV-C I understand there is risk of developing scurvy (a vitamin C deficiency disease) if I do not continue taking oral vitamin C as prescribed by the doctor. I agree to follow my doctor's advice closely in this regard, as well as the prescribed lifestyle changes.*

5. ALTERNATE: I understand that the treatment projected, like all treatment, has some risks. I, however, prefer not to be acquainted with the

specific risks and accept the judgement of Dr._____ as to the acceptability of any such risks. Even so, I do_____(Please check) agree to follow my doctor's advice closely for a specified time period before and following IV-C, especially as it relates to necessary changes in my diet and lifestyle, since this is important to the outcome of the treatment.

6. I have been afforded time and opportunity to discuss this proposed treatment and alternatives and risks with Dr._____

Signature of Patient_____
Date (month/day/year)_____
Signature of Witness _____

If under age or disabled, the signature of your legal guardian or disability sponsor is required:

Legal Guardian _____
Relationship to Patient_____
Date (month/day/year)_____

(or)

Disability Sponsor_____
Relationship to Patient_____
Date (month/day/year)_____

(To be completed by the patient at the time of treatment)

IV-C Mercury Tox Program®
SHARED RESPONSIBILITY: PLEASE READ, SIGN, and WITNESS

Doctor, I have completed the Patient Medical History and Risk Analysis, as well as the Lifestyle Questionnaire, and I have given my Informed Consent for **The IV-C Mercury Tox Program** in writing.

I understand fully the commonly reported reactions to intravenous vitamin C (sometimes referred to by the doctor as IV-C). This includes thirst, a slight chill, and lightheadedness. I have prepared myself accordingly with adequate clothing and, should I feel lightheaded, someone is with me who can accompany me home. Most importantly, I understand that I must continue to take oral vitamin C supplements for a prescribed period of time or risk the chance of scurvy-like symptoms; and I attest to the fact that **I DO NOT HAVE** any of the high risk conditions listed on the Patient Medical History form which, under normal conditions, would disqualify me as a candidate for **The IV-C Mercury Tox Program**. I also understand that any medium risk conditions must be dealt with appropriately, perhaps through consultation and additional testing. At the very least, the slightest increased risk will require me to make necessary diet and lifestyle adjustments before and immediately following IV-C. To improve the chances for a successful treatment outcome I have been following specific lifestyle changes prescribed by the doctor, and I have agreed to follow my doctor's advice closely in this regard.

Signature of Patient _____

Date (month/day/year)_____

Signature of Witness   _____

If under age or disabled, the signature of your legal guardian or disability sponsor is required:

Legal Guardian _____

Relationship to Patient_____

Date (month/day/year)_____

(or)

Disability Sponsor _____

Relationship to Patient_____

Date (month/day/year)_____

Step 6: Patient Counseling

Properly informed and sufficiently motivated, the patient is now ready to proceed with **The IV-C Mercury Tox Program**. The steps that have been presented leading up to the actual administration of IV-C do not represent hard and fast rules. At best, they serve as a model upon which the serious practitioner or researcher can base his efforts toward developing a safer and more effective treatment protocol. Upon this spirit of flexibility and scientific evolvement is based **The IV-C Mercury Tox Program**.

While this book is designed primarily to direct doctors in the treatment of chronic mercury toxicity, it is also a source book for the administration of IV-C in general. Thus, regardless of the indication, whether IV-C is to be administered for chronic mercury toxicity or for some other disease condition, it is recommended that the counseling session be begun by making the required lifestyle behavioral changes that address the patient's particular risk category as described in Chapter 6.

For those patients with no history of renal insufficiency, gout, hyperuricemia, or uricosuria, who presently are free of a urinary tract infection, and who are not presently taking an antibiotic or an antibacterial for a urinary tract infection, instruct the patient to follow the minimum lifestyle behavioral changes as described in Chapter 6. These changes should be in force for a minimum of 36 hours (preferably a week) prior to implementing the steps in Chapter 2 for ridding the body of cadmium or mercury. Low risk patients can be instructed to begin immediately taking their 3 g per day of vitamin C supplements. Medium risk and high risk patients should be asked to delay taking oral vitamin C until there has been a chance to evaluate the effect of their lifestyle adjustments.

CAUTION: Datyner and Cox[5], in treating a mercury-toxic patient who was also suspected of having chronic lead toxicity, warned that EDTA should not be administered first to these people. EDTA, they report, has the disadvantage of causing nephrotoxicity, and has been shown by Glomme and Gustavson to increase the mortality of rats poisoned with mercury.[6] The patient with concomitant lead and chronic mercury toxicity should first adopt the lifestyle regimen proposed in Step 1, Chapter 2, but should not undergo chelation therapy with EDTA prior to addressing the mercury issue. For these reasons, the patient's mercury problem should be addressed first, before EDTA is administered.

Once the lifestyle behavioral changes have been made relative to minimizing whatever health risk that IV-C may present, the mercury-toxic patient should be instructed to then follow the lifestyle program outlined in Step 3 of Chapter 2. For low risk patients the transition is made quite simply, since there is a very small difference in the two dietary regimens.

It will be found that patients who are sufferers of chronic mercury toxicity will often have difficulty eating. This is evidenced by the fact that they are so often mentally impaired, of poor health, underweight, and malnourished. Thus, at first it may only be possible to partially implement the program. If so, the patient will not likely be able to consume the amount of protein and fat required to transport mercury through and out of the body. So the doctor will have to do the best he can in this regard. The administration of IV-C (Protocol Step 7, Chapter 9) won't at first be as effective in these people as is preferable, but progress by any measure is still progress. Following the initial IV-C there will be enough progress measured so that the patient will be better able to eat and to follow the recommended lifestyle. This will be discussed more in Protocol Step 8 (Chapter 10, Evaluating The Patient). A second IV-C can then be administered with expectations of better cooperation as the patient's outlook and general health improve.

LITERATURE CITED

[1] L. Goldfrank and E. Bresnitz, "Mercury Poisoning," *Hospital Physician*, 38-46, June 1980.

[2] K.M. Jaffe, et al., "Survival After Acute Mercury Vapor Poisoning," *Am J Dis Child*, 137: 749-751, August 1981.

[3] H. Schulte-Wissermann and E. Straub, "Effect of L-Thyroxine on Renal Excretion of Water and Electrolytes in Both Normal and Mercury-Intoxicated Rats," *Urol Res*, 8: 189-96, 1980.

[4] E.A. Friedman, et al., "Charcoal-Induced Lipid Reduction in Uremia," *Kidney Int*, 13 (Suppl 8): S-170-76, 1978.

[5] M.E. Datyner and P.A. Cox, "Inorganic Mercurial Poisoning," *Anaesth Intens Care*, 9: 266-70, 1981.

[6] J. Glomme and K.H. Gustavson, "Treatment of Experimental Acute Mercury Poisoning by Chelating Agents BAL and EDTA," *Acta Med Scand*, 164: 175-82, 1959.

CHAPTER 9

The Administration of
Intravenous Vitamin C

"There is no more contradiction between the science of medicine and the art of medicine than between the science of aeronautics and the art of flying."

~Francis Weld Peabody [1881-1927]

Because there is no other source book available for the general administration of intravenous vitamin C—for chronic mercury toxicity, or otherwise—Chapter 9 provides the necessary information for administering IV-C. In so doing, this chapter is structured to answer those questions most often asked by doctors regarding the administration of IV-C:

Is there a difference between ascorbic acid and sodium ascorbate? What effect does sodium ascorbate have on a sodium-free diet?

What methods of preparation are used in the manufacture of IV-C? Which method is best? What do I ask for when obtaining IV-C? Is one brand better than another?

How do I determine the dosage? How was that dosage first arrived at?

What about other indications for IV-C? How does the method for administering IV-C differ for indications other than chronic mercury toxicity?

What parenteral fluid is best used? How does one justify infusing a hyperosmolar solution?

How do I prepare the injectable for I.V. administration? What paraphernalia do I need, and what should be the rate of administration?

What about IV-C's use in dentistry? At what point should it be administered to the mercury-toxic patient relative to amalgam replacement?

Is IV-C in the **IV-C Mercury Tox Program** intended as a one-time treatment, or does the program require multiple infusions?

These are all valid questions which are necessary considerations to the safe and effective administration of IV-C, regardless of its indicated use. These questions—and others—will be answered in the following.

ASCORBIC ACID VS. SODIUM ASCORBATE

Due to the extremely acid nature of ascorbic acid, doctors generally state they prefer sodium ascorbate as a source of IV-C. However, an interview with Dr. Dennis Adair—a pharmacologist at the veterinary branch of Schering/Plough (a major producer of IV-C)—informs that while the risk of acidity from IV-ascorbic acid presents a valid concern, pure ascorbic acid has never been an optional IV-C source.

"All IV-C preparations manufactured today for use in both humans and animals," says Adair, "are essentially sodium ascorbate, even those that are labeled as ascorbic acid. You wouldn't inject pure ascorbic acid for two reasons: The acidic nature of ascorbic acid makes it much too insoluble, and you would be asking the patient's body to provide the buffer needed to bring it to the optimal pH (about 7.4). To do so would cause much pain." In addition, the patient, having had to use his own buffering capacity, could possibly be in danger of acidosis. Thus, even when IV-C is made directly from ascorbic acid, the pH must be adjusted with an alkalizing agent before it can be administered.

There are several methods used in the preparation of IV-C. Regardless of the method employed, the IV-C endproduct is sodium ascorbate. "In fact," says Dr. Gerald Brunzie, "90 to 99 percent of ascorbic acid is converted to ascorbate as a consequence of the neutralization process," so no matter what the label reads, the two products are, in the end, very close to the same.

Adair goes on to explain, "The chemistry used in adjusting the pH of IV-C is similar to any acid/base reaction." For instance, in a sample acid/base reaction, hydrochloric acid (HCl) added to sodium hydroxide (NaOH), yields sodium chloride (a neutral salt) plus water:

$$HCl \quad + \quad NaOH \quad \longrightarrow \quad NaCl \quad + \quad H_2O$$

$$[Acid] \quad + \quad [Base] \quad \longrightarrow \quad [Neutral\ Salt] \quad + \quad Water$$

"In the manufacture of IV-C," says Adair, "ascorbic acid suffices for the acid, and ordinary baking soda (sodium bicarbonate) provides the base, together they yield sodium ascorbate (the neutral salt) plus water (and an equivalent amount of carbon dioxide)."*

$$\text{Ascorbic Acid} \quad + \quad \text{Sodium Bicarbonate} \quad \longrightarrow \quad \text{Sodium Ascorbate} \quad + \quad \text{Water} \quad + \quad \text{Carbon Dioxide}$$

$$[Acid] \quad + \quad [Base] \quad \longrightarrow \quad [Neutral\ Salt] \quad + \quad Water$$

* The manufacturer could also incorporate sodium carbonate or sodium hydroxide as the base, but ordinary baking soda is more desirable—mostly because there is less CO_2 released. Even when baking soda is the base the doctor should be made aware of the potential for headspace pressure (the pressure that builds in the IV-C vials) due to residual CO_2, which can cause considerable force on the plunger of the syringe used for extracting the concentrated solution. In practice, the manufacturer will remove excess carbon dioxide before filling vials; no further CO_2 buildup occurs since the reaction is complete. Yet they recommend vials be kept under normal refrigeration to minimize headspace pressure from whatever residual CO_2 cannot be removed.

What About the Sodium in Intravenous Sodium Ascorbate?

Each gram of sodium ascorbate contains approximately 5 mEq of sodium, which must be considered when IV-C is used in patients on salt-restricted diets. However, the study by Elliott[1] (Chapter 5) suggests that the sodium contributed either by oral sodium ascorbate or IV-C may not have an additive effect as expected. While no one, as yet, has attempted to confirm or dispute these findings, Elliott's report suggests that megadose sodium ascorbate actually causes a net loss of body sodium rather than the suspected net gain. The recent findings of Kurtz's team,[2] which were likewise discussed in Chapter 5, shed new light on the salt/high blood pressure issue. The researchers determined that the anionic component of an orally-administered sodium salt is the real determinant of the salt's capacity to cause high blood pressure. Sodium chloride, they found, was the only form of sodium that raised blood pressure, while sodium citrate did not. Thus, while there remains no acceptable, alternate form of IV-C (other than sodium ascorbate), these findings ironically tend to support rather than conflict with the goals of a sodium-free diet.

METHODS OF PREPARATION

In the preparation of IV-C the manufacturer must first consider the reducing redox potential of vitamin C. As discussed in Chapter 4, vitamin C is healthfully engaged in a reversible oxidation/reduction reaction—an event that proceeds normally as long as the equilibrium of the reducing redox potential favors a left shift, which can only occur when certain conditions are met. Ascorbic acid must first be supplied in such quantity to support its predominance. Then factors that encourage oxidation must be held to a minimum. For example, the adjusted pH must range from neutral to moderately acid, since the reduction of dehydroascorbate to sodium ascorbate can occur only in an acid environment and is inhibited by alkalinity.

Thus, the manufacturer uses hydrochloric acid, when necessary, to readjust the pH of sodium ascorbate downward to a point that promotes stability. The product would otherwise expire too quickly, and would probably not perform as expected. In fact, manufacturers generally prefer that their IV-C products carry as low a pH as is currently permissible, to better ensure stability. The acceptable pH range of 5.5 to 7.0 was therefore arrived at to satisfy the requirements of stability, while also being within the buffering capacity of normal venous blood. (Although pH 7.4 is the approximate normal for arterial blood, pH 5.5 is still within the buffering capacity of human blood, providing the solution is infused slowly.)

In satisfying this need there are two recognized methods of manufacturing IV-C—by the direct and the indirect methods.

The Direct Method

The direct method for producing IV-C as sodium ascorbate from powdered ascorbic acid is accomplished through a process similar to that used for making oral sodium ascorbate. Both oral sodium ascorbate and IV-sodium ascorbate are synthesized by adding sodium bicarbonate* (an alkalizing agent)

---

* Sometimes—in the making of oral vitamin C—calcium, magnesium, or potassium buffer is substituted for sodium, in which case the end product may be either calcium ascorbate, magnesium ascorbate, or potassium ascorbate. In general, this is how the oral product discussed by Cathcart was formulated (Chapter 2).

and sterile water to powdered ascorbic acid. In this reaction, an equivalent of sodium bicarbonate (pH 8.3) is added to an equivalent of ascorbic acid (pH range of 2.3 to 2.5) @ 25° C, and the resulting solution is adjusted to within the pH range of 5.5 to 7.0.

Even when IV-C is made directly from ascorbic acid, the manufacturer does not allow total transformation of pH to occur, since the final product would then be too alkaline. A 10 percent solution of sodium ascorbate, for instance, would have a final pH range of 7.4 to 7.7, which would interfere with product stability (in solution).

The Indirect Method

In producing IV-C by the preferred indirect method, the manufacturer begins by reconstituting dry sodium ascorbate with sterile water. The pH is then adjusted to a range of 5.5 to 7.0, using sodium bicarbonate and hydrochloric acid, after which a trace amount (0.025%) of edetate disodium (EDTA) is added to stabilize the ascorbate (not to stabilize the pH, as is often assumed). Because spoilage of vitamin C occurs more quickly in solution, due to oxidation, the threat of oxidation by this method is somewhat less than if IV-C were prepared directly from ascorbic acid (the direct method requires more time in solution), perhaps explaining why the final pH tends to be a little higher (in the range of 6.0 to 7.0).

This may also explain why doctors who regularly administer IV-C believe that IV-C made by this method causes the patient noticeably less pain and discomfort from mild tetany than IV-C prepared using the direct method. This is also the likely reason why doctors tend to voice a preference for sodium ascorbate as the IV-C source, and why they prefer one brand over another.* The sources that provide pain-free IV-C are more likely to have been prepared using the indirect method. However, because the potential for pain is mostly a function of pH—it is possible to have a pain-free product made by either method, simply by adjusting the final pH upwards. Ultimately, therefore, because the final pH makes a decided difference in the patient's response, perhaps it would be to the doctor's advantage to contact the IV-C manufacturer and express a preference for a product that has a pH ranging from 6.0 to 7.0, or 6.5 to 7.0 rather than 5.5 to 7.0. Dr. Cathcart, for instance, has gone on record stating that, if technically possible, he would prefer his IV-C buffered to 7.4.[3]

Other than simply informing the manufacturer of a preference, there are steps that can be taken now to help improve the pH. Dr. Levin, for instance, suggests adding sodium bicarbonate to the IV-C/parenteral fluid mixture, and checking with nitrozine paper—adjusting the pH to 6.5—just before administering the IV-C. The only drawback is the risk of over-alkalizing the IV-C, which could then cause the product to become ineffective. The remaining steps are otherwise risk-free: Prepare the IV-C only as needed, never in advance. To prevent spoilage, always store the concentrated IV-C vials in the refrigerator at 2° - 8° C (36° - 46° F), and away from light. Then, if you wish to

---

* While there are several manufacturers of low-dose ampules of vitamin C in the U. S. today, mostly for intramuscular use, I am only aware of two major U.S. manufacturers who prepare IV-C in the dosage required by the **IV-C Mercury Tox Program**—Steris Laboratories and Schering/Plough. (Complete addresses are listed in Appendix E.) Hopefully, from the interest generated by this book, other reputable pharmaceutical firms will soon enter this market. The research that naturally accompanies such action would help solve the technical problems previously cited.

bring the cold IV-C solution to room temperature before administering it, do so in a darkened cabinet.

Arm Pain, Achy Muscles, and Mild Tetany:
A Problem with pH, or a Consequence of the Chelating Action of Vitamin C?

Because IV-C made directly from ascorbic acid is more susceptible to oxidation, the final pH of IV-C is adjusted to fall within a range of 5.5 to 7.0, which in turn creates another potential problem. IV-C made by this method tends to fall within the lower range of pH acceptability—closer to 5.5 than 7.0, causing the patient to suffer some pain and discomfort or mild tetany, such as an achy upper arm and shoulder with tight muscles.

The mild tetany-like effect on the patient's arm is likened to the anoxic condition in heart muscle following a coronary—in which case calcium gluconate and sodium bicarbonate are administered to restore normal rhythm and cardiac contraction. Just as the sudden drop in arterial pH during a coronary contributes to severe arrythmia and the risk of cardiac arrest, the localized transient drop in blood pH due to IV-C can cause the protein muscle fibers of the arm to denature, or rotate on their axes. In both situations the proteins denature either in response to the increased acidity of the blood, or to a reduction in the buffering capacity of the patient's blood, or both. As the difficulty progresses, the cell membrane receptors located within the muscle fibers—which are primarily protein—become less and less accessible to the nutrients and hormones that are intended to direct the action of muscle tissue. The cell receptors for calcium rotate also—making the receptors for calcium less accessible. Eventually, the process hinders calcium from engaging effectively in its many important functions; one of which is to enhance the contraction and relaxation phase of striated muscle. Thus, when administering IV-C having a pH closer to 5.5 than 7.0, a mild localized transient tetany may occur. Hence doctors who regularly administer IV-C try to avoid this by adding calcium gluconate directly to the IV-C, or by requesting that their source of IV-C be prepared by the indirect method.

The absence of arm pain, and the absence of pain at the infusion site, is a good indication that the pH of the product meets the criteria discussed, regardless of the method employed in its preparation. Of course, if arm pain persists at the slower rate of infusion, quite the opposite is likely true, indicating that the product's pH is simply too acid, and requiring that the IV-C be infused much slower than normal. There's another possible explanation, however, for the transient symptoms of tetany, pain, and muscular aches, which involves the chelating action of vitamin C on calcium and magnesium.

Klenner was first to report that an occasional patient may develop a transient, localized, mild tetany while IV-C is being administered. Because vitamin C is known to chelate (and excrete in the urine) certain metals when they are present in excess—such as copper, iron, zinc, and manganese—he reasoned that it probably had the capacity to chelate calcium and magnesium as well, thus accounting for the mild tetanic reaction that particular patients experienced.

Klenner's 1 in 10 Rule: Calcium Added to IV-C. To test his point, Klenner began adding calcium gluconate to the IV-C infusion, and found that 1 gram of calcium gluconate per 10 grams of IV-C entirely did away with the symptoms of mild tetany in otherwise susceptible people. Thereafter, the addition of calcium gluconate to IV-C became standard practice, though it is not added today at the same high dosage.

Doctors who administer IV-C today take exception to Klenner's 1 in 10 rule. Wright, for instance, who regularly administers IV-C for conditions other than chronic mercury toxicity, offers the following advice, "There are problems with Klenner's 1 in 10 rule," says Wright, "It's sometimes too bold, especially in the patient at risk to cardiac arrythmia. I may want to administer 50, 60, or even 70 grams in these and other patients and, in addition, it doesn't consider the patient's need for magnesium. Such a rule would require 5, 6, or 7 grams (respectively) of calcium gluconate, and without the simultaneous addition of magnesium in a ratio that ranges somewhere between 2:1 and 1:1 the patient may develop a dangerous heart rhythm. A 1:1 (Ca:Mg) ratio in a patient receiving 60 grams IV-C, for instance, would require 6 grams of calcium glu-conate and 6 grams of magnesium sulfate, or magnesium chloride. This amount of magnesium can make the patient quite uncomfortable. It is known, for instance, that 2 grams magnesium sulfate infused in less than 30 minutes can make the patient warm, hot, and vasodilated. It probably won't hurt him, but it can become quite uncomfortable for the patient. So as a rule of thumb I tend to add calcium and magnesium to IV-C at a ratio of 2:1, and I withhold even that until the IV-C consists of at least 20 grams, as mild tetany is not likely to occur until the IV-C dosage reaches 30 to 40 grams." Dr. Warren Levin tends to agree. When administering 30 grams of IV-C or more it is his practice—in order to prevent tetany—to add 10 ml calcium gluconate and 5 ml magnesium sulfate, in sterile distilled water, along with enough sodium bicarbonate to bring the solution to pH 6.5.

Dr. Wright: "When the risk of cardiac arrythmia becomes a valid concern, I prefer adding the calcium and magnesium at a ratio of 1:1. My rule per 60 grams IV-C (infused in sterile distilled water) is to add 4 to 5 grams of calcium (as calcium gluconate) plus 3 to 4 grams of magnesium (as magnesium sulfate). I rarely exceed this, however, even when the IV-C consists of 70 grams or more. As for side effects, they are few.* The most serious (side effects) I've observed have followed the administration of 70, 80, and 90 grams.† During that evening and the next day the patient may complain of flu-like symptoms, feeling 'under the weather' and a fever that peaks at 100° to 102° F. While they soon go away, the symptoms are clearly a signal (to me) to back off. Other than this, IV-C has had an exceptional record of safety here."

Dr. Cathcart takes exception to Klenner's 1 in 10 rule. Using his proto-col, he claims that patients do not complain of tetany, and there's no need to add calcium—his success being credited to a slower rate of administration (3 to 4 hours per 500 ml rather than the usual 2–1/2 to 3 hours) and to his choice of parenteral fluid—lactated Ringer's rather than sterile distilled water.

Doctors who administer IV-C to mercury-toxic patients likewise take exception to Klenner's 1 in 10 rule, but for different reasons, citing the work of Galin and Obstbaum.[4] While studying the effect of mercury on eyesight, Galin

---

* As stated in Chapter 5, Dr. Wright makes it a practice to guard against kidney stones by testing for UGOT and UGPT enzymes beforehand, among other practices. When below 22 IU he administers an oral supplement of glutamic acid to the patient which, as reported by Israeli researchers, serves as an inhibitor of calcium oxalate stones. His 100% safety rate, he believes, can be credited to this and other aspects of his IV-C protocol.

† Before administering this large a dosage of IV-C, it is recommended that you consult first with Dr. Wright, with a clinical pharmacologist familiar with IV-C, or with Barbara Hannah, R.N., (Dr. Wright's nurse) for guidance. (See Appendix E.)

and Obstbaum learned that mercury exerts its damage by denaturing the protein within particular cell membranes of the eye, thereby causing calcific deposits in the cornea. The defect caused decreased vision as well as elevated ocular rigidity, which led to an increase in intraocular pressure and an increased risk of glaucoma. The detriment of calcium excess, these doctors believe, goes beyond its effect on the eye; the mercury/calcium interaction causes the denaturing of protein in other tissues as well; and an undue amount of calcium added to the IV-C may hinder the treatment program. Dr. Huggins, for instance, believes that the chelating action of IV-C on excesses of calcium may be one of the many ways in which IV-C improves the symptoms of the mercury-toxic patient. This, coupled with the recognition that calcium is nevertheless needed in the IV-C, is the basis for the varied protocols for administering IV-C.

Dr. Levin, as you'll recall, has found that as little as 10 ml of calcium gluconate and 5 ml magnesium sulfate added to the IV-C (in sterile distilled water) is satisfactory to prevent tetany when administering 30 grams or more. Dr. Cathcart prefers using lactated Ringer's to avoid having to add any additional calcium, since lactated Ringer's normally contains a small amount of calcium, along with other electrolytes. A question that arises is whether the rare occasion of tetany due to IV-C is truly related to vitamin C's capacity to chelate calcium, or whether the symptoms are simply a consequence of introducing an acidic IV-C infusion in which pH is at the outer limit of the buffering capacity of the patient's blood. Both may be correct, of course, but pH is probably the greatest determinant. In either case the debate doesn't stop with the pH of IV-C and the IV-C's potential for chelating calcium. It also includes the influence of the effect of osmolality. We will consider this under **THE CHOICE OF PARENTERAL FLUIDS**.

Facts To Consider When Ordering IV-C

When ordering IV-C made by the indirect method, the product will most likely be listed in the catalogue as ascorbic acid. It is not likely to be found as sodium ascorbate because sodium ascorbate doesn't currently match USP (United States Pharmacopeia) titles. Sample headings will be "ascorbic acid (as sodium ascorbate)", and "ascorbic acid injection (equivalent to sodium ascorbate)." These are available in vials containing 7.5 and 25 grams. The doctor will need both dosage sizes on hand.

However, simply finding it under the heading of "sodium ascorbate" still doesn't let one know by what method it was prepared, or to what pH the IV-C was finally adjusted. A letter or phone call to the manufacturer would readily reveal this. If a satisfactory product is unavailable, administer whatever IV-C source is available at a slower rate, extending the initial 2-1/2 to 3 hour infusion time to 3-1/2 to 4 hours.

DETERMINING THE DOSAGE

Scientists began administering megadose oral and intravenous vitamin C in the late 1930's, shortly after ascorbic acid was first made available for experimentation. In each case the dosage was arrived at by adjusting the dosage level to get the desired effect. Dey,[5] for instance, studied the effectiveness of megadose vitamin C in countering strychnine poisoning. He first determined that 100 mg per kilogram of body weight was the dosage required—in animals—to attain a 50 to 60 percent survival rate, while half this amount offered the animals little or no protection. On the other hand, when the dosage was increased ten-fold to one gram/kg body weight (this equates to 70 grams for an average adult human), none of the animals died. Only at this exceptional dosage were the animals totally protected from strychnine poisoning.

Dey found that dosages required to counter the effects of the tetanus toxin were even more exceptional. From animal studies, he found that complete neutralization of the toxin required one gram of vitamin C/kg body weight twice daily for 3 days (the equivalent of 140 grams of vitamin C/day for a 150 lb human).[6] A comparably high dosage was required to neutralize bacteria and viruses (as discussed in Chapter 4). Similarly, Mittler found that 50 to 70 grams were required to counter the effects of ozone,[7] and 35 grams for nitric oxide.

These early successes served as strong influences on the medical career of the noted Canadian psychiatrist, Dr. Abram Hoffer. Dr. Hoffer, in 1971, attested to having successfully treated more than 1,000 mental patients using megadose vitamin C—with dosages ranging from 3 to 30 grams/day.[8] Subsequently, Pauling coined the term "orthomolecular medicine." Based upon Hoffer's treatment concept, a collective group of psychiatrists formed the Society for Orthomolecular Psychiatry. They had jointly agreed on the importance of megadose vitamin C in the practice of psychiatric medicine. Later, after completing his work on elucidation of the protein helix, Pauling would dedicate his research efforts to understanding how vitamin C relates to the treatment of cancer, the common cold, and disease in general, arriving at dosages by adjusting the dosage level to get the desired effect.

To an even greater extent than these, Klenner provided an exceptional collective file on dosage, effectiveness, and safety. During his 30 years of use of megadose vitamin C in medicine and surgery, Dr. Klenner determined from animal studies that the human equivalent of 35 grams every 8 hours (105 grams per day) accelerated the healing process in patients with severe burns, and that a total of 54 grams was effective against barbiturate poisoning when administered during the first 24 hours.[9] In fact, he found it effective in detoxifying nearly every agent harmful to man, at dosages ranging from 5 to 200 grams per day.

In addition to these pioneering works, two other factors were important in arriving at the IV-C dosage that is now being used for treatment of chronic mercury toxicity. The first of these include the finding of Galin and Obstbaum which showed that excess calcium in the eye of patients poisoned with mercury was capable of denaturing ocular proteins—thereby contributing to poor vision. This finding, combined with earlier reports of the effective treatment of glaucoma using 50 to 70 grams of vitamin C, led to the assumption that many people with glaucoma, band keratopathy, and related eye pathology, probably had chronic mercury toxicity at the root of their problem.

More importantly, however, it suggested that micromercurialism in general, regardless of its manifested form, would respond to a like dosage schedule (50 to 70 grams IV-C). From these observed results an intravenous dosage of 700 mg/kg body weight (48 grams of IV-C per 150 lb person) was decided upon as the optimally effective dosage for the average mercury-toxic patient; and 800 mg/kg body weight (54 grams of IV-C per 150 lb person) for the patient with severe chronic mercury toxicity. Any additional vitamin C needed would be provided orally.

Calculating IV-C Dosage for the Average Mercury-Toxic Patient
To determine the dosage required when titrating to bowel tolerance, or for the vitamin C flush:
Divide weight in pounds by 2.2 and multiply by 0.7 g.
The average mercury-toxic patient requires 16 to 20 grams orally.

Example
For a 110 lb person:
110 lbs ÷ 2.2 = 50 kg
50 kg x 700 mg (0.7 g) = 35 g IV-C for average toxicity

Calculating IV-C Dosage For Patients with Severe Chronic Mercury Toxicity
Those who required 32 to 50 grams or more of oral vitamin C when titrated to bowel tolerance, or to complete the vitamin C flush.
Divide weight in pounds by 2.2 and multiply by 0.8 g.

Example
For a 110 lb person:
110 lbs ÷ 2.2 = 50 kg
50 kg x 800 mg (0.8 g) = 40 g IV-C for severe toxicity

Table 9:1 gives some sample dosages, using the same procedure. By using the method of calculation above, it becomes very easy to determine exact dosage for a patient.

THE CHOICE OF PARENTERAL FLUIDS

Klenner, in administering IV-C to thousands of patients with various conditions, used either normal saline, sterile distilled water, or dextrose 5% in water. Yet interviews conducted for this book revealed that today's doctors are more selective and critical of these former practices. Dr. Cathcart, for instance, prefers lactated Ringer's. (He previously used sterile distilled water but found that the patient's veins were more comfortable with lactated Ringer's.) He finds lactated Ringer's especially helpful for the patient who's fragile, frail, or recovering from a lengthy illness. He limits dosage to 60 grams IV-C per 500 ml lactated Ringer's. Whatever additional IV-C that's required is added to a second bottle of lactated Ringer's, or to sterile distilled water.

Table 9:1

Weight (in lbs.)	Grams needed for Average Toxicity	Grams needed for Severe Toxicity
120	38	44
130	41	47
140	45	51
150	48	54
160	51	58
170	54	62

Even then the dosage is limited to 60 grams IV-C per 500 ml, or no more than 10 grams IV-C per 100 ml. A higher dosage in either vehicle, Cathcart believes, has the potential for destroying the vein and causing much pain in the process.

Lactated Ringer's is Dr. Huggins' first choice of parenteral fluids—for all mercury-toxic patients, regardless of their condition—for the first 48 grams of IV-C (contrasting only slightly with Dr. Cathcart's method). Sterile distilled water is reserved for the average mercury-toxic patient for whatever additional IV-C is required beyond 48 grams—5 grams IV-C minimum per 100 ml, with a maximum of 7.5 grams IV-C per 100 ml sterile distilled water. A second bottle of lactated Ringer's is used for the severely mercury-toxic patient (when more than 48 grams IV-C is required). Drs. Levin and Wright, on the other hand, rely almost entirely on sterile water, regardless of the patient's diagnosis. They contend that sterile distilled water is the only logical vehicle for IV-C, feeling that it should not be mixed into a vehicle that is isotonic to begin with, such as 5% dextrose, normal saline, or lactated Ringer's.

All the doctors share an identical concern that the dosage of IV-C required for the **IV-C Mercury Tox Program** always necessitates infusing a hyperosmolar solution. The only alternative—giving the treatment dosage as an isoosmolar solution—would require infusing too great a volume of fluid in most cases. An explanation of this requires a discussion of osmolality.

Osmolality

A review of the basics of the practical application of plasma osmolality is necessary, although most doctors and health professionals will likely have had some training, and some will probably be well-acquainted with the subject. I also wish to present the perspective that the osmolality of IV-C in solution has a physiological effect that often differs considerably from other I.V. solutions of equal osmolality.

Osmolality, properly defined, is that property of body fluids or any infused solution which determines the flow of fluid between cells, cell membranes, and the extracellular environment. The flow of fluid across the osmotic partition (the plasma cell membrane) follows a path from the lesser to the greater concentration. When plasma osmolality is normal, the intracellular and extracellular concentration of osmotically active particles are equal.* A hypoosmolar infusion, on the other hand, causes cells to expand in size. This occurs when the intracellular concentration of osmotically-active particles is greater than the resulting extracellular concentration. The opposite occurs when one administers a hyperosmolar solution, such as IV-C. The cells in this case tend to shrink, as the extracellular concentration of osmotically-active particles is initially greater than the intracellular concentration (even if the effect is only transient). It is the latter scenario that naturally concerns the doctor who administers IV-C, simply because IV-C, to be effective, must be administered as a hyperosmolar solution.

The doctor's initial uneasiness to administer IV-C as a hyperosmolar infusion rather than an isoosmolar infusion is understandable. It is well documented, through animal studies, that an extremely hyperosmolar infusion, given rapidly, may cause any number of ill effects including CNS dysfunction,

---

* A normal reading of plasma osmolality on the osmometer is 285-310 mOsm/liter water, or mmol/liter, when measured by the freezing-point depression method—the freezing point being dependent upon the number of particles, molecules, or ions in solution.

mental disturbances, coma as the result of shrinkage of brain cells, and severe cardiovascular alterations.[10],[11]   Yet, as Quiros and Ware demonstrated,[12] these severest of conditions do not develop until the infused, hyperosmolar solution exceeds 6 to 10 times normal (1800 mOsm/liter and up), and is given rapidly. This fact is important since hyperosmolar IV-C administered in water ranges normally between 600 and 900 mOsm/liter; while IV-C in lactated Ringer's, when used as recommended, ranges normally from 700 to 1200 mOsm/liter; and, when given slowly, its effect on blood osmolality is minimal and transient.

At the opposite extreme, the body often <u>benefits</u> from smaller, transient rises in osmolality. Transient changes in plasma osmolality, for instance, account for fifty percent of the positive effect on bile formation by plasma sodium.[13] It also influences blood pressure through a sensitive osmoreceptor mechanism in the brain, which regulates the release of vasopressin. In addition, a transient, hyperosmolar condition develops normally as a means of countering hypoxic stress, such as during severe exercise[14] and during hemorrhagic hypotension.[15]

The effect of a hyperosmolar I.V. infusion, therefore (whether good or bad), will always lie somewhere between these two extremes—the outcome determined mainly by the rate of infusion, the choice of parenteral fluids, and the patient's preexisting state of health.

To better understand the physiological effect of infusing a hyperosmolar solution, one needs only to observe patients who suffer from trauma, cancer, or malnutrition. Each condition has essentially the same effect on the patient's plasma osmolality as a hyperosmolar I.V. infusion of sodium chloride.[16] Trauma, cancer, and malnutrition cause extracellular fluid to increase, especially in skeletal muscles, with significant vasodilation of affected organs (related to severity of involvement). This same effect can be observed when hyperosmolar I.V. sodium chloride is administered, as Read, et al.[17] readily demonstrated. When infused quickly enough, the researchers found that every organ and tissue type responded with significant vasodilation. Yet the effect was only transient and much less extensive when sodium chloride and other hyperosmolar solutions were infused slowly. So the first general rule, derived from Read's experience, is to <u>decrease the rate of infusion as the dosage and osmolality of IV-C increases</u>.

The Physiological Osmolar Effects of Parenteral Fluids don't Always Compare Equally. The latest research suggests that a distinct difference exists in the physiological effect of various I.V. solutions of equal osmolality. Referring once again to the findings of Kurtz, the capacity of sodium chloride to increase blood pressure in his five subjects indicated that its effect was a function of the anionic, chloride component—not the sodium component. Kurtz' findings clearly demonstrated that sodium chloride increases plasma volume and thereby increases blood pressure, while an equal osmolar solution of sodium citrate has no effect. Support for these findings was added by the team's animal model studies, in which they found that an expanded plasma volume (with an increase in blood pressure) occurs only when sodium is administered as the chloride salt. Neither plasma volume nor blood pressure increase when sodium is administered as bicarbonate, phosphate, glutamate, glycinate, aspartate, or the ascorbate salt.[18],[19]

The findings of Kurtz suggests that hyperosmolar IV-C (as sodium ascorbate) administered in sterile distilled water exerts a physiological effect or effects that are more consistent with health than an equal osmolar infusion of sodium chloride. While the paradox will require additional research for a full understanding, the facts even today illustrate that sodium chloride definitely should not be considered as a parenteral fluid for administering IV-C. IV-sodium ascorbate administered in sterile water seems the logical choice.

Potential Benefits From Hyperosmolar IV-C. Elliott's work suggests that hyperosmolar IV-C actually promotes a net loss of sodium, which is counter to the hyperosmolar effect of sodium chloride. This, and the fact that IV-C promotes diuresis, further supports the contention that hyperosmolar IV-C exerts a physiological effect that opposes the expected, negative effects of infusing other hyperosmolar solutions. Additional support for this phenomenon is available from the doctors who have the most clinical experience with IV-C. They generally concur that the blood pressure of a hypertensive patient tends to normalize during, and for a short time following, the administration of hyperosmolar IV-C. So the potential for benefit from infusing hyperosmolar IV-C is significantly greater than the risk.

In addition, there are those patients with either hyperglobulinemia or hyperlipidemia whose plasma osmolality tends to be lower than normal prior to treatment. These people, who are generally at increased risk to ischemia, tend to benefit more from hyperosmolar IV-C than they might from isoosmolar IV-C. It is perhaps this action that has accounted for some of the improvement of symptoms reported by the thousands of patients who've received IV-C therapy. The finding of Sawchuk, et al.,[20] unobtrusively suggests a plausible explanation. The transient volume expansion that accompanies the hyperosmolar infusion, however slight, may temporarily correct tissue ischemia—as long as the patient has sufficient blood sugar to support anaerobic metabolism. Thus, the scientific and extensive clinical evidence available today suggests that hyperosmolar IV-C, when infused as suggested here, is beneficial to the patient in many ways. Particularly, it's a safe and effective therapeutic for chronic mercury toxicity. If, however, you choose to deviate from this protocol, or should you desire a more thorough understanding for calculating osmolality, I suggest that you confer either with a clinical pharmacologist, or with Barbara Hannah, R. N., Pat Hayes, R. N., The McGuff Medical Products Company, or Dr. Warren Levin. (See Appendix E.)

Before Administering Hyperosmolar IV-C: A Few Precautions. A patient with hyperglycemia (poorly controlled insulin-dependent diabetes mellitus), whose resting plasma osmolality may be 360 mOsm/liter, or higher, should not receive hyperosmolar IV-C because of the risk of developing nonketotic coma due to a further rise in plasma osmolality. Once the patient is thoroughly hydrated and his blood sugar is controlled, then it is probably alright to administer hyperosmolar IV-C (as long as the patient's diabetic specialist has been notified). Otherwise, rather than administer the usual recommended dosage, the dosage should be reduced to conform with the formula for an isoosmolar solution. A similar rule would apply equally for the high-risk patient with azotemia, or altered kidney function; and for the high-risk patient with a history of red blood cell fragility, anemia, or G-6-PD deficiency.

Lactated Ringer's is Particularly Useful for the Weak and Severely Ill Patient.

It is understandable, and perfectly acceptable, that the osmolality issue would cause most doctors to rely strictly on sterile distilled water as the parenteral fluid of choice for IV-C, regardless of the patient's condition. Sterile distilled water, after all, is necessary to optimize the osmolality of IV-C, and it's the only logical choice if one desires to keep the osmolality of the infusion as close to the osmolality of blood as possible (approximately 300 mOsm/liter). Yet, there are good reasons why some doctors choose lactated Ringer's for administering IV-C to the mercury-toxic patient, and to patients with other conditions as well.

Lactated Ringer's provides the electrolytes necessary for normal cardiac function, including traces of sodium, chloride, potassium, and calcium (but not so much calcium that it interferes with the treatment for chronic mercury toxicity); it's a source of water for hydration; and, depending on the patient's clinical condition, it is capable of inducing diuresis. IV-C is likewise capable of inducing diuresis. So when given together, lactated Ringer's and IV-C tend to cooperate in normalizing plasma osmolality by inducing diuresis. Finally, and perhaps most importantly, this solution also contains sodium lactate, which—acting together with the electrolytes—produces a metabolic alkalizing effect. Referring to the package insert, sodium lactate is a racemic salt. The *levo* form is oxidized by the liver to bicarbonate, and the *dextro* form is converted to glycogen—both reactions depending on oxidative cellular activity. In the formation of bicarbonate, l-lactate is slowly metabolized to carbon dioxide and water, accepting one hydrogen ion in the process. This is beneficial to the high-risk and severely ill patient whose blood is often acidic, thereby serving to reduce both the risk of acidosis and kidney stones.

There are, of course, contraindications to the I.V. administration of lactated Ringer's, as well as warnings and precautions. A thorough accounting of these can be found in the I.V. package insert. Ringer's is contraindicated for patients with severe liver disease, or for those suffering from severe anoxia, shock, or cardiac failure. In addition, Richard Veech, M. D., who represents the Foundation for Advanced Research in the Medical Sciences, has hypothesized drawbacks to the present formula for lactated Ringer's and to parenteral acetate solutions.[21]

In a review of the toxicity of parenteral solutions, Veech warns that acetate solutions should not be used to replace solutions containing bicarbonate. (This is mentioned here only because acetate Ringer's solution is becoming increasingly popular, especially in Europe.) Acetate Ringer's solution has the potential of causing diabetes and promoting the uptake in the brain of heavy metals, among other drawbacks. Veech argues further that the d,l-lactate presently a part of lactated Ringer's should be replaced by the manufacturers with l-lactate:pyruvate and other constituents, each in a physiologically balanced ratio. He contends that with present technology and research capabilities there is no justification for the continued use of d,l-lactate, given its known neurotoxic potential. Yet until an improved formula becomes available, the d,l-lactated Ringer's remains important for administering IV-C to severely ill patients. "The IV-C itself," says Dr. Huggins, "being of special benefit to mercury-toxic patients having neurological involvement, has been shown in our clinic to override the potential for neurotoxicity from d,l-lactated Ringer's."

PREPARING THE IV-C SET-UP

It's important to have on hand 500 ml bags or bottles of both lactated Ringer's and sterile distilled water. Lactated Ringer's is the parenteral fluid of first choice for the mercury-toxic patient, up to 48 grams of IV-C in 500 ml. Sterile distilled water is reserved for the average mercury-toxic patient—for whatever dosage of IV-C is required beyond 48 grams. This additional IV-C is added to the sterile distilled water at the rate of 5 to 7.5 grams per 100 ml. A second bottle of lactated Ringer's is reserved for the severely mercury–toxic patient, for whatever dosage is required beyond 48 grams IV-C. Before the concentrate is added, however, decant and dispose of enough of the parenteral fluid to accommodate the number of milliliters of IV-C needed. This is done by first attaching an I.V. solution administration set (I.V. line) to the outlet on each of the infusion bottles. Once attached, hang the I.V. line(s) and bottle(s), attached, upside down from an I.V. stand (pole or standard) and drain into the sink an amount of lactated Ringer's equivalent to the amount of IV-C to be added. If the dosage exceeds 48 grams—in which case the additional IV-C will be added to a second bottle—also drain the predetermined amount of the second bottle of parenteral fluid into the sink. In the process, make sure all the air is out of the I.V. lines and, by giving the filter/windows a soft squeeze, fill the filter/windows about half way so the rate of infusion can be observed and controlled. When the desired quantity of fluid is decanted, halt the flow with the clamp attached to the I.V. line.

> NOTE: If treating a condition other than chronic mercury toxicity, you will likely be using only sterile distilled water. Decant whatever additional amount of parenteral fluid is necessary to allow for the ml of calcium gluconate, magnesium sulfate, or other parenteral nutrition to be added. Before commencing, however, do consult with one of the source people previously mentioned who can assist in titrating the I.V. solution to an acceptable osmolality for that patient.

An infusion set of your choice is then ready for attachment to the tip of the lactated Ringer's administration set. A 21-23 gauge 3/4" butterfly will suffice, although more elaborate and secure setups are available. Then, using aseptic technique, transfer the IV-C to the parenteral fluids via 16 gauge needle and a 50 ml single use syringe. Instructions will accompany the IV-C vial. Afterwards, mix gently and return the solution to the I.V. stand.

> CAUTION: It is very important to make certain that the IV-C has indeed been added to the sterile distilled water. Otherwise, the zero osmolality of sterile water will cause hemolysis, a hemolytic crisis, or perhaps patient death. Keep in mind: IV-C concentrate is clear, just as water, but slightly yellow. The fluid that's about to be infused should also have some yellow.

Before the infusion begins make certain that the patient has read, signed, and witnessed the **Shared Responsibility Form** (Chapter 8), and that he has an understanding of what's expected of him. Afterwards, record on the **Patient Record Form** (a sample of which follows) the patient's pre- and post-IV-C vital signs, especially the blood pressure and heart rate. There is room for other pertinent notes as well.

While prepping the patient, check to see that he is comfortable, and has had an opportunity to use the restroom beforehand. Have a few pre-torn strips of adhesive handy to secure the infusion set and the I.V. line.

Infuse the IV-C in lactated Ringer's first. "Piggy-back" the second bottle, if needed, just before completion of the first. In that manner only one needle has to be inserted. Once the IV-C is started, adjust the rate to approximately 60 drops/minute, with an acceptable range of 45 to 70 drops/minute. This rate assumes the patient is receiving no more than 48 grams IV-C per 500 ml infusion fluid. (In general, the higher the dosage the higher the osmolality, which necessitates a slower rate of infusion.) If infiltration is suspected, question the patient at once. Infiltration will quickly cause the patient to suffer a burning sensation at or above the needle site. If only a slight tingle is noted, slow the rate of infusion. The tingle generally goes away in a matter of minutes, in which case the infusion rate can then be returned to normal. Should the tingle again return, repeat the process. The need to repeat this procedure would indicate either that the needle needs to be adjusted, the IV-C is too acidic, or both.

During the IV-C <u>do</u> provide the patient with all the water he wants, adding a few drops of lemon juice as his condition (risk for kidney stones) warrants. The patient should also be encouraged to use the restroom whenever he wishes, taking the I.V. paraphernalia with him. Halfway through the IV-C note how the patient is feeling. If the rate of infusion is too fast he will report being dizzy, faint, or hypoglycemic,* on rare occasions feeling nauseated. Thirst, however, is to be expected. While it's not an adverse sign, <u>do</u> encourage him to drink water to help offset the transient, hyperosmolar condition due to the IV-C. In most cases he will report being more relaxed and hopeful than he has been in some time. This is especially true of the mercury-toxic patient who, midway through the IV-C, often becomes decidedly more receptive to—and emotionally desirous of—further lifestyle counseling.

---

* Dr. Cathcart counters this by slowing the rate of infusion and encouraging the patient to eat or drink natural juices during the IV-C.

IV-C Mercury Tox Program®
PATIENT RECORD FORM

For Office Use Only

Blood Pressure   Heart Rate

Pre IV-C _____ _____ IV-C started by: _____ time: _____

Post IV-C _____ _____ IV-C ended by: _____ time: _____

Midtest Observations

Initials: _____

Time: _____

Date: _____

Immediate Post-test Observations

Initials: _____

Time: _____

Date: _____

12 Hour Follow-Up

Initials: _____

Time: _____

Date: _____

24 Hour Follow-Up

Initials: _____

Time: _____

Date: _____

36 Hour Follow-Up

Initials: _____

Time: _____

Date: _____

48 Hour Follow-Up

Initials: _____

Time: _____

Date: _____

IV-C AND DENTAL AMALGAM REPLACEMENT

When opinions were sought on the value of IV-C, and what was considered the best timing for the administration of IV-C in mercury-toxic patients undergoing dental amalgam replacement, Huggins replied, "From observations of patients...and how they tolerate dental procedures...the optimum time to use IV-C would be during the first appointment of amalgam removal. Megadose IV-C reduces the amount of unwanted reaction, and the patient's feeling of well-being is usually greater after IV-C than would be after the conventional procedure without it. I look at it as protective and therapeutic both. It's value is such that every patient undergoing amalgam removal should receive IV-C simultaneously.

"There is an enormous amount of exposure to the patient during the removal of fillings. Studies that were done by Duane Cutwright showed that the average mercury level in the brains of mice, when exposed to amalgam mist just a few inches away from where an amalgam was being cut, went from around 50 nanograms (ng) up to 400 ng within an hour, and that the mercury level in the heart increased to over 4000 ng. So the exposure to amalgam replacement gives the patient a serious, toxic challenge, for which IV-C is not only protective, but therapeutic. It serves as a transport ligand that escorts the excess mercury out through the urine. This has not been reported in the literature, but it can easily be documented. What's not so easily documented is the form taken by excreted mercury. My contention is that it's most likely excreted as mercury ascorbate, much like lead is excreted as lead ascorbate. I've found that the amount of urine mercury excreted during amalgam replacement closely parallels the vitamin C excretion curve, so I believe this explanation would certainly make sense."*

Burton A. Miller,† a dentist in Anchorage, Alaska, together with John D. Walsh, D. D. S., has pulled together a medical team which I believe is the ideal partnership for documentation, treatment, and evaluation of the mercury-toxic patient. Dr. Miller says, "I solicit the help of our registered nurse therapist to start the IV-C infusion fifteen minutes before I'm scheduled to begin [dental amalgam replacement], and to adjust the rate so the IV-C drips continuously while I'm working, usually 2-1/2 to 3 hours. Using this standard protocol, our mercury-toxic patients seem to improve quickly." (Much more so, I believe, than if IV-C were administered afterwards, or before amalgam replacement). The team findings of Dr. Miller's group seem to agree with the findings of other clinicians that mercury-toxic patients respond much more quickly to the total treatment plan—dramatically, in some cases—when IV-C is administered during dental amalgam replacement.

In speaking with Pat Hayes, R. N., Walsh's/Miller's therapist, it became evident that there are two divergent protocols for administering IV-C to the mercury-toxic patient. Both involve the use of supportive, oral megadose vitamin supplementation, in addition to an amended lifestyle which begins a few days or weeks prior to administering IV-C. In the first protocol, however

* Dr. Huggins' observations are, as yet, unpublished.

† Drs. Miller and Walsh coordinate their treatment of mercury-toxic patients with a medical team that includes Robert Rowan, M.D. (a family practitioner and specialist in chelation therapy) Roger Clyne, Ph.D. (clinical psychologist), and Pat Hayes, R.N., among other health care specialists.

(which I recommend because of simplicity) the only nutrition that is added to the parenteral fluid is IV-C. In the second, which is the one advocated by the team of Miller and Walsh, et al., the nurse therapist adds parenteral B-complex vitamins and minerals to the parenteral fluid and IV-C.

Hayes explained that she, working with Dr. Rowen, has developed a modified formula for a nutritional IV for dental patients. The formula calls for the addition of 1 ml vitamin B-complex, plus 1 ml extra vitamin B_6 and 1 ml vitamin B_5 (pantothenic acid) to the IV-C and parenteral fluid, as well as the addition of minerals, as indicated by the patient's blood, urine, and hair analysis beforehand. "Most people who are mercury-toxic," Hayes explains, "are deficient in essential trace minerals. The additional nutrition helps support the patient's immune system, and support their metabolic and enzymatic functions. The additional vitamin B_5 may especially be important (to the mercury-toxic patient), since its active form (coenzyme A) is required in many of the body's repair processes.

"As for speed, the IV-C usually takes about 3 hours...whatever is needed to carry the patient through the drilling time. This usually means 60 drops per minute, sometimes slower, but never any faster than 70 to 80 drops per minute. We believe the dental patient's improvement is greatly accelerated by following this protocol, rather than relying completely on oral megadose vitamins. The patient may not be capable of absorbing orally administered nutrients, in which case his recovery would be slowed. In our method, in which we combine oral supplements with megadose parenteral nutrition, the patient is better able to correct nutritional and hormonal imbalances, and simultaneously prevent kidney stones." The doctor who follows this course, however, must be especially aware of the procedure for balancing and calculating osmolality. If this is your choice, you will want to consult first with Ms. Hayes. (See Appendix E.)

Is IV-C in the IV-C Mercury Tox Program Intended as a One-Time Treatment, or does the Program Require Multiple Infusions?

Most people who are mercury-toxic will require only one IV-C infusion in conjunction with the **IV-C Mercury Tox Program**. When administered to the mercury-toxic patient who is having his dental amalgam fillings replaced, a single infusion is indicated for each day of drilling. The regimen thereafter will focus on prevention, diet, and lifestyle behavioral changes, along with whatever additional supportive therapy the doctor believes necessary. Those who have suffered the longest from chronic mercury toxicity are likely to require additional IV-C infusions, but this won't be difficult for them to accept. Once patients have experienced the benefit of their first IV-C, it won't be hard to motivate them for a second treatment, should the doctor believe it's needed. It's not unusual, in fact, for a patient to request it himself.

IN SUMMARY, THE IV-C Mercury Tox Program SHOULD INCLUDE THE FOLLOWING PROTOCOL:

- Lactated Ringer's Injection, USP, is the parenteral fluid of choice for administering 48 g or less of IV-C. (If you prefer sterile distilled water, contact one of the source people who can guide you in its use.)

- No more than 48 g IV-C should be added to 500 ml lactated Ringer's.

- Sterile water is the parenteral fluid of choice for any additional IV-C beyond 48 g, administered to the average mercury–toxic patient. A second bottle of lactated Ringer's is recommended for any additional IV-C beyond 48 g, administered to the severely mercury–toxic patient.

- If lactated Ringer's is your choice, then any additional parenterally administered nutrition must be omitted.

- If parenteral supplemental nutrition is to be added other than IV-C then sterile distilled water is the only choice. In this case, follow the procedure(s) suggested by either Drs. Levin (10 ml calcium gluconate and 5 ml magnesium sulfate added to any dosage of 30 g IV-C or more, plus sodium bicarbonate to adjust to pH 6.5) or Miller, Walsh, and Rowen, and Pat Hayes.

- If lactated Ringer's is contraindicated for the patient's condition, then, again, sterile distilled water is the only choice.

- *Remember Dr. Cathcart's Advice (Chapter 2):* Have the patient continue taking oral vitamin C during the infusion, but restrict the oral vitamin C once the infusion is down to 100 ml. Otherwise, the patient will get diarrhea—sometimes even before the infusion is discontinued. To avoid headaches and many other adverse effects, Cathcart also advises the doctor to follow the IV-C by again titrating to bowel tolerance with oral vitamin C.

A WORD OF CAUTION: When administering IV-C in sterile distilled water be very certain that you have indeed added the IV-C before starting the infusion. IV-sterile distilled water, given alone, will certainly cause hemolysis, a hemolytic crisis, and perhaps death. Keep in mind: IV-C concentrate is clear, just like water, but slightly yellow. The fluid that's about to be infused should likewise have some yellow.

A cloud of mystery and heresy has for many years blanketed the administration of IV-C. Many of these false notions have now been dispelled, such as the former belief that IV-C could be administered either as sodium ascorbate or ascorbic acid. Sodium ascorbate is the only choice. Now that most of the issues have been covered in this and preceding chapters, there remains a need to standardize the IV-C protocol, which can only be resolved through research and clinical experience. Hopefully, the information presented here will help to lay the groundwork for establishing a protocol for administering IV-C that's acceptable to everyone. Only then, I believe, will IV-C gain its proper place in the healing arts—important not only in the treatment of chronic mercury toxicity, but in treating nearly every disease that commonly afflicts man.

LITERATURE CITED

[1] H.C. Elliott, "Effects of Vitamin C Loading on Serum Constituents in Man," *Proc Soc Exp Biol Med*, 169: 1982.

[2] T.W. Kurtz, H. A. Al-Bander, and R.C. Morris, Jr., " 'Salt-Sensitive' Essential hypertension In Men: Is the Sodium Ion Alone Important?" *N Eng J Med*, 317 (17): 1043-8, October 22, 1987.

[3] R.F. Cathcart, "Vitamin C In The Treatment Of Acquired Immune Deficiency Syndrome (AIDS)," *Med Hypo* , 14: 426, 1984.

[4] M.A. Galin and S.A. Obstbaum, "Band Keratopathy in Mercury Exposure," *Annals of Ophthalmology*, 1257-61, December 1974.

[5] P.K. Dey, "Protective Action of Ascorbic Acid and Its Precursors on the Convulsive and Lethal Actions of Strychnine," *Indian J Exper Biol*, 5: 110-112, 1967.

[6] P.K. Dey, "Efficacy of Vitamin C in Counteracting Tetanus Toxin Toxicity," *Naturwissenschaften*, 53: 310, 1966.

[7] S. Mittler, "Protection against Death due to Ozone Poisoning," *Nature*, 181: 1063-4, 1958.

[8] A. Hoffer, "Ascorbic Acid and Toxicity," *N Eng J Med* , 285: 635-6, 1971.

[9] F.R. Klenner, "Observations on the Dose and Administration of Ascorbic Acid When Employed Beyond the Range of a Vitamin in Human Pathology," *J Applied Nutrition:*, 23: 61-88, 1971.

[10] J.M. Atkins, et al., "Cardiovascular Responses to Hyperosmotic Mannitol in Anesthetized and Conscious Dogs," *Am J Physiol* 225: 132-7, 1973.

[11] J. Järhult, et al., "Circulatory Effects Evoked by Physiological Increases of Arterial Osmolality," *Acta Physiol Scand*, 93: 129-34, 1975.

[12] G. Quiros and J. Ware, "Cardiovascular and Lymph Flow Changes Caused by Physiological Hyperosmolar Provocation in Unanesthetized Rats," *Eur Surg Res*, 16: 69-76, 1984.

[13] O. Mathisen and M. Raeder, "Role of Sodium, Bicarbonate, and Plasma Osmolality in Biliary Secretion," *Scand J Gastroenterol*, 18: 825-32, 1983.

[14] J. Lundvall, et al., "Fluid Transfer Between Blood and Tissues During Exercise," *Acta Physiol Scand*, 85: 258-69, 1972.

[15] S.E. Bergentz and D.D. Brief, "The Effect of pH and Osmolality on the Production of Canine Haemorrhagic Shock," *Surgery, St. Louis,* 58: 412-9, 1965.

[16] A. Stillström, et al., "Postoperative Water and Electrolyte Changes in Skeletal Muscle: a Clinical Study with Three Different Intravenous Infusions," *Acta Anaesthesiol Scand,* 31: 284-8, 1987.

[17] R.C. Read, et al., "Vascular Effects of Hypertonic Solutions," *Circulation Res,* 8: 538-46, 1960.

[18] T.W. Kurtz, and R.C. Morris, Jr., "Dietary Chloride as a Determinant of "Sodium-Dependent" Hypertension," *Science,* 222: 1139-41, 1983.

[19] S.A. Whitescarver, et al., "Salt-Sensitive Hypertension: Contribution of Chloride," *Science,* 223: 1430-2, 1984.

[20] A. Sawchuk, et al., "A Comparison between Fructose 1,6-diphosphate, Glucose, or Normal Saline Infusions and Species-Specific Blood Exchange Transfusions in the Treatment of Bowel Ischemias," *Surgery,* 100 (4): 665-70, October 1986.

[21] R.L. Veech, "The Toxic Impact of Parenteral Solutions on the Metabolism of Cells: a Hypothesis for Physiological Parenteral Therapy," *AJCN* ,44: 519-51, October 1986.

CHAPTER 10

Follow-Up and Evaluation:
A Logical Basis For
Continued Lifestyle Counseling

"The physician, the patient, the medicine, and the attendants (nurses) are the four essential factors of a course of medical treatment. Even a dangerous disease is readily cured, or it may be expected to run a speedy course in the event of the preceding four factors being respectively found to be qualified, self-controlled, genuine and intelligently watchful."

~Sushruta [5th Cent. ? B.C.]

In concluding this book, the final chapter is concerned with evaluating both the patient's progress and the effectiveness of the **IV-C Mercury Tox Program.** The distinction is necessary since the patient's progress may be due to a placebo effect—a phenomenon which exists in any treatment program. As in all therapies the treatment may indeed improve the patient's health without addressing the suspected cause, specifically chronic mercury toxicity.

The intent of the **IV-C Mercury Tox Program** is two-fold: to detoxify mercury (reducing the total body burden of mercury to the point where chronic mercury toxicity is no longer manifested); and to repair the bodily injury caused by mercury and other heavy metals. It is the latter outcome that makes this treatment program unique, and universally necessary.

To help in assessing the treatment outcome, and to justify the means for attaining the best possible outcome, this chapter has a dual purpose. First we'll review the established methods of evaluating improvement in the mercury-toxic patient, while also suggesting newer methods of evaluation.* Then, we'll demonstrate the importance of continued lifestyle counseling as a means of maximally reducing the patient's total body burden of mercury and ultimately restoring the body to health. The keys for accomplishing the desired outcome are commitment, goal-setting, and motivation.

THE EVALUATION PROCEDURE

Because of past proven successes of IV-C in the treatment of a wide range of diseases and disease conditions, one might logically question any specific claim of efficacy. Is the patient's improvement a reflection of IV-C in general, without any effect on chronic mercury toxicity? Should the observed, healthful results be credited to the treatment's specific effect in detoxifying mercury? Or are both possible? There are, unfortunately, no tests today that offer absolute answers to such questions, with the possible exception of the experimental porphyrin fingerprint. So until objective tests <u>do</u> become available, the doctor's evaluation must be based on positive, indirect evidence of symptoms, structured to the following three-stage process:

1. The <u>pretest evaluation</u>, which starts with initial doctor/patient contact.

* A sample **Patient Evaluation Form** will be found at the end of this chapter.

2. The <u>midtest evaluation</u>, embracing all possible events (good and bad) that surround the administration of IV-C, most of which were covered previously.
3. The <u>post-test evaluation</u>, which takes place once the treatment program has been completed.

In practice, the evaluation process is continuous and involves the doctor, patient, therapist, and entire medical staff. All participants should be alerted to possible feedback, as with any treatment program. The staff must be ready to observe and record any symptoms that may occur during or immediately following completion of the IV-C, and throughout the first few days after administration. The patient must likewise be made aware of the varied responses that can be expected. This is why a "patient call-back" (via telephone, house-call, or in-house interview) becomes a vital part of the treatment program.

The patient call-back will keep the doctor informed, as he will want to know of any and every change in bodily function. There are other benefits to this arrangement as well. Staying in touch will provide the patient with the assurance that the symptoms experienced are not of a serious nature, and if they <u>do</u> become serious, the informed doctor is better prepared to deal with it. In fact, because of the need to reassure the patient and periodically make therapeutic and lifestyle adjustments, the communicative channels opened by patient call-backs lay the foundation of trust needed to ensure the success of the **IV-C Mercury Tox Program**. Additionally, it provides the basis by which the doctor can later effectively implement an ongoing program of lifestyle counseling.

Pretest Evaluation: Preparing for Treatment

The pretest evaluation includes whatever testing is necessary to make the diagnosis of chronic mercury toxicity. Once the diagnosis is documented, a broader, second, pretest analysis can be initiated for the purpose of evaluating the patient's progress later on. The protocol followed by Dr. Miller and Dr. Walsh of Anchorage, provides an excellent working model. They work closely with a medical diagnostician and a clinical psychologist. At some point before the treatment begins—after the patient has been evaluated by the dentists— these two professionals also conduct an evaluation. Particularly, the clinical psychologist performs a pretest psychological and personality inventory analysis, while the medical diagnostician performs a physical examination that includes blood, hair, and urine chemistries. If necessary, the patient is referred elsewhere for a chiropractic examination, or to yet another health specialist as his condition warrants. The patient then receives IV-C in conjunction with his dental treatment.

(*Author's note: The patients are allowed to enter this system at any of several points, whether they are first seeking the advice of a clinical psychologist, physician, or dentist. To ensure that the system works efficiently as well as effectively, each doctor has only to become familiar with the symptoms of chronic mercury toxicity relative to his or her own health specialty.*)

Midtest Evaluation: What To Look For Immediately Following IV-C

Some of the symptoms known to occur within the first 8 to 36 hours following IV-C administration include headache, nausea, constipation, and diarrhea (reflecting patient individuality), as well as subtle changes in the menstrual cycle or some other hormone-mediated event. These are symptoms that the patient more than likely did not experience previous to the IV-C treatment.

Rarely, anxiety attacks and heightened neuromuscular reactions might also be expected.

Most of these symptoms, however discomforting to the patient, should not be considered negative features. After all, the **IV-C Mercury Tox Program** was designed to diminish the body burden of mercury as much as possible while restoring normal cellular function. If one considers the removal of mercury from plasma cell membranes a "good" event, then perhaps the symptoms that subsequently follow are equally good, due to the return of cell membrane health, even if the initial manifestation is sorely unpleasant. As you'll recall from Chapter 2, when normalcy is restored to a dysfunctioning cell, the cell membrane can again carry out its six primary functions, one of which is the release of pent-up cellular waste. The subsequent dumping of waste into the blood stream may very well account for the patient's feeling of fatigue and lethargy for a day or so afterwards. It may also account for a plenitude of other symptoms which, to the uninformed observer, may incorrectly be considered unfavorable.

An example of the process that the patient often goes through in his recovery was volunteered during an interview with Sandra Denton, M. D., a board certified emergency physician who—after 14 years in her chosen profession—decided to limit her practice to the treatment of mercury-toxic patients, and other nutritional/biochemical disorders. Dr. Denton observed that victims of chronic mercury toxicity often present with headaches, as well as with various other symptoms. They have difficulty with mental concentration, memory, and are visibly without energy. In the first few hours and days following the detoxification program (which includes removal and replacement of mercury dental fillings) her patients often complain that their symptoms get worse, especially the headache. Yet, after a couple of weeks the headache goes away, short term memory improves, and their energy levels pick up noticeably. Of particular importance, she believes, is the patient's perception of these events. If they understand what to expect, largely dependent upon the counseling they and their families have received ahead of time from the doctor and staff, they demonstrate improvement much more quickly, and are far less likely to become anxious during the period of transition from sickness to health.

Drs. Miller and Walsh have studied the urine mercury excretion rate of two patients during and shortly following IV-C.* In one patient the midtest urine level doubled from 1.2 to 2.3 micrograms of mercury/liter, the second patient showed a 10-fold increase. Both patients demonstrated a higher excretion rate for the first 24-hour specimen following therapy, than for a similar period prior to treatment. Beyond the first 24 hours, however, they found that the amount of urine mercury excreted largely depends upon the patient's willingness to continue following instructions. Their finding adds credence to the effectiveness of IV-C and the **IV-C Mercury Tox Program** in ridding the body of mercury.

Once IV-C has been administered, it is important to remind the patient that the **IV-C Mercury Tox Program** is not yet completed. He or she must continue to share the responsibility of the treatment program, by supplying the doctor and staff with feedback, and subsequently, correctly following lifestyle directives. This quality of intimacy will determine the ultimate success or failure of the treatment's outcome. Likewise, a relationship of mutual trust provides the basis for continued lifestyle counseling. This is highly important because only through such a relationship can the mercury-toxic patient fully expect to recover and eventually lead a healthful, productive, and happy life.

---

* The doctors plan soon to publish the results of their study.

Post-Test Evaluation: Early Indices of Improvement
    We have seen that a change in cell membrane fluidity (away from normal) is a common, fundamental event in all diseases, resulting in cell membrane stress, fatigue and, ultimately, cellular dysfunction. Consideration of this process provides a basis for using the following parameters to evaluate the patient's response to treatment.
    Chronic Stress. A reduction of chronic stress provides the earliest clinical indices of improvement. An abatement of the stress level of the mercury-toxic patient is observed at every stage of the **IV-C Mercury Tox Program**, but its validity is most apparent some three to six weeks following the IV-C. A method of determining the extent of improvement of chronic stress, by comparing the pretest and post-test levels of blood cortisol, has been suggested by Robert S. Eliot, M. D., a cardiologist who heads the Life Stress Simulation Lab and Clinic in Phoenix, Arizona. In the book, *Is It Worth Dying For?*,[1] Dr. Eliot differentiates between two types of stress—short-term alarm stress, and long-term vigilance stress. Alarm stress, he explains, is the healthful 'fight or flight' response, in which the body reacts to sudden emergencies by causing transient increases in the level of blood adrenaline and noradrenaline. When the emergency is over the alarm hormones return to normal levels. Vigilance stress is an unhealthy response to chronic stress, highlighted by an increase in blood cortisol.
    Blood cortisol, the vigilance hormone, normally rises while the patient is awake, and declines during sleep. The gradual rise of blood cortisol just before daybreak is a factor in waking and becoming hungry, giving it the name "vigilance hormone." However, during chronic stress it remains elevated during sleep, thereby preventing the body's repair mechanisms from functioning normally. The level of blood cortisol is thus an indication of the extent of a patient's reaction to chronic stress, and becomes an indicator of improvement.
    Judging from Eliot's work, in which he has found that blood cortisol rises in response to chronic stress, and subsides in response to his stress reduction program, a significant reduction in blood cortisol three to six weeks following IV-C may likewise indicate improvement of the mercury-toxic patient (as a reduction of chronic stress). Yet, as Degkwitz has shown,[2] megadose vitamin C alone may lower blood cortisol, so reliance upon blood cortisol for evaluation is limited to the patient's progress, since it is a nonspecific measure of the program's effect on chronic mercury toxicity.
    A lowering of total serum cholesterol (TSC) during this period is another important indicator of reduced cellular stress. As cell membrane fluidity returns to normal during mercury removal from the cell membrane, there is a coincidental tendency for a reduction of TSC. However, because factors other than mercury are known to influence cell membrane fluidity and TSC, the lack of a significant, post-test reduction of TSC should not be considered an indication of failure to respond to the treatment program. In fact, because of the potential for a magic bullet effect in some patients, mentioned in earlier chapters, the initial response to improved cell membrane fluidity may be manifested by an elevated TSC.
    Conversely, there are positive factors other than the **IV-C Mercury Tox Program** that could plausibly account for a patient's improved condition. One such factor is hope, which may account as well for the reduction of post-test cortisol, and the plus or minus change in TSC. To what extent hope is a factor is not known, but the experience of Norman Cousins, as described in *Anatomy of an Illness*, demonstrates that the simple act of giving a patient hope—even with-

out the promise of improvement—is often quite enough to initiate the body's healing mechanisms.[3] Hence, while it is difficult to credit the patient's improvements in the post-test level of blood cortisol and the plus or minus changes in TSC to the treatment program, post-test readings of each are potentially important determinants of the extent of reduction of cellular stress.

Chronic Fatigue. Chronic fatigue is the exaggerated symptom of prolonged cellular stress in which the level of blood cortisol is correspondingly elevated, suggesting that—similarly to chronic stress—a reduction of post-test TSC and blood cortisol would indicate improvement. Here too, however, the tests are inconclusive and of general value only, since chronic fatigue characterizes not only toxic exposure to mercury, but cadmium and lead toxicity as well. Hence, a reduction in chronic fatigue won't necessarily indicate a reduction in chronic mercury toxicity. If a mercury-toxic patient, who is suffering from lead and cadmium toxicity as well, receives an iron supplement before IV-C is administered, the regimen will likely relieve the patient's cadmium and lead-related fatigue without addressing chronic mercury toxicity specifically. This is one of the reasons why it was recommended in earlier chapters that iron supplementation not be allowed until after the initial post-test evaluation in order to retain the value of using fatigue as a means of evaluation. A positive change in chronic fatigue may then be considered an indicator of general health improvement, although not specifically an indicator of reduction of chronic mercury toxicity.

Bowel Tolerance To Megadose Vitamin C. The amount of oral vitamin C that a patient can tolerate without developing diarrhea is a reliable indicator of the patient's general health. When the need for vitamin C decreases proportionately to the decrease in toxicity of the disease, a reduction in bowel tolerance levels can be expected following vitamin C therapy in general, and specifically following the **IV-C Mercury Tox Program**. Among mildly ill patients, for instance, the doctor can expect a decrease from 40 grams pretest to 25-30 grams post-test; and, among severely ill patients from 100-200 grams pretest to 50-100 grams or less post-test. Thus, while bowel tolerance is incapable of specifically indicating a decrease in chronic mercury toxicity, its value is unmatched as an indicator of general health improvement, requiring only that the doctor maintain accurate pretest and post-test records of the patient's bowel tolerance.

Appetite Restored with Weight Gain. The work of Drs. Charles Lapin and Dean Carter,[4] of the Toxicology Program at the University of Arizona, suggests that in patients whose levels of stress and fatigue have been reduced, the doctor is likely to note also an increase in appetite and a gain in body weight. Their observation was made from studying the eating habits and diet of rats poisoned with methylmercury, before and after a standard treatment. The earliest and most pronounced change in response to effective therapy was the rats' improved appetites and positive weight gain. To what extent a possible reduction of food allergies contributed to the rat's change in appetite is not known, but it is likely that a lessened sensitivity to foods of high nutritional density played a role both in the rats' weight gain and improved appetites (in response to mercury poisoning therapy). Yet if we can construe these animal findings to human expectations, the recording of pre- and post-treatment notes to indicate food sensitivities, body weight, and appetite, will likely play an important role in the patient's evaluation.

Changes in Other Test Parameters. A number of tests that may be used to evaluate patient improvement were discussed in Chapter 3. Yet because of the many possible combinations of symptoms due to chronic mercury toxicity, only a few examples are included here:

- Electrodiagnostic studies
- Electroencephalogram
- Mercury levels of
  - Blood
  - Hair
  - Urine
- Porphyrin fingerprint (experimental) of
  - Blood
  - Urine

When asked how he might objectively evaluate a patient's progress, Dr. Hal Huggins commented, "Evaluating whether there is improvement is quite easy to do. It's a matter of watching for changes in chemistries and other blood indices. If somebody has a white blood cell count of 50,000 and it comes down to 10,000, that's a big improvement. These and other immune parameters, such as T-lymphocytes and B-lymphocytes, are the ones that change the quickest, and the most dramatically."

Choosing other blood parameters, says Huggins, for patient evaluation, is strongly connected to the position of sulfhydryl groups. For instance, if the bulk of mercury is bound to hemoglobin, and as a consequence the patient is fatigued as a result of poor oxygen transport, then the evaluation can focus on changes in alkaline phosphatase and lactic dehydrogenase (LDH).

An increase in urine mercury can be observed shortly after its release from hemoglobin (partially explaining Miller's finding that the average excretion of urine mercury following IV-C increases ten-fold) and, as the mercury-toxic RBC's are broken down, a simultaneous increase in alkaline phosphatase and LDH is observed as well. This happens because, as Huggins believes, the spleen and the liver are breaking down the red blood cells more rapidly. (Yet as Elliott demonstrated in chapter 5, the elevation in LDH may partially be accounted for independently by the action of megadose vitamin C.) Eventually, as homeostasis occurs (usually requiring three to six weeks), the alkaline phosphatase and LDH will return to normal.

Psychiatrists and clinical psychologists, in evaluating mental disorders, often recommend the use of personality and psychological inventory tests, while cardiologists might rely upon the electrocardiogram, or changes in the patient's blood fat profile. Particularly, in patients with Type II hyperlipoproteinemia whose TSC is most often in excess of 275 dl/l, the cardiologist might initially note a rise in TSC, followed by a drop in TSC a few weeks or months later. This phenomenon, the magic bullet effect, occurs due to the sudden improvement in cholesterol turnover.

In concluding a discussion of evaluation methods, it is important to emphasize that today chronic mercury toxicity has become endemic among the world's population. It is therefore a threat to the health of every living person, and it will be treated by virtually every health practitioner, whether its existence is acknowledged or not. Consequently, there are as many ways of evaluating improvement from the **IV-C Mercury Tox Program** as there are ways of documenting the symptoms that the patient may manifest. The potential for ways of indirectly measuring patient improvement, therefore, depends upon an attending doctor's specialty, patient symptoms before and afterwards, and the ability of science to measure and interpret such changes. To simplify matters, however, the facts just covered indicate that certain indicators are characteristically better parameters of improvement than others. Let's summarize these:

<u>Indicators of patient improvement after the **IV-C Mercury Tox Program**</u>
A decrease in:
- chronic stress and fatigue
- fasting blood cortisol levels
- TSC levels
- bowel tolerance to megadose oral vitamin C
- hair and blood mercury levels

An increase in:
- alkaline phosphatase levels
- LDH levels (which may be due to the effect of vitamin C alone)
- TSC levels (a transient rise lasting 3 to 9 weeks, followed by a decrease, is often observed in patients with arterial disease)
- urine mercury levels (a transient rise followed by a decrease)
- appetite
- body weight

Positive changes in:
- the porphyrin fingerprint (currently under development)
- the blood fat profile
- the electrocardiogram (EKG)
- the electroencephalogram (EEG)
- the personality and psychological inventory test
- the white blood count
  - the white blood cell differential
    - T-lymphocyte count
    - B-lymphocyte count

In spite of the many indirect ways of evaluating a patient's progress, and the program as well, it is desirable to know what effect the **IV-C Mercury Tox Program** has on the total body burden and excretion of mercury. To date, the available means of doing this are less than ideal. While a post-test rise in urine mercury can be documented, it is much more difficult to test for fecal mercury, which is nevertheless the preferred test because the intestines are the primary route of exiting methylmercury. Even the value of determining a change in urine mercury is questioned, not so much in theory as in practice. There is some suspicion, for instance, that the comparison of urine mercury determinations may be flawed by differences in the type of collection bottle used. It is possible that the mercury gradually erodes faster or slower from one container than another, making study comparisons difficult.

Areas such as this need to be researched before one can accurately interpret a change in the excretion of urine mercury. And again, this is one of the reasons for the book—to stimulate thought and promote interest in further research. Until this necessary research is organized and completed—including the research required for making the porphyrin fingerprint a valid, operational test—the task of gathering and comparing indirect data remains the doctor's number one means of evaluating the patient's response to the **IV-C Mercury Tox Program**.

CONTINUED LIFESTYLE COUNSELING:
A BY-PRODUCT OF PATIENT EVALUATION

While chronic mercury toxicity is fast becoming a recognized, though seldom diagnosed, health problem, some people who <u>are</u> diagnosed complain of little more than unexplained allergies, chronic nervous tension, or infrequent bouts of irritability and mental depression. Still others have conditions that are life-threatening, such as hypercholesterolemia, heart disease, cardiac arrythmia, ALS, multiple sclerosis, or one of the many congenital diseases—cerebral palsy, for instance. In either case the patient's total recovery will likely require a long period of time, judging from the observations of doctors who regularly treat the full range of chronic mercury toxicity, and from observing my own case history. This is true as well for those who initially suffered acute mercurial poisoning, or who were exposed repeatedly to a high level of mercury over an extended time frame. In years past the recognition of subacute symptoms that followed significant mercury exposure, which bordered more on poisoning than chronic mercury toxicity, was the only way that the condition was recognized. Back then the symptoms that failed to fit the syndrome of classic mercury poisoning were dismissed as mysterious, "non-disease entities." Although the same holds true even today, these symptoms are increasingly being recognized as chronic mercury toxicity.

The extended period of time required for symptoms to emerge in some people complicates the diagnosis of chronic mercury toxicity, its treatment, and evaluation. This is especially true in low-level exposure where the symptoms tend to be delayed by months, years, or even decades following initial contact with mercury. Some of those who are mercury-toxic become hypersensitized to further mercury exposure, thereafter reacting to smaller, subsequent exposures than before. These are the patients who are biologically unique—people in whom mercury-sensitive tissues seem to have a stronger affinity for mercury, causing symptoms well below the usual dose/response curve. So, regardless of the type of chronic mercury toxicity, whether due to a single high-level exposure, hypersensitivity, or repeated contact with mercury, the affected patient will express symptoms that handicap his every attempt to lead a normal life. From the viewpoint of these people, <u>any</u> improvement is a big improvement.

The **IV-C Mercury Tox Program** is designed to support the body's natural healing processes while enhancing the means by which mercury is detoxified and eliminated naturally. This program is not a "quick fix," but rather a way of life coupled with supportive, megadose nutrition that will hopefully speed the healing process and in time reduce the body burden of mercury. Some mildly affected patients are expected to make substantial progress following a single IV-C treatment. Others will require continued supervision, counseling and, perhaps, multiple IV-C treatments. Both groups, however, will require periodic evaluations and lifestyle counseling if they expect to fully recover.

Whatever method the doctor uses to determine improvement, it is likely that the patient will have offered beforehand his own subjective opinion as to whether or not his condition has improved. The success of the treatment, as perceived by the patient, leaves a greater impact on his willingness to continue the program than the documented results of scientific tests. Those patients expressing milder symptoms are the ones most likely to abandon the program once symptoms have subsided, even when their improvement is well documented. The tendency is to turn away from further lifestyle counseling and mistakenly consider themselves cured, only to be faced with additional mercury-related health problems weeks or months later. These people, in addition to those who are more severely affected, require continued lifestyle counseling. Whether the doctor determines that the treatment plan will require additional IV-C infusions (among other treatment considerations), or whether the patient needs only to continue with his diet, lifestyle, and physical rehabilitation program—along with supportive medical therapy—the need for additional counseling will require very little encouragement on the part of severely affected patients. The mildly affected patients, however, may call for additional motivation.

Motivation, commitment, and a cooperative spirit are exactly what is needed if <u>any</u> patient is to fully recover, whether his symptoms were initially mild or severe. During rehabilitation, the patient must become totally committed to learning those lifestyle and nutritional practices required of the **IV-C Mercury Tox Program** that are necessary for optimal recovery. The patient and doctor are challenged, as well, to continue their close association; it all but demands that the patient remain with the cooperative shared responsibility concept for planning and executing the treatment plan.

Being adequately motivated, therefore, is the ultimate key to a patient's recovery.

So How Does the Doctor Motivate a Patient?

In truth, no one person can singlehandedly motivate another. The spark of motivation is found in the subconscious mind of each of us. Every patient (regardless of temporary or permanent disability) already has this capability in the form of his goals and needs. When brought before the conscious mind, these desires give him a reason to act—reason to work as hard as needed in order to regain health. While doctors and their assistants cannot, alone, motivate patients to continue, they can do much to help these patients discover their goals, or acknowledge their needs. The doctor and staff can help bring forth a patient's awareness of his own reasons to persist when faced with pain, discomfort, and/or mental anguish.

Pain, discomfort, and mental anguish are the usual driving forces that bring the patient to seek his doctor's help. The desire for relief is usually motivation enough for the first doctor/patient encounter. However, as the patient's condition improves, his perception of need changes accordingly. At some point, therefore, as his symptoms become less critical, his perceived needs will change, and he will begin to feel he has no further reason to act. This could be detrimental to his overall health improvement, if he stops consulting his doctor before being completely healed. Therefore, one of the most important roles of the health care doctor is to assist the patient in motivating himself toward optimal health.

Before contracting to continue, patients of both categories (mildly and severely affected) must come to realize that the attainment of optimal health is not an end in itself, but rather a means to the end. A person doesn't really want to overcome a health problem for the simple purpose of being healthy. Rather, he wants to be healthy in order to achieve his other goals. Optimal health is important to patients only to the extent that it will allow them to realize their dreams and reach their life goals. At some point in a patient's treatment program, as his motivation shows signs of wear, the doctor is advised to question the patient regarding his or her most immediate goals and interests.

The doctor must use a patient's wants, desires, and wishes to reinforce reasons for continuing with the lifestyle counseling sessions: Optimal health will help him attain these goals and pursue his ambitions and dreams with the enthusiasm and energy that's expected (and within the realm) of a healthy body. Once these motivations are established, the patient and doctor can then work toward setting a series of short- and long-term health goals.

Goal Setting is a Remarkable Experience

"Remember in *Alice in Wonderland*, when Alice comes to the junction in the road that leads in different directions and she asks the Cheshire Cat for advice?
'Chesire-Puss...would you tell me please, which way I ought to go from here?'
'That depends a good deal on where you want to get to' said the Cat.
'I don't much care where...' said Alice.
'Then it doesn't matter which way you go' "[5]

It does not surprise anyone to hear that every normal person has his or her own set of dreams, desires, and wishes. Yet we find it surprising when told that few people ever make those dreams a reality. Why not? The answer, I believe, can be found in the words of Denis Waitley, a behavioral psychologist who in recent years has become a noted author, speaker, and crusading advocate of the notion that all humans, regardless of their disabilities, have the potential to accomplish great deeds. "The reason so many individuals fail to achieve their goals in life is that they never really set them in the first place."[6]

The average person, says Waitley, simply never gets beyond the dream stage. He hasn't yet learned that by sequentially setting attainable, short-term goals, his dreams and desires will eventually become a reality.   This also can be applied to setting and reaching health goals. The secret to successful goal-setting is to be specific and to develop a road map for getting there—a mile, a foot, even one step at a time. If the planners (in our case, the doctor and patient) are persistent, they will eventually reach goals, even if roadblocks and detours are found along the way. Before beginning, they must have first determined where they are headed; and must break the journey into miles and steps traveled each year, month, week, day and, in some cases, hour and minute. In other words, persistence is the key. The patient, especially, must constantly bear in mind that each step—however small—represents significant progress, taking him one step closer to the freedom he seeks for ultimately pursuing his life goals.

A Positive Attitude is Necessary for Optimal Success

Actually reaching the goals set by the doctor and patient requires a particular state of mind. Each must develop the mental habit of putting into practice what Dr. Norman Vincent Peale has referred to as the power of positive thinking,[7] and Dr. Robert H. Schuller calls possibility thinking.[8] What these three authors (Waitley, Peale, and Schuller) have to say is of such importance that I highly recommend their books to all doctors and staff members who are interested in lifestyle counseling. Dr. Waitley's *Seeds of Greatness*, *The Power of Positive Thinking* by Dr. Peale, and Dr. Schuller's book *Move Ahead with Possibility Thinking* might be read by each participant from cover to cover. I would also suggest Norman Cousins' *Anatomy of an Illness*. Copies should be recommended or made available to every patient. After having read these books, everyone involved in counseling will have developed the correct mind-set necessary for achieving optimal health: Focusing on the solution rather than the problem, and finding ways of reaching that solution.

Wilma Had That Positive Attitude

Denis Waitley tells a story that illustrates the concept perfectly. Wilma was a little girl who started out her life with many health disadvantages. A premature baby who was stricken with scarlet fever, and twice contracted double pneumonia, she was also affected by polio which had caused her left leg to be crooked and in braces. By the age of six she was dreaming of traveling and making a contribution to the world. When she told her mother of her dreams, she was reassured with "Honey, the most important thing in life is for you to believe it and keep on trying." Already—at six—Wilma had the two most important means of achieving her dreams: She had a specific goal in mind, and the support of someone else who encouraged her. Notice that her goal was <u>not</u> simply to become well.

By the time Wilma was 11, she knew she would be able to remove her braces one day. Her doctor, on the other hand, wasn't so sure, but told her to exercise her legs a little. Wilma was determined to walk, and decided to take this a step further. Whenever her parents would leave the house, her brothers and sisters would act as lookouts while she took her braces off and, in much pain, walked around the house for hours at a time.

This went on for a year before her guilt overwhelmed her, and she decided to "come clean" during a visit to the doctor. The doctor—surprised by her being able to walk without braces—told her it would be all right to walk around 'occasionally' without them. That was all she needed to hear. She never wore them again.

As Wilma grew older, she decided she would conquer athletics. At the age of 12, her father got her on the school's girls' basketball team. This was not an ideal situation for Wilma, but she was thrilled to be a part of the team in any case. Determined to be successful, she went to her coach and told him, "If you will give me ten minutes of your time, and only ten minutes—every day—I will give you in return a world-class athlete." Her coach laughed at her, but agreed to give it to her, although he reminded her that most of the time he would be busy with *real* athletes.

Undaunted by this, Wilma began to master the game, and the following year was selected for the team on her own. During all this time she was bent on doing her very best, while never losing sight of her goals of being able to travel and make a contribution to the world.

At 14, Wilma began training after school and on weekends with the Tigerbelles of Tennessee State University, the prestigious girls' track team. She started to win races, and by the end of that first summer, she had won several in the junior division at the national AAU meet in Philadelphia.

After two years, Wilma was able to realize her goal of travel: The Olympics were to be held in Australia and she had qualified. At the 1956 Olympics in Melbourne, at the age of 16, Wilma won a bronze medal for the women's team 400-meter relay. While she was happy, she was also disappointed in her performance, knowing her capability was greater. She vowed that next time she would do better.

In 1960, in Rome, Wilma won three gold medals: for the 100- and 200-meter dashes, and as part of the women's team 400-meter relay. Not only that, but each race was to break a world's record!

Not bad for a crippled girl with a dream! Wilma Rudolph had become a champion, overcoming tremendous health difficulties and so-called permanent disabilities with the aid of her goals, some hard work, and perseverance. Her goal had not been to get well. Her goals, even as a child, had been to travel and make a contribution to the world. Having these goals drove her to overcome all odds and get well. Achievement of health became the means to the end, and not the end in itself. And if she could do this, any patient with a temporary or permanent disability can overcome the odds as well.

Illness Has Many Aspects

There is no doubt that a positive mental attitude can help the course of healing. The three before-mentioned authors fill their books with inspiring stories such as this one. Not only that, but they all give many practical solutions and plans for achieving the same results in all individuals. The books are excellent for both doctor and patient in that they provide the proper frame of mind for healing. Many good doctors have begun recommending these authors to their patients, with excellent results.

A physician of Dr. Peale's acquaintance once told him: "I have found that a high percentage (of my patients) do not need medicine but better thought patterns. They are not sick in their bodies so much as they are sick in their thoughts and emotions. They are all mixed up with fear thoughts, inferiority feelings, guilt, and resentment. I found that in treating them I needed to be about as much a psychiatrist as a physician, and then I discovered that not even those therapies helped me fully to do my job. I became aware that in many cases the basic trouble with people was spiritual. So I found myself frequently quoting the Bible to them. Then I fell into the habit of 'prescribing' religious and inspirational books, especially those that give guidance in how to live."[9]

Dr. Carl R. Ferris, former president of the Jackson County Medical Society of Kansas City, Missouri, declared that in treating human ills the physical and spiritual are often so deeply interrelated that there is often no clearly defined dividing line between the two.[10]

Dr. Flanders Dunbar, author of *Mind and Body*, says, "It is not a question of whether an illness is physical or emotional, but how much of each."[11]

Does this mean I am suggesting that patients are not really sick and don't need doctors? Of course not! What I am saying is that there is a great deal of mental and emotional involvement in an illness, and the doctor is the ideal professional to be able to help patients overcome all aspects of sickness. A patient who has had prior success with the medical profession will trust his doctor more than anyone else for health advice, and if some spiritual and motivational inspiration should come from him as well, so much the better if it aids in the healing process. The doctor has the scientific knowledge and expertise to treat illness. The patient has the mental capacity to speed that healing process, and the doctor can encourage this. Dr. Albert Schweitzer told Norman Cousins, "Each patient carries his own doctor inside him. They come to us not knowing that truth. We (doctors) are at our best when we give the doctor who resides within each patient a chance to go to work."[12] This process will result in a much-improved health outcome for the patient, and he will have even more praise for his physician's part in the success.

Putting it into Practice

Once the patient has spent the time and effort to examine his dreams, and goals are set, he will have all the motivation he needs to get well. This will not be an automatic solution; he will need to review these often, and be encouraged and motivated by health personnel.

Dr. Peale suggests that if a patient feels defeated; if he's lost confidence in his ability to deal with his illness; then the doctor should instruct him to sit down with pencil and paper and make a list—not of the factors that are against him—but of those that are _for_ him in dealing with his health problem. By so doing the patient learns to look for possible solutions rather than pity and reasons to quit trying. This mode of thinking teaches one to become solution-oriented, to focus on the solution rather than the problem and—particularly when searching for answers to health problems—it's as useful to the doctor as it is to the patient.

Possibility thinking (as opposed to impossibility thinking, where the participants see little hope) tends to give the patient incredible courage, the doctor the confidence needed to learn this new aspect of the trade, and the faith for both to persist, allowing them to accomplish tasks together that otherwise may seem totally impossible given the circumstances.

By putting into practice the aforementioned way of thinking, the doctor and patient alike will come to realize that there are no 'incurable' diseases. There is only a lack of awareness of the roles played by diet and lifestyle in health and disease, and there are only diseases for which an answer has not yet been found. Believe me when I say that the only reason I'm alive today, after having become a victim of severe chronic mercury toxicity, is because I became a disciple of these same principles. I came to accept the thesis that all successful doctors and patients come to accept: Every step taken to improve health through diet, lifestyle, and supportive medical therapies takes them that much closer to a possible solution, whether they're concerned with treating or preventing disease. The **IV-C Mercury Tox Program** was developed over many years through the process of trial and error.

The mercury-toxic patient's ultimate recovery is made possible only by applying the correct thought processes to the **IV-C Mercury Tox Program**, by the continuation of lifestyle counseling, and by the doctor's and patient's persistence. Beyond chronic mercury toxicity it leaves the doctor and patient with a process by which they can logically work together toward preventing other diseases as well, heart disease included. The concept, as I'm sure you'll agree, is what has been needed all along.

"Body and soul cannot be separated for purposes of treatment, for they are one and indivisible. Sick minds must be healed as well as sick bodies."

~C. Jeff Miller [1874-1936][13]

IV-C Mercury Tox Program®
EVALUATION

PARAMETER	PRETEST		POST-TEST								IMPROVEMENT (+/−)							
	Patient	Doctor	3 wk.		6 wk.		6 mo.		1 yr.		3 wk.		6 wk.		6 mo.		1 yr.	
			P	D	P	D	P	D	P	D	P	D	P	D	P	D	P	D
Chronic Stress																		
Chronic Fatigue																		
TSC																		
Blood Cortisol																		
Hair Hg+ +																		
Blood Hg+ +																		
Bowel Tolerance																		
Alk. Phosphatase																		
Blood LDH																		
Urine Hg+ +																		
Appetite																		
Body Weight																		
Porphyrin Fingerprint																		
Blood Fat Profile																		
EKG																		
EEG																		
Personality Inventory																		
Psychological Inventory																		
WBC																		
WBC differential																		
T-lumphocytes																		
B-lymphocytes																		
Other																		

DIRECTIONS: Using a subjective scale of 1-10, indicate evaluation for each category. For the first 2 parameters, both patient (P) and doctor (D) observations should be noted.

LITERATURE CITED

[1] R.L. Eliot and D.L. Breo, *Is It Worth Dying For?*, Bantam Books, New York, pp. 27-34, 1984.

[2] E. Degkwitz, "Some Effects of Vitamin C May Be Indirect, Since It Affects the Blood Levels of Cortisol and Thyroid," *Ann NY Acad Sci*, 498: 470-72, 1987.

[3] N. Cousins, *Anatomy of An Illness*, Bantam Books edition, New York, 1981; copyright W.W. Norton & Co., 1979

[4] C.A. Lapin and D.E. Carter, "Early Indices of Methyl Mercury Toxicity and their Use in Treatment Evaluation," *J Tox Environ Health*, 8: 767-76, 1981.

[5] D. Waitley, *Seeds of Greatness*, Pocket Books, Simon and Schuster, New York, 1983, p. 114.

[6] D. Waitley, ibid., p. 116.

[7] N.V. Peale, *The Power Of Positive Thinking*, Random House edition, ninth printing, 1984, copyright Prentice-Hall, 1952.

[8] R.H. Schuller, *Move Ahead With Possibility Thinking*, 12th printing, 1986, Doubleday & Company, Inc., New York, 1967.

[9] N.V. Peale, op. cit., p. 148.

[10] N.V. Peale, ibid.

[11] N.V. Peale, ibid., p. 159.

[12] N. Cousins, op. cit., p. 69.

[13] M.B. Strauss, ed., *Familiar Medical Quotations*, Little, Brown and Company, Boston, 1968.

Appendixes

APPENDIX A

The American Dental Association's (ADA) Official Position on Mercury Amalgam Fillings

The communications that follow were obtained directly from the ADA: from a telephone interview conducted in the spring of 1987 with the ADA's Manager of Media Services, Mr. Richard Asa; and as a part of their packet of information issued in December 1983 and intended for the news media.

NEWS RELEASE I:
Experts to Review Safety of Metals in Dentistry

Chicago — Dental amalgam, the silver filling material commonly used to restore damaged or decayed teeth, was developed in France during the 1820's and introduced in the U. S. shortly thereafter. Since that time it has been continually studied by dental researchers, who have found it to be safe for use in the general population. But recent reports suggesting a potential hazard linked to dental amalgams have sparked renewed interest in the safety of this restorative material.

"Although there is no evidence of a health threat, we will pursue the question of safety until the matter is resolved to the satisfaction of the American people," said Edgar W. Mitchell, Ph.D., secretary to the American Dental Association's Council on Dental Therapeutics.*

Dental amalgam is produced by combining mercury with silver, copper, and tin and sometimes zinc. Mercury is used to facilitate hardening of the filling compound once it has been placed in the tooth. It is the use of mercury that concerns some dental patients, fueled chiefly by claims that link amalgams to health problems ranging from multiple sclerosis to epileptic seizures.

"These claims have no basis in scientific fact," said John Stanford, Ph.D., a biochemist and secretary to the ADA Council on Dental Materials,

*Author's note: Following Dr. Mitchell's declaration—at the ADA's urging—the National Institute of Dental Research (NIDR), a component of the federal National Institutes of Health, hosted a 1984 Workshop on The Safety and Biocompatibility of Metals in Dentistry.[1] The experts who reviewed the current knowledge of metals in dentistry generally and officially agreed that mercury is indeed released from amalgam fillings. Yet they maintained that such a small amount could not possibly cause health problems, with the exception of people who were already hypersensitive or allergic to mercury. To my knowledge, no further research (funded by either the ADA or NIDR) has been started, or even planned, as a result of this workshop. In protest of the official consensus statement, however, a group of dentists, physicians, and scientists formed the International Academy of Oral Medicine and Toxicology (IAOMT) to study the problem independently. Their critique of the 1984 NIDR/ADA workshop, which was published as an educational service, can be obtained by requesting a copy in writing [IAOMT, 5400 Hernando Drive, Orlando, FL, 32806].)

---

[1] NIDR Workshop, "Biocompatibility of Metals in Dentistry," *JADA*, 109 (3): 469-71, 1984.

Instruments and Equipment. "There is no evidence relating dental amalgam to these diseases and afflictions. To our knowledge, no cause-effect relationship has ever been established."

The safety of dental amalgam has been questioned largely because of a recent advance in technology. Researchers are now able to measure extremely small quantities of mercury vapor in a patient's exhaled breath. Research on this topic has been conducted at the University of Iowa, under the direction of Dr. Carl W. Svare who measured mercury vapor exhaled after patients have chewed gum and also following the removal and insertion of silver fillings.

The average level of mercury vapor detected in research subjects with amalgam fillings was only about one-fifth the National Institute of Occupational Safety and Health recommended maximum allowable level of 50 micrograms (one-millionth of a gram) of mercury vapor per cubic meter of air for persons exposed eight hours a day, five days a week.* Moreover, the study did not indicate whether the breath was exhaled through the nose or mouth. If through the mouth, there is no evidence that the mercury vapor was from the lungs or from the oral cavity.

Dr. Mitchell predicted that mercury vapor in exhaled air would be a principal topic of discussion for next year's NIDR workshop on metals in dentistry. He added, "We wish the public to be as certain as we are that dental amalgam is safe, and we will pursue this matter until that certainty is assured."

Author's note: The difference, however, is that OSHA's standards were based on a 40-hour work week, while mercury amalgam fillings are with a person 24 hours a day, 168 hours per week. On this basis alone, the mercury amalgam filling would contribute four-fifths of the maximum allowable level. What then would be the combined effect of mercury on a single individual who ate fish regularly, who was exposed to OSHA's maximum allowable limit in the workplace, and who had mercury amalgam fillings that contributed an additional four-fifths of that amount?

NEWS RELEASE II:
ADA President Underscores Safety of Dental Fillings

Chicago — Contrary to scattered media reports, the material dentists commonly use to fill decayed teeth presents no known general health threat to dental patients, the president of the American Dental Society said here today.

Several sources have attempted to link dental amalgam (silver fillings) to various health hazards, but without supporting scientific evidence. These reports have suggested that the mercury contained in dental fillings can affect the general health of the patient, and they have spurred a barrage of questions from a concerned public.

"We wish to assure the American people that dental amalgam is safe," said Dr. Donald E. Bentley, ADA president. "It has been used without incident in this country for about 150 years. For nearly a century, dental filling materials have been continually evaluated for safety and tolerance, and at no time have we ever seen any proof that they pose a health risk to the general population."

In support of his statement, Dr. Bentley pointed to a report published in the April 1983 issue of the *Journal of the American Dental Association*, which concluded that dental amalgam is safe for patients. Produced jointly by the

Association's Council on Dental Therapeutics and council on Dental Materials, Instruments, and Equipment, this comprehensive review of accepted scientific knowledge notes that dental amalgam is used in about 75 percent of all tooth repairs requiring fillings.

It acknowledges, however, that in extremely rare cases patients may develop a hypersensitivity or allergy from contact with mercury, a condition that usually turns up as skin rash and is similar to other common allergies.

"The fact that a very small percentage of the population is hypersensitive to mercury should not be cause for alarm," said Dr. Bentley. "Obviously, if an allergic reaction is discovered, we recommend that some other restorative material be used, usually gold. But there is no reason the average patient should seek to have amalgam restorations removed, unless hypersensitivity is evident."*

For nonallergic patients, he added, the effect of removing silver fillings and replacing them with some other material could do more harm than good, possibly jeopardizing the patient's oral health and often resulting in the needless loss of teeth.

"The dental profession is continually studying the safety of its methods and materials" the president concluded. "It should go without saying that we would shun any treatment procedure that would jeopardize the health of a patient."

  * *Author's note: In the interview with Richard Asa, he explained that a dentist would normally include questions regarding allergies on the patient's medical history— if they've had a past reaction to metals. If so, the patient is referred to a dermatologist or an allergist, as the dentist is neither trained nor qualified to perform such testing. Patients are normally not tested in any way if an allergy or sensitivity has not previously manifested itself, because reactions of this sort are believed to be rare (occurring in less than 1% of the population).*

NEWS RELEASE III:
Dentists, Staff Members Healthy, Despite Daily Contact with Mercury

Chicago — Dentists and their assistants, people who are regularly exposed to pure mercury as part of their daily work, are a generally healthy group of individuals.

"If the mercury used in dentistry posed any real health threat, it stands to reason that the professionals who handle it each day would suffer adverse effects," said Gordon Schrotenboer, Ph. D., Chief of the American Dental Association's Division of Scientific Affairs. "The fact is, dental professionals are a generally healthy group of individuals who show no ill effects from their contact with mercury."

In support of that statement, Dr. Schrotenboer cited results of the ADA's own mercury testing program, a service the Association offers its members and their office aides as an outgrowth of a health assessment program started in 1975.

The Mercury Testing Service has been in operation since January 1982. As of November 1983, 776 dentists and dental staff members had enrolled in the program, which employs urinalysis to measure levels of mercury in the human system. An average urinary level of 14.6 micrograms (one-millionth of a gram) per liter has been found from the first 2,575 urine samples tested. This figure is understandably higher than the level found in the general population (about three micrograms per liter) but well below the level at which neurological symptoms are normally first detected—about 500 micrograms per liter of urine.

"The Mercury Testing Service has shown that dentists and their staff members have mercury levels well within the safety zone of acceptability," said Dr. Schrotenboer. "And the mercury levels we detect in dental patients are considerably lower than those found in dentists. To put it bluntly, patients are in no danger."

When asked if he had any concluding remarks that he would like passed along to our mixed audience of health professionals, Richard Asa quickly commented that..."dental amalgam is safe. The epidemiological evidence of the past 100 years," he said, "clearly demonstrates that dentists do not manifest the symptoms that are being credited to dental amalgam fillings. This observation is made in spite of the fact that dentists have four to five times more exposure to mercury than their patients. The claim that dental amalgam fillings represent a significant health concern among the general population is unsubstantiated, undocumented, and unproven."

APPENDIX B

Addresses:
A partial listing of key doctors and organizations who oppose the use of amalgam dental fillings, who promote mercury-free dentistry, and who may be willing to provide information. If you would like your name or organization added to this list please write to us.

UNITED STATES
Sandra Denton, M. D.
Tahoma Clinic
24030 132nd Ave. Southeast
Kent, Washington, 98042
Telephone (206) 631-8920

Richard Holden, D. D. S.
1767 S. 8th Street
Colorado Springs, Colorado, 80906

Hal A. Huggins, D. D. S.
P. O. Box 2589
Colorado Springs, Colorado, 80901

Roy Kupsinel, M. D.
P. O. Box 550
Oviedo, Florida, 32763

Burton E. Miller, D. D. S.
550 W. 7th Avenue, Suite 1390
Anchorage, Alaska, 99501

Jerry Mittleman, D. D. S.
263 West End Avenue #21
New York, New York, 10023

John D. Walsh, D. D. S.
550 W. 7th Avenue, Suite 1390
Anchorage, Alaska, 99501

Michael F. Ziff, D. D. S.
The International Academy of Oral Medicine and Toxicology
5400 Hernando Drive
Orlando, Florida, 32806

The American Academy of Environmental Medicine
P. O. Box 16106
Denver, Colorado, 80216

American College of Advancement in Medicine
Formerly, The American Academy of Medical Preventics
Suite 204
23121 Verdugo Drive
Laguna Hills, California 92653
Telephone: 1-800-LEAD OUT

Bio-Probe, Inc.
4401 Real Court
Orlando, Florida 32808
Educational material available for a small fee. The Bio-Probe Newsletter is published bi-monthly @ $65.00 per year. The new expanded edition of The Toxic Time Bomb: Can The Mercury In Your Dental Fillings Poison You?, by Sam Ziff, can be obtained for $10.95.

The Holistic Dental Association
P.O. Box 817
Lombard, Illinois, 60148
Dr. Stanley Tylman, President

The Holistic Medical Association
2727 Fairview Ave., East
Seattle, Washington, 98102

Toxic Testing, Inc.
Suite 232, 303 E. Altamonte Drive
Altamonte Springs, Florida, 32701

CANADA
Dr. F. L. Lorscheider
Department of Medical Physiology
Calgary University Faculty of Medicine
Calgary, Alberta, Canada, T2N 4N1

Murray J. Vimy, D. D. S.
The International Academy of Oral Medicine and Toxicology (Canada)
615-401 9th Avenue, SW
Calgary, Alberta, Canada, AB T2F 3C5

Roel J. Wyman, D. D. S.
7084 Airport Road
Mississauga, Ontario, Canada, L4T 2G9

NORWAY
Dr. Dag Brune
Scandinavian Institute of Dental Materials
Forskningsveien 1
Oslo 3, Norway

Dr. Dag M. Evje
Scandinavian Institute of Dental Materials
Forskningsveien 1
Oslo 3, Norway

SWEDEN
Dr. Dowen Birkhed
Department of Cardiology
School of Dentistry
Carl Gustafs väg 34
S-21421 Malmö, Sweden

Dr. Toare Dërand
Department of Oral Technology
University of Lund
School of Dentistry
S-21421 Malmö, Sweden

Dr. Stig Edwardsson
Oral Microbiology Department
University of Lund
School of Dentistry
S-21421 Malmö, Sweden

Dr. Ulf Heintze
Department of Cardiology
School of Dentistry
Carl Gustafs väg 34
S-21421 Malmö, Sweden

Patrick Störtebecker, M. D., Ph. D.
Störtebecker Research Foundation
Akerbyvägen 282
S-183 35 Täby, Stockholm, Sweden

APPENDIX C

High Risk Professions:
Potential Occupational Exposures to Mercury
(Modified With Permission: From Goldfrank, Bresnitz, and Weisman, Hospital Physician 38-46, June, 1980.)

Acetic acid makers
Amalgam makers
Bactericide makers
Barometer makers
Battery makers
Bronzers
Calibration instrument makers
Caustic soda makers
Carbon brush makers
Ceramic workers
Chlorine makers
Dental amalgam makers
Dental office workers
Dentists
Direct current meter workers
Disinfectant makers
Drug makers
Dye makers
Electric apparatus makers
Electroplaters
Embalmers
Explosive makers
Farmers
Fingerprint detectors
Fireworks makers
Fungicide makers
Fur processors
Gold extractors
Histology technicians
Ink makers
Insecticide makers
Instrument calibration technicians
Jewelers
Laboratory workers
  clinical
  chemical
Lamp makers
  fluorescent
  mercury arc
Manometer makers
Mercury workers
  miners
  refiners
Neon light makers

Paint makers
Paper pulp workers
Percussion cap makers and loaders
Pesticide workers
Photographers
Printers
Pressure gauge makers
Seed handlers
Silver extractors
Tannery workers
Taxidermists
Thermometer makers
Vinyl chloride makers
Wood preservative workers

APPENDIX D

The Vitamin D Connection in Heart Disease

Research from the past few years indicates that vitamin D excess may serve as an angiotoxin, causing the initial aberration in arterial lesions, and providing a basis whereby calcium may accumulate in arterial plaque.

While for 30 years there has been some evidence of the reality of this mechanism, until 1980 it had been difficult to demonstrate. During experimentation with rabbits, Imai, et al.,[1] at Albany Medical College, New York, learned that oxidized derivatives of cholesterol (of which vitamin D is one), rather than cholesterol *per se*, caused cell degeneration and induced atherosclerosis. The researchers found that these oxidized forms of cholesterol are present in the beef tallow used in preparation of french fries (fast-food chain style), in powdered milk products and powdered eggs, and also in crystalline cholesterol (a common source of cholesterol used in both human and animal experiments). Oxidized vitamin D, they found, was one of the most lethal forms of oxidized cholesterol. This suggested to them that the unrestricted and indiscriminate use of vitamin D supplements in foods may be a contributing factor in human atherosclerosis, and perhaps many other degenerative human diseases as well.

While the mechanism of how oxidized cholesterol derivatives contribute to disease is incompletely understood, it appears that cell membrane fluidity is affected (Chapter 2). Membrane fluidity depends upon the order of placement within the cell membrane of phospholipids and cholesterol. Lecithin is the main phospholipid, comprising phosphorous and fatty acids. While the cell does require calcium, a special feature of the cell membrane is its lack of permeability to calcium and other cations. Yet there are several means of getting calcium into the inner chamber. This may include ion gradient (nonhormone dependent) and receptor-mediated (hormone dependent) routes. Calling upon these mechanisms through a variety of hormonal and dietary circumstances, special channels open and close within the membrane to allow calcium to enter and exit. Vitamin D excess, however, serves to upset this control mechanism, by upsetting membrane fluidity.

The extent to which excess vitamin D is involved in this aberration was demonstrated by Shepherd,[2] and Holmes.[3] Studying *25 (OH) vitamin D* (the oxidative product of vitamin D), they found that during severe hypervitaminosis D (an excess of dietary vitamin D, not sunshine) in both test animals and man, there was more than a fifty-fold increase in the level of serum *25 (OH) vitamin D,* and that this was accompanied by severe soft tissue calcification along with substantial increases in tissue vitamin D and the oxi-

---

[1] H. Imai, et al., *Science*, 207: 651-653, 1980.

[2] R.M. Shepherd, and H.F. DeLuca, *Arch Biochem Biophys*, 202: 43-53, 1980.

[3] R.P. Holmes; *Chemical, Biological and Clinical Endocrinology of Calcium Metabolism*; A.W. Normal, K. Normal, D.V. Schaeffer, D.V. Herrath, and H.G. Grigoleit, eds.; Walter De Gruyter, NY, NY; 567-579, 1982.

dized sterols. Arterial smooth muscle cells, in particular,[1] were found to be most susceptible to the damaging effect of derivatives of vitamin D, thereby indicating that any program for preventing heart disease should include restriction of vitamin D (which should not exceed 400 IU for most people). The significance of these findings are such that the doctor who treats heart disease or who wishes to advise his patients in the prevention of heart disease, should become aware of the many ways that vitamin D is included in his patients' diets.

Nearly all manufacturers of dietary calcium supplements, for instance, feel it is their duty, singlehandedly, to make sure that people get all the vitamin D they need from their calcium supplements. So nearly every calcium supplement program will contain 100 percent of the RDA. This is in addition to diet. Milk and milk products, for instance, are consistently supplemented with vitamin D, as are breakfast cereals. This, added to the vitamin D that one gets from meat, eggs, and a wide variety of food supplements, including fish oil, easily and quickly can amount to a vitamin D excess. It seems that the food industry, lacking a coordinated effort, has designed to contribute in each of their products the RDA for vitamin D without regard to the potential total contribution from all sources. It is therefore necessary for doctors to assist their patients in monitoring total vitamin D intake. Doing so not only will support whatever treatment program the doctor chooses, it will also support any program the doctor and patient choose for the prevention of heart disease, and the prevention of other degenerative diseases as well.

---

[1] A. Kamio and F.A. Kummerow, *Arch Pathol Lab Med*, 101: 378-381, 1977.

APPENDIX E

Addresses:
A list of individuals, companies, and organizations who were mentioned throughout the book

---

INDIVIDUALS

Dennis Adair, Ph. D., Manager, Animal Health Formulations Research
Schering/Plough
Galloping Hill Road
Kenelworth, New Jersey, 07033
Telephone (201) 298-4000
Manufacturers of large dose I.V. Vitamin C for non-human use

Gerald F. Brunzie, Ph. D., Director Documentation Control
Steris Laboratories
620 N. 51st Avenue, P. O. Box 23160
Phoenix, Arizona, 85063-3160
Telephone (602) 278-1400
A reliable source of the legality of use of IV-C, and how it relates to indications for use, as well as warnings, labeling, package insert, and the manufacturing of IV-C.

Robert F. Cathcart, III, M. D.
Allergy, Environmental & Orthomolecular Medicine
127 2nd Street
Los Altos, California, 94022
A specialist in Nutritional Medicine; and perhaps the most active user today of I.V. Vitamin C in medicine.

E. Cheraskin, M. D., D. M. D.
MetriScience
2435 Monte Vista Drive
P. O. Box 20287
Vestavia Hills, Alabama 35216-0287
Telephone (205) 934-4750
An internationally recognized authority in nutritional medicine; chairman for 17 years of the department of Dentistry at the University of Alabama School of Dentistry; co-author of over 500 journal articles on medicine, nutrition, and dentistry; author of 13 books on health and disease. Of significance to the doctor who must treat the mercury-toxic patient who exhibits signs of erethism, I highly recommend his book, Psychodietetics, co-authored by Drs. Cheraskin and W. M. Ringsdorf, Jr., with Arline Brecher; available from Bantam Books.

Sandra Denton, M. D.
Tahoma Clinic
24030 132nd Ave. Southeast
Kent, Washington, 98042
Telephone (206) 631-8920
A board-certified emergency physician, and an associate of Dr. Jonathan Wright, she limits her practice to treatment of mercury-toxic patients and other nutritional/biochemical disorders. For this purpose she has formed her own cooperative with dentists and other medical specialists, and is most interested in teaching fellow physicians to recognize and treat the mercury-toxic patient.

Howard C. Elliott, Ph. D.
Baptist Medical Center Montclair
Department of Pathology
800 Montclair Road
Birmingham, Alabama, 35213
A clinical researcher of Vitamin C kinetics.

Bengt Fellström, M. D., Ph. D.
Associate Professor of Nephrology
Department of Internal Medicine
University Hospital
S-751 85, Uppsala, Sweden
An internationally recognized authority on kidney stones.

Barbara Hannah, R. N.
24030 132nd Ave. Southeast
Kent, Washington, 98042
Telephone (206) 631-8920
A source person for calculating osmolality. She oversees the administration of IV-C for Dr. Wright's medical group.

Pat Hayes, R. N.
615 East 82nd Street
Anchorage, Alaska 99518
Telephone (907) 344-7775
A source person for calculating osmolality. She regularly administers IV-C for Drs. Rowen, Miller, and Walsh.

Hal A. Huggins, D. D. S.
Huggins Diagnostic Center
P. O. Box 2589
Colorado Springs, Colorado, 80901
Telephone (303) 473-4703
Outside Colorado 1-800-331-2303 (M-F; 8:00 a.m. to 6:00 p.m., MST)
Specializes in the treatment of chronic mercury toxicity. RE: Hal A. Huggins and Sharon A. Huggins, It's All In Your Head, a private publication. Copies may be obtained by contacting the Huggins Diagnostic Center.

Warren M. Levin, M. D. FAAFP, FACN
World Health Medical Group
444 Park Avenue South
New York, New York, 10016
Telephone (212) 696-1900
An authority in chelation therapy, and experienced in administering IV-C to thousands of patients, Dr. Levin is an authoritative source of various, alternative methods of treating chronic mercury toxicity. See Appendix H.

Burton A. Miller, D. D. S.
550 W. 7th Avenue, Suite 1390
Anchorage, Alaska, 99501
Together with John D. Walsh, D. D. S., Dr. Miller has pulled together a medical team which I believe is the ideal partnership for documentation, treatment, and evaluation, of the mercury-toxic patient.

Walter J. Murphy, Jr., Esquire
Welch, Murphy & Welch Law Offices
Suite 703
Wheaton Bldg; Plaza N
Wheaton, Maryland, 20902
Specialist in Medical Legal Affairs and an authority on the topic of Informed Consent. If you have any medical/legal questions surrounding the administration of IV-C you might want to consult with him.

Linus Pauling, Ph. D.
Linus Pauling Institute of Science and Medicine
440 Page Mill Road
Palo Alto, California, 94306
The leading researcher in the use of IV-C as a treatment for cancer. Twice the recipient of a Nobel Prize, he is also a leading proponent in the use of megadose oral vitamin C as a means to optimal health and a longer life.

Robert Rowen, M. D.
615 East 82nd Street
Anchorage, Alaska 99518
Telephone (907) 344-7775
Has formed a working partnership with Drs. Miller and Walsh for documentation, treatment, and evaluation, of the mercury-toxic patient.

Patrick Störtebecker, M. D., Ph. D.
Akerbyvagen 282
S-183 35, Taby/Stockholm, Sweden
Author of The Effect of Mercury On The Brain, *(privately published). You may obtain a copy by addressing your inquiry to the above address.*

Kenneth E. Warner, M. D.
Chief Medical Examiner
P. O. Box 2411
Tuscaloosa, Alabama, 35403
Telephone (205) 348-5060
Formerly held the same position in Albuquerque, New Mexico, during which time he reported the relationship between body size and violent death.

John D. Walsh, D.D.S.
550 W. 7th Avenue, Suite 1390
Anchorage, Alaska, 99501
Together with Burton A. Miller, D. D. S., Dr. Walsh has pulled together a medical team which I believe is the ideal partnership for documentation, treatment, and evaluation, of the mercury-toxic patient.

James S. Woods, Ph. D.
Senior Research Scientist
Battelle Seattle Research Center
4000 N.E. 41st Street
Seattle, Washington 98105
Telephone (206) 525-3130; Cable BATSEA
Is conducting research to establish the porphyrin profile (fingerprint) method for assessing toxicity from mercury exposure. Once established, he sees no reason why this test couldn't be employed in monitoring mercury-toxic patients to evaluate their treatment response to the **IV-C Mercury Tox Program.**

Jonathan V. Wright, M. D.
Tahoma Clinic
24030 132nd Ave. Southeast
Kent, Washington, 98042
Telephone (206) 631-8920
Conducts "Seminars in Clinical Applications of Nutritional Biochemistry," semi-annual seminars on the practice of nutritional medicine, during which time he also instructs doctors in the use of I.V. Vitamin C. A 21-hour tape set and course syllabus are available also. You may inquire, or have your name added to their mailing list—which will inform you of the next seminar—by writing to Wright/Gaby Seminars; 4215 Lowell Drive; Baltimore, MD 21208, or by telephoning 301/486-9490.

COMPANIES AND ORGANIZATIONS

American College of Advancement in Medicine
Suite 204
23121 Verdugo Drive
Laguna Hills, California 92653
Telephone: 1-800-LEAD OUT
Formerly, The American Academy of Medical Preventics

American Heart Association
National Center
7320 Greenville Avenue
Dallas, Texas, 75231
Telephone (214) 750-5300
Cable AMHEART Dallas, Texas

Arizona Instrument Corporation
P.O. Box 336
Jerome, Arizona, 86331
Telephone (800) 952-2566, (602) 634-4263
TELEX: 165-083
Manufacturer of the Mercury Vapor Analyzer.

Bio-Probe, Inc.
4401 Real Court
Orlando, Florida, 32808
Educational material available for a small fee. The new expanded edition of The Toxic Time Bomb: Can The Mercury In Your Dental Fillings Poison You?, by Sam Ziff, Aurora Press, can be obtained from them.

Bronson Pharmaceuticals
4526 Rinetti Lane
La Canada, California 91011
Distributor of vitamin C as mixed ascorbates, and distributor of food supplements in general.

CRC Press, Inc.
2000 Corporate Blvd. NW
Boca Raton, Florida 33431
Telephone (305) 994-0555; Telex 568689
Books available on Biocompatibility Testing. RE: Techniques in Biocompatibility Testing, Volumes I and II, Edited by David F. Williams, Ph.D., D.Sc., Institute of Medical and Dental Bioengineering, University of Liverpool, England: From the CRC series in Biocompatibility.

(The) International Academy of Oral Medicine and Toxicology
c/o Michael F. Ziff, D. D. S.   c/o Murray J. Vimy D. D. S.
5400 Hernando Drive   615-401 9th Avenue, SW
Orlando, Florida, 32806   Calgary, Alberta, Canada, AB T2F 3C5
Can provide dentists with information concerning dental material alternatives. The Academy officially recommends "that the governments of the United States and Canada declare an immediate prohibition on the further use of dental silver-mercury fillings until primary scientific documentation can be provided proving that the mercury released from dental fillings is not harmful to the public."

Klaire Laboratories, Inc.
P.O. Box 618
Carlsbad, California, 92006
Distributor of Vital Dophilus—a non-dairy supplemental source of Lactobacillus acidophilus.

Meridian Valley Laboratories
24030 132nd Ave. Southeast
Suite E
Kent, Washington 98042
Telephone (206) 631-8922
Can provide UGOT/UGPT determinations. All that's needed is a test tube of urine, securely stoppered, and sent by Express Mail, but it's advisable to contact the laboratory by phone before shipping.

Merit Pharmaceutical Company
2622 Humboldt Street
Los Angeles, California, 90031
Distributor of I.V. Vitamin C

The McGuff Company
Medical Products
3625 W. MacArthur, Suite 306
Santa Ana, CA 92704
Telephone: (800) 854-7220; (714) 545-2491
This manufacturer will gladly provide doctors and nurses with additional information on calculating osmolality. When enquiring, ask for their Revised Osmolarity Table.

Neo-Life/Shelton's Health Products
113 W. Woodard
P.O. Box 201
Denison, TX 75020
(214) 463-4635
A major distributor of Neo Life Enteriodophilus—a nondairy supplemental source of Lactobacillus acidophilus, L. bifidus, and L. bulgaricus; Salmon oil capsules; Calcium supplements that are free of vitamin D; and all natural food supplements in general.

Steris Laboratories
620 N. 51st Avenue
P.O. Box 23160
Phoenix, Arizona, 85063-3160
Telephone (602) 939-7565
Manufacturers of large dose I.V. Vitamin C.

ToxSupply, Inc.
Glenn Brickley, President
P.O. Box 5088
Greeley, Colorado, 80631
Telephone (303) 356-4374
Distributor of patch tests for Mercury and Nickel Sensitivity.

APPENDIX F

For the Researcher: A Brief Summation of the Vitamin C Biosynthesis Capabilities of Various Animals

This book has been purposefully designed to answer many of the questions demanded of researchers for developing a research protocol. To this end, the information that follows will provide useful background information. Specifically, this information is essential if science is to ever learn why some animals produce such a large quantity of ascorbic acid daily, while others do not. By seeking these answers, I believe we will one day prove that the need for vitamin C in man's diet goes far beyond the present RDA.

Dr. Robert Jenness, of the Primate Research Institute of New Mexico State University, explains that GLO catalyzes the last step in the synthesis of L-ascorbic acid from D-glucose. He and his colleague, Dr. Elmer Birney at Minnesota, have examined 43 species of bats, while Indian workers have examined an additional two species for GLO. While Dr. Jenness cannot say there are no bats that synthesize GLO (there are over 900 species), GLO—in all 45 of the species tested to date—was either absent or extremely low. Jenness, Birney, and their students have examined over 100 species of mammals other than bats or primates. All have significant levels of GLO activity except for the snowshoe hare, in which the embryos and newborn young have the enzyme, but older animals have either none or very low levels.

Mullin, a former student of Jenness's, and Pollock (*Am J Phys Anthropology* 73: 65-70, 1987) have reported substantial levels of GLO in the livers of 14 species of prosimian primates (such as galagos and lemurs, as opposed to anthropoid primates, in which GLO is lacking).

Some animal species other than mammals lack GLO, just as man and other anthropoid primates do. Among these are four species of India's bulbuls (an Asiatic nightingale bird of the order Passeriformes). Of 60 species of North American birds tested by Jenness and colleagues, all except three species of swallows, the brown creeper, and one species of wren, produce substantial levels of GLO in either kidney or liver tissues. Thus, the inability of some animals to synthesize ascorbic acid is not exclusively limited to a select group of mammals. It would be interesting to observe how these animals fare in their resistance to stress and disease as compared with similar species that produce GLO.

APPENDIX G

A Bibliographic Guide to the Treatment of Acute Poisoning Due to Mercury

As was explained in the Glossary, and has been highlighted throughout this book, IV-C is not indicated for acute mercurial poisoning. If the doctor suspects acute poisoning rather than chronic mercury toxicity, the following bibliography will prove to be helpful in deciding a course of therapy.

Discussion of General Protocol

J. M. Arena, ed., and R. H. Drew, as. ed., *Poisoning*, Fifth Edition, Charles C. Thomas, Springfield, Illinois, p 198-209, 1985.

R. H. Dreisbach, *Handbook of Poisoning: Diagnosis and Treatment*, 6th edition, Lange Medical Publications, Los Altos, CA, 1969.

R. E. Gosselin, R. P. Smith, and H. C. Hodge, eds., *Clinical Toxicology of Commercial Products*, Fifth Edition, Williams & Wilkins, Baltimore/London, p III 262-275, 1984.

Accepted Therapies

Penicillamine

N. Ishihara, et al., "Selective Enhancement of Urinary Organic Mercury Excretion by D-Penicillamine," *Brit J Indus Med*, 31: 245-49, 1974.

H. Persson, "Aspects on Antidote Therapy in Acute Poisoning Affecting the Nervous System," *Acta Neurol Scand*, 70 (suppl 100): 203-13, 1984.

Comparison of BAL & Penicillamine

M. E. Datyner and P. A. Cox, "Inorganic Mercurial Poisoning," *Anaesth Intens Care*, 9: 266-70, 1981.

S. B. Elhassani, "The Many Faces of Methylmercury Poisoning," *J Toxicol Clin Toxicol*, 19 (8): 875-906, 1983.

M. M. Jones, et al, "Comparison of Standard Chelating Agents for Acute Mercuric Chloride Poisoning in Mice," *Res Com in Chem Path and Pharmacol*, 27 (2): 363-72, February 1980.

C. A. Lapin and D. E. Carter, "Early Indices of Methyl Mercury Toxicity and their Use in Treatment Evaluation," *J Toxicol Environ Health*, 8: 767-76, 1981.

Experimental Agents/Therapies

2,3-Dimercaptopropane-1-sulphonate (DMPS)

A. Wannag and J. Aaseth, "The Effect of Immediate and Delayed Treatment with 2,3-Dimercaptopropane-1-Sulphonate (DMPS) on the Distribution and Toxicity of Inorganic Mercury in Mice and in Foetal and Adult Rats," *Acta Pharmacol Et Toxicol*, 46: 81-88, 1980.

NOTE: DMPS is not an approved drug in the U. S. In Europe, it is marketed by the Heyl Coerzallee (Company) under the brand name, Dimaval (recommended dosage: 1 tablet, 3 times/day). For further information direct inquiries to:
> Heyl Coerzallee - 253
> D-1000, Berlin 37, West Germany
> Telephone (038) 8-17-60-52

N-Acetyl-D, L-penicillamine (NADP)

H. V. Aposhian, and M. M. Aposhian, "N-Acetyl-DL-Penicillamine, a New Oral Protective Agent against the Lethal Effects of Mercuric Chloride," *J Pharmacol Exp Ther*, 126:131-35, 1959.

D. O. Hryhorczuk, et al., "Treatment of Mercury Intoxication in a Dentist with N-Acetyl-D, L-penicillamine," *J Toxicol Clin Toxicol*, 19 (4): 401-08, 1982.

NOTE: NADP is presently unavailable in North America.

N, N' -di-phenyl-p-phenylenediamine (DPPD)

S. O. Welsh, "The Protective Effect of Vitamin E and N, N'-di-phenyl-p-phenylenediamine (DPPD) against Methyl Mercury Toxicity in the Rat," *J Nutr*, 109: 1673-81, 1979.

Polymercaptal Microspheres

S. Margel and J. Hirsh, "Chelation of Mercury by Polymercaptal Microspheres: New Potential Antidote for Mercury Poisoning," *J Pharmaceutical Sciences*, 71 (9): 1030-34, September 1982.

Thiol Antidote

E. Giroux, and P. J. Lachmann, "Thiol Antidote to Inorganic Mercury Toxicity with an Uncharacteristic Mechanism," *Toxicol and Applied Pharmacol*, 67: 178-83, 1983.

Methicillin

K. Twardowska-Saucha, "Evaluation of the Chelating Action of Methicillin in Prolonged Experimental Metallic Mercury Poisoning," *Brit J Indus Med*, 43: 611-14, 1986.

2,3-Dimercaptosuccinic Acid (DMSA).

P. J. Kostyniak, "Methylmercury Removal in the Dog During Infusion of 2,3-Dimercaptosuccinic Acid (DMSA)," *J Toxicol Environ Health*, 11: 947-57, 1983.

J. H. Graziano, "The Role of 2-3 DMSA in the Treatment of Heavy Metal Poisoning," *Medical Toxicology*, 1: 155-162, 1986.

NOTE: DMSA is expected to be marketed in the U. S. in late 1987, or early 1988. It is believed to be an orally effective chelating agent.

Hemoperfusion

T. J. Pellinen, et al. "Letter to the Editor: Hemoperfusion in Mercury Poisoning," *J Toxicol Clin Toxicol*, 20 (2): 187-9, 1983.

Neonatal Extracorporeal Hemodialysis

P. J. Kostyniak, et al., "An Extracorporeal Complexing Hemodialysis System for the Treatment of Methylmercury Poisoning. I. *In vitro* Studies of the Effects of Four Complexing Agents on the Distribution of Dialyzability of Methylmercury in Human Blood," *J Pharmacol Exp Ther*, 192: 260-9, 1975.

M. E. Lund, et al., "Treatment of Acute Methylmercury Ingestion by Hemodialysis with N-Acetylcysteine (Mucomyst) and Infusion 2, 3-Dimercaptopropane Sulfonate," *J Toxicol Clin Toxicol* 22:31-49, 1984.

S. B. Elhassani, et al., "Exchange Transfusion Treatment of Methylmercury-Poisoned Children," *Environ Sci Health* 13: 63-80, 1978.

NOTE: Dr. Elhassani reports that exchange transfusion removes six percent of the body burden of methylmercury compared to one percent through normal excretory pathways.

Therapeutics Compared

F.W. Sunderman, "Clinical Response to Therapeutic Agents in Poisoning From Mercury Vapor," *Clinical and Laboratory Science*, 8 (4): 259-68, 1980.

APPENDIX H

Alternative Therapies for the Treatment of Chronic Mercury Toxicity

To assist the doctor in evaluating alternatives, other than IV-C, for the treatment of chronic mercury toxicity, the following information from Warren M. Levin, M. D., FAAFP, FACN, is quite helpful. Dr. Levin, whose credentials include that of Diplomate of the Board of Family Practice; Diplomate of the Board of Chelation Therapy; Advisor to the Board of College of Advancement in Medicine; Treasurer of the American Board of Chelation Therapy; and Fellow, American Academy of Environmental Medicine (Clinical Ecology), has had extensive training and experience in alternative treatments of chronic mercury toxicity (see Appendix E).

Calcium DiSodium EDTA

EDTA is known for its chelating property and is used therapeutically to remove lead and other toxic minerals. *In vitro*, EDTA binds mercury even more tightly than lead, so it has been very disappointing to chelation specialists to learn that it is ineffective in clinical practice as a treatment for chronic mercury toxicity. It appears that once the mercury has been cleared from the bloodstream into the body's cells it resists removal by the EDTA. "However, if the patient is to have his or her dental amalgams replaced," said Levin, "I recommend administering IM-EDTA one-half hour to two hours beforehand—a preventive measure that's intended not to be a long-term approach to detoxification of mercury,* but an attempt to counter the immediate increase in mercury load as a result of mercury vapor absorption in the dentist's chair. With all proper precautions taken there is still inevitably some mercury vapor released into contact with mucous membranes so that it is absorbed into the bloodstream. The purpose of the pre-administration of EDTA is so that the mercury released during the drilling process will be chelated out of the body. My dosage recommendation (which follows) for this purpose is similar for all patients weighing fifty pounds or more.

* Dr. Levin's point here is qualified because of my own theoretical concerns about nephrotoxicity from EDTA. There is evidence that EDTA may be a cause of nephrotoxicity in patients with chronic mercury toxicity[1,2] whose condition coexists with lead toxicity. My concern is that these people are seldom screened for lead toxicity first, although every human is contaminated with lead to some degree, so that doctors really can't be confident that nephrotoxicity won't develop in any particular patient in response to IM-EDTA treatment. In response, Dr. Levin adds, "Speaking with much clinical experience, this does not happen at the dosage that I'm recommending (and for the indication I've discussed), even in lead-toxic patients, unless they have significant impairment of renal function as manifested by very high creatinine levels."

---

[1] M.E. Datyner and P.A. Cox, "Inorganic Mercurial Poisoning," *Anaesth Intens Care*, 9: 266-70, 1981.

[2] J. Glömme and K.H. Gustavson, "Treatment of Experimental Acute Mercury Poisoning by Chelating Agents BAL and EDTA," *Acta Med Scand*, 164: 175-82, 1959.

1 ampoule (5 cc) of Calcium Disodium EDTA
(Calcium Disodium Versenate™ -Riker)
+ 1 ampoule (2 cc) 2 percent procaine or xylocaine
(for local anesthesia, as IM-EDTA can be painful
Mixed in 1 syringe and given deep intramusculaly in 1 or 2 sites

"The only drawback is the need for decent kidney function, without which EDTA therapy may cause harm. That's why I recommend checking the patient's BUN and serum Creatinine first, similarly as you would do if administering IV-C. If normal, proceed; if not, then the doctor should consider alternatives other than EDTA or IV-C."

2, 3-Dimercapto propane - 1 - sulphonate (DMPS)

DMPS, marketed by Heyl Coerzallee of West Germany (Appendix G), under the name Dimaval, is accepted for use in Europe but not in the U. S. It has been used for treating both mercury poisoning and chronic mercury toxicity. While its claim of effectiveness in chronic mercury toxicity is unsubstantiated, its ease of administration (1 tablet 3 times/day) and its purported lack of side effects is a feature which, as a therapeutic, appears quite attractive.

2,3-Dimercapto succinic acid (DMSA)

DMSA, like DMPS, has shown much promise as a treatment for mercury poisoning. The research of Joseph H. Graziano, Ph. D.,[1] a pharmacologist at Columbia University College of Physicians and Surgeons, indicates that DMSA also is of value in treating the mercury-toxic patient. If all goes well, orally administered DMSA should be available in the U. S. sometime in 1988.

Nutritional Support

"Other than the measures indicated in this book," said Dr. Levin, "special emphasis should be given to the supplementation of megadose zinc, manganese, and selenium, in addition to foods high in pectin and other types of nondigestible fiber, as getting rid of mercury requires good intestinal action. Glutathione (GSH), especially, should be supplemented in the diet, along with cysteine, and vitamins E and C. When these four are adequately provided, GSH plays a role in the antioxidant recycling process, thereby stabilizing the cellular and aqueous level of free radical scavengers. This is important when addressing chronic mercury toxicity—as mercury tends to create an unusual demand for antioxidant activity."

Sam Ziff makes an additional point. In his book, *The Toxic Time Bomb: Can The Mercury In Your Dental Fillings Poison You?*,* Ziff recommends supplementing with pantothenic acid (vitamin B$_5$). Because coenzyme A (which is required in the synthesis of steroid hormones, among other stress-reducing functions) is the physiological active form of vitamin B$_5$, and because mercury interferes with enzyme activity, supplementing with vitamin B$_5$ is likely to be important to the patient's recovery.

* See Appendix E for ordering information.

---

[1] J.H. Graziano, "The Role of 2-3 DMSA in the Treatment of Heavy Metal Poisoning," *Medical Toxicology*, 1: 155-162, 1986.

APPENDIX I

Information on HEART TALK and *The Doctor's Guide for Lifestyle Counseling*
These publications present up-to-date, reliable scientific information of a general nature related to health, and is intended for health and medical professionals only. Lay readers should be aware that these are not intended to provide individual medical advice. Such advice must be obtained from a qualified doctor/practitioner.

The Doctor's Guide for Lifestyle Counseling is a book series published by QUEEN AND COMPANY HEALTH COMMUNICATIONS, INC. Its aim: To assist doctors of every health care specialty toward enhancing the quality of their health care services through nutrition and lifestyle counseling; to encourage doctors of every health specialty to accept responsibility for becoming the central providers of health information, as they are best qualified for this role; to facilitate improvement of the doctor/patient relationship by applying the concepts of informed consent and shared responsibility; to propose in each book a program for treatment of a specific disease condition (consistent with the stated requirements for optimal health); and to develop further in each book a diet and lifestyle program for the prevention and treatment of heart disease.

HEART TALK is a quarterly newsletter for health professionals which supports the aim of the book series. Registered with the National Library of Congress (ISSN 0882-1836), **HEART TALK** presents current scientific information related to health, with emphasis given to heart health. Matters of controversy are included in each issue. The Mid-Winter issue informs, interprets, and gives significance to the annual Scientific Sessions of the American Heart Association, translating their findings to lifestyle. The same type of coverage will be given the annual proceedings of the Federation of American Societies for Experimental Biology (FASEB), reported in the Summer issue. The Spring and Fall issues provide timely update reports. **HEART TALK is not a publication of AHA or FASEB.** The analysis and opinions are those of H.L. "Sam" Queen, QUEEN AND COMPANY HEALTH COMMUNICATIONS, INC., or an assigned agent.

The cost of a year's subscription to **HEART TALK** is $25.00. Prices of individual books in the Lifestyle Series will be determined at the time each is published.

To order **HEART TALK** or indicate your interest in continuing to receive the Lifestyle Series, you may contact us directly at:

Queen and Company health communications, inc.
Post Office Box 49308
Colorado Springs, Colorado, 80919-9938

or you may fill out the attached, postage-paid reply card and return it to us. You may also place your Mastercard or Visa order by calling:

1-800-2-HEART-2
(1-800-243-2782)

Office hours are from 9:00 a.m. to 5:00 p.m. Mountain Time. You may, however, call at any other time and leave a message on the answering machine; your call will be returned.

Index

About
QUEEN AND COMPANY
HEALTH COMMUNICATIONS, INC.

QUEEN AND COMPANY HEALTH COMMUNICATIONS, INC. was formed for the purpose of communicating to doctors and other health professionals accurate and up-to-date information regarding the roles that diet and lifestyle play in health and disease—particularly heart disease—as well as in the prevention of disease. Through independent, secondary research, the company is able to evaluate the essential research that these professionals just do not have the time to study, and consolidate it into a format that's easily understood, and easily passed along to the patient during lifestyle counseling sessions. We've committed ourselves to providing whatever specialized training the doctor needs to accomplish this.

Our work is drafted within the premise that doctors have the best possible educational background for lifestyle counseling, but lack only the specialized training. There is an ongoing need of the patient to rely on a lifestyle professional he can trust, and, in recent years, he has increasingly relied on health information from outside the medical profession. We believe that the average patient would prefer to get health information from his doctor, if he could be sure that information was truly the best available.

Our goal, as QUEEN AND COMPANY HEALTH COMMUNICATIONS, INC., is to be able to say that our publications have made a positive impact on the quality and type of health care that people can expect from their doctors. Believing that we are able to formulate and make available the most comprehensive program to date for attaining optimal health and avoidance of heart disease, our central goal is to encourage doctors of every health specialty to accept responsibility for becoming the central providers of health information [as opposed to solely medical treatment]. A secondary, but cardinal, goal is to encourage patients to seek their doctors' advice concerning health matters, since we believe doctors are best qualified for this role.

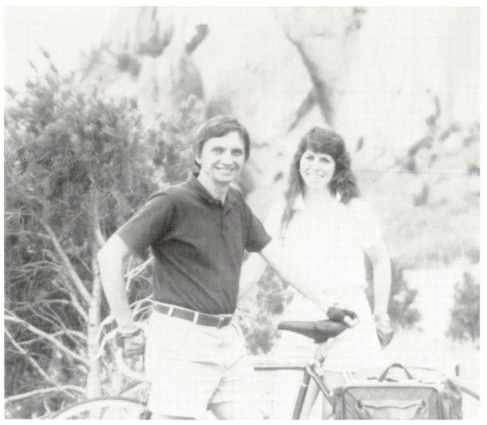

The author, H.L. "Sam" Queen, with his wife and managing editor, Betty A. Queen, enjoying their Rocky Mountain lifestyle at Garden of the Gods, near their home in Colorado Springs, Colorado.

About the Author

H.L. Queen is a health care educator, secondary researcher, and an investigative medical writer with an M.A. in Health Care Education. His 30 years in the health care field includes hands-on experience with administering intravenous vitamin C. This book is his first in a series of books that relate health and disease to lifestyle, and which give the doctor a basis for lifestyle counseling. His other credits include editor and publisher of **HEART TALK** (ISSN:0882-1836)—a newsletter about lifestyle for the health care professional. He has contributed to a medical reference book, *Nutrition and Heart Disease* (CRC Press, Ronald R. Watson, editor, 1987), on the topic of "Diet as a Potent Modifier of Cardiovascular Risk: Has Something Been Overlooked?", as well as to *Professional Pilot* magazine with articles pertaining to health. His critical assessment of the accepted diet/heart viewpoint, and the government's interpretation of the LRC-CPPT Study, earned for him the position of moderator of the Wallace Genetic Foundation Lipid Research Conference, 1984, Scottsdale, Arizona.

Order Form

We would like to have your feedback on **Chronic Mercury Toxicity: New Hope Against an Endemic Disease**. Please use the following postage paid card to give us your opinion, suggest a topic for research, and/or send the name of someone you feel would like to have information on any of these publications.

If you would like to order **HEART TALK**, or extra copies of this book, you may contact:

Queen and Company health communications, inc.
Post Office Box 49308
Colorado Springs, Colorado, 80919-9938

1-800-2-HEART-2
(1-800-243-2782)

For more information regarding *The Doctor's Guide for Lifestyle Counseling* series, and **HEART TALK** newsletter, please see Appendix I of this book.

I enjoyed reading **Chronic Mercury Toxicity: New Hope Against an Endemic Disease**. My comments on this book and/or suggestions for future editions are:

_____

_____

_____

_____ Please inform me when the next book in the **Doctor's Guide for Lifestyle Counseling** series is ready for distribution.

Additionally, I would like to recommend **HEART TALK** and **The Doctor's Guide for Lifestyle Counseling** series to the following :

Name_____

Address_____

City_____ State_____ Zip_____

Telephone_____

Professional Specialty_____

Your   Name_____

Address _____

City_____State _____Zip_____

Telephone_____

Professional Specialty_____

- -

- -

I enjoyed reading **Chronic Mercury Toxicity: New Hope Against an Endemic Disease**. My comments on this book and/or suggestions for future editions are:

_____

_____

_____

_____ Please inform me when the next book in the **Doctor's Guide for Lifestyle Counseling** series is ready for distribution.

Additionally, I would like to recommend **HEART TALK** and **The Doctor's Guide for Lifestyle Counseling** series to the following :

Name_____

Address_____

City_____ State_____ Zip_____

Telephone_____

Professional Specialty_____

Your   Name_____

Address _____

City_____State _____Zip_____

Telephone_____

Professional Specialty_____

BUSINESS REPLY MAIL
FIRST CLASS MAIL PERMIT NO. 827, Colorado Springs, CO

POSTAGE WILL BE PAID BY ADDRESSEE

**Queen and Company
health communications, inc.
P.O. BOX 49308
Colorado Springs, CO 80919-9938**

BUSINESS REPLY MAIL
FIRST CLASS MAIL PERMIT NO. 827, Colorado Springs, CO

POSTAGE WILL BE PAID BY ADDRESSEE

**Queen and Company
health communications, inc.
P.O. BOX 49308
Colorado Springs, CO 80919-9938**

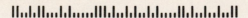